AF094626

Current Perspectives on the Treatment of Obstructive Sleep Apnea—Part II

Current Perspectives on the Treatment of Obstructive Sleep Apnea—Part II

Editor

Yüksel Peker

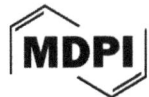

Basel • Beijing • Wuhan • Barcelona • Belgrade • Novi Sad • Cluj • Manchester

Editor
Yüksel Peker
Koc University
Istanbul
Turkey

Editorial Office
MDPI AG
Grosspeteranlage 5
4052 Basel, Switzerland

This is a reprint of articles from the Special Issue published online in the open access journal *Journal of Clinical Medicine* (ISSN 2077-0383) (available at: https://www.mdpi.com/journal/jcm/special_issues/Apnea_Sleep).

For citation purposes, cite each article independently as indicated on the article page online and as indicated below:

Lastname, A.A.; Lastname, B.B. Article Title. *Journal Name* **Year**, *Volume Number*, Page Range.

ISBN 978-3-7258-2273-7 (Hbk)
ISBN 978-3-7258-2274-4 (PDF)
doi.org/10.3390/books978-3-7258-2274-4

© 2024 by the authors. Articles in this book are Open Access and distributed under the Creative Commons Attribution (CC BY) license. The book as a whole is distributed by MDPI under the terms and conditions of the Creative Commons Attribution-NonCommercial-NoDerivs (CC BY-NC-ND) license.

Contents

Samuel Knoedler, Leonard Knoedler, Helena Baecher, Martin Kauke-Navarro, Doha Obed,
Cosima C. Hoch, et al.
30-Day Postoperative Outcomes in Adults with Obstructive Sleep Apnea Undergoing Upper
Airway Surgery
Reprinted from: *J. Clin. Med.* 2022, *11*, 7371, doi:10.3390/jcm11247371 1

Robert Stansbury, Toni Rudisill, Rachel Salyer, Brenna Kirk, Caterina De Fazio,
Adam Baus, et al.
Provider Perspectives on Sleep Apnea from Appalachia: A Mixed Methods Study
Reprinted from: *J. Clin. Med.* 2022, *11*, 4449, doi:10.3390/jcm11154449 23

Agnieszka Polecka, Natalia Olszewska, Łukasz Danielski and Ewa Olszewska
Association between Obstructive Sleep Apnea and Heart Failure in Adults—A Systematic Review
Reprinted from: *J. Clin. Med.* 2023, *12*, 6139, doi:10.3390/jcm12196139 37

Servet Altay, Selma Fırat, Yüksel Peker and The TURCOSACT Collaborators
A Narrative Review of the Association of Obstructive Sleep Apnea with Hypertension: How to
Treat Both When They Coexist?
Reprinted from: *J. Clin. Med.* 2023, *12*, 4144, doi:10.3390/jcm12124144 70

Ki Hwan Kwak, Young Jeong Lee, Jae Yong Lee, Jae Hoon Cho and Ji Ho Choi
The Effect of Pharyngeal Surgery on Positive Airway Pressure Therapy in Obstructive Sleep
Apnea: A Meta-Analysis
Reprinted from: *J. Clin. Med.* 2022, *11*, 6443, doi:10.3390/jcm11216443 82

Ning Zhou, Jean-Pierre T. F. Ho, René Spijker, Ghizlane Aarab, Nico de Vries, Madeline J. L.
Ravesloot and Jan de Lange
Maxillomandibular Advancement and Upper Airway Stimulation for Treatment of Obstructive
Sleep Apnea: A Systematic Review
Reprinted from: *J. Clin. Med.* 2022, *11*, 6782, doi:10.3390/jcm11226782 91

Almala Pinar Ergenekon, Yasemin Gokdemir and Refika Ersu
Medical Treatment of Obstructive Sleep Apnea in Children
Reprinted from: *J. Clin. Med.* 2023, *12*, 5022, doi:10.3390/jcm12155022 107

Yeliz Celik, Yüksel Peker, Tülay Yucel-Lindberg, Tilia Thelander and Afrouz Behboudi
Association of TNF-α (-308G/A) Gene Polymorphism with Changes in Circulating TNF-α Levels
in Response to CPAP Treatment in Adults with Coronary Artery Disease and Obstructive Sleep
Apnea
Reprinted from: *J. Clin. Med.* 2023, *12*, 5325, doi:10.3390/jcm12165325 124

Yukako Tomo, Ryo Naito, Yasuhiro Tomita, Satoshi Kasagi, Tatsuya Sato and Takatoshi Kasai
The Correlation between the Severity of Obstructive Sleep Apnea and Insulin Resistance in a
Japanese Population
Reprinted from: *J. Clin. Med.* 2024, *13*, 3135, doi:10.3390/jcm13113135 136

Sébastien Bailly, Monique Mendelson, Sébastien Baillieul, Renaud Tamisier
and Jean-Louis Pépin
The Future of Telemedicine for Obstructive Sleep Apnea Treatment: A Narrative Review
Reprinted from: *J. Clin. Med.* 2024, *13*, 2700, doi:10.3390/jcm13092700 146

Christina Gu, Nicole Bernstein, Nikita Mittal, Soumya Kurnool, Hannah Schwartz, Rohit Loomba and Atul Malhotra
Potential Therapeutic Targets in Obesity, Sleep Apnea, Diabetes, and Fatty Liver Disease
Reprinted from: *J. Clin. Med.* **2024**, *13*, 2231, doi:10.3390/jcm13082231 . . . . **156**

Oren Cohen, Vaishnavi Kundel, Philip Robson, Zainab Al-Taie, Mayte Suárez-Fariñas and Neomi A. Shah
Achieving Better Understanding of Obstructive Sleep Apnea Treatment Effects on Cardiovascular Disease Outcomes through Machine Learning Approaches: A Narrative Review
Reprinted from: *J. Clin. Med.* **2024**, *13*, 1415, doi:10.3390/jcm13051415 . . . . **168**

Wouter P. Visscher, Jean-Pierre T. F. Ho, Ning Zhou, Madeline J. L. Ravesloot, Engelbert A. J. M. Schulten, Jan de Lange and Naichuan Su
Development and Internal Validation of a Prediction Model for Surgical Success of Maxillomandibular Advancement for the Treatment of Moderate to Severe Obstructive Sleep Apnea
Reprinted from: *J. Clin. Med.* **2023**, *12*, 503, doi:10.3390/jcm12020503 . . . . **184**

Yvonne Chu and Andrey Zinchuk
The Present and Future of the Clinical Use of Physiological Traits for the Treatment of Patients with OSA: A Narrative Review
Reprinted from: *J. Clin. Med.* **2024**, *13*, 1636, doi:10.3390/jcm13061636 . . . . **200**

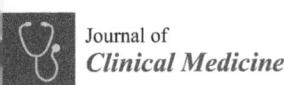

Article

30-Day Postoperative Outcomes in Adults with Obstructive Sleep Apnea Undergoing Upper Airway Surgery

Samuel Knoedler [1,2,*,†], Leonard Knoedler [3,†], Helena Baecher [1], Martin Kauke-Navarro [4], Doha Obed [2,5], Cosima C. Hoch [6], Yannick F. Diehm [2,7], Peter S. Vosler [8], Ulrich Harréus [9], Ulrich Kneser [7] and Adriana C. Panayi [2,7,*]

1 Department of Plastic, Hand and Reconstructive Surgery, University Hospital Regensburg, 93053 Regensburg, Germany
2 Division of Plastic Surgery, Department of Surgery, Brigham and Women's Hospital, Harvard Medical School, Boston, MA 02115, USA
3 Division of Plastic and Reconstructive Surgery, Massachusetts General Hospital, Harvard Medical School, Boston, MA 02114, USA
4 Department of Surgery, Division of Plastic Surgery, Yale New Haven Hospital, Yale School of Medicine, New Haven, CT 06510, USA
5 Department of Plastic, Aesthetic, Hand and Reconstructive Surgery, Hannover Medical School, 30625 Hannover, Germany
6 Department of Otolaryngology, Head and Neck Surgery, Rechts der Isar Hospital, Technical University Munich, 81675 Munich, Germany
7 Department of Hand-, Plastic and Reconstructive Surgery, Microsurgery, Burn Trauma Center, BG Trauma Center Ludwigshafen, University of Heidelberg, 67071 Ludwigshafen, Germany
8 Head and Neck Cancer Center, Sarasota Memorial Health Care System, Sarasota, FL 34239, USA
9 Department of Otolaryngology, Head and Neck Surgery, Asklepios Hospital, 83646 Bad Toelz, Germany
* Correspondence: samuel.knoedler@stud.uni-regensburg.de (S.K.); apanayi@bwh.harvard.edu (A.C.P.)
† These authors contributed equally to this work.

Abstract: Background: Obstructive sleep apnea (OSA) is a chronic disorder of the upper airway. OSA surgery has oftentimes been researched based on the outcomes of single-institutional facilities. We retrospectively analyzed a multi-institutional national database to investigate the outcomes of OSA surgery and identify risk factors for complications. Methods: We reviewed the American College of Surgeons National Surgical Quality Improvement Program (NSQIP) database (2008–2020) to identify patients who underwent OSA surgery. The postoperative outcomes of interest included 30-day surgical and medical complications, reoperation, readmission, and mortality. Additionally, we assessed risk-associated factors for complications, including comorbidities and preoperative blood values. Results: The study population included 4662 patients. Obesity (n = 2909; 63%) and hypertension (n = 1435; 31%) were the most frequent comorbidities. While two (0.04%) deaths were reported within the 30-day postoperative period, the total complication rate was 6.3% (n = 292). Increased BMI ($p = 0.01$), male sex ($p = 0.03$), history of diabetes ($p = 0.002$), hypertension requiring treatment ($p = 0.03$), inpatient setting ($p < 0.0001$), and American Society of Anesthesiology (ASA) physical status classification scores ≥ 4 ($p < 0.0001$) were identified as risk-associated factors for any postoperative complications. Increased alkaline phosphatase (ALP) was identified as a risk-associated factor for the occurrence of any complications ($p = 0.02$) and medical complications ($p = 0.001$). Conclusions: OSA surgery outcomes were analyzed at the national level, with complications shown to depend on AP levels, male gender, extreme BMI, and diabetes mellitus. While OSA surgery has demonstrated an overall positive safety profile, the implementation of these novel risk-associated variables into the perioperative workflow may further enhance patient care.

Keywords: obstructive sleep apnea (OSA); airway surgery; head and neck surgery; big data

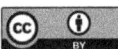

1. Introduction

Obstructive sleep apnea (OSA) is a chronic disorder defined as increased pharyngeal airway resistance during sleep with subsequent repetitive collapse of the upper airway [1,2]. With over one billion people affected worldwide, OSA represents a highly prevalent and continually increasing disorder. OSA patients suffer from different symptoms, including sleep fragmentation, hypoxia, and increased cardiovascular morbidity [3–6].

Positive airway pressure (PAP) therapy represents the gold standard in non-surgical OSA management [7]. A wide array of surgical treatment options exist, including (i) uvulopalatopharyngoplasty (UPPP); (ii) other soft tissue reduction procedures, such as tonsillectomy, glossectomy, and epiglottidectomy; (iii) skeletal surgeries, such as maxillomandibular advancement (MMA), genioglossus advancement (GA), and hyoid myotomy and suspension (HMS); and (iv) upper airway bypass procedures, including tracheostomy for severe OSA [1,3].

In most cases, OSA surgeries are performed in non-academic facilities [8]. Outcome research on complication rates and risk-associated factors for OSA is often derived from retrospective analyses of single-surgeon, single-institution, or technique-specific medical records, which can reduce research transferability and significance to the scientific community [9]. By pooling patient data with geographical and institutional variation, an analysis of multicenter national databases can help identify more robust risk-associated factors and provide a panoramic view of postoperative outcomes in OSA patients.

The American College of Surgeons (ACS) National Surgical Quality Improvement Program (NSQIP) provides an extensive and diverse patient cohort by collecting validated data from more than 700 US hospitals. We, therefore, query this database to fill the research gap regarding the outcomes and occurrence of adverse events of OSA procedures in larger, mostly academic hospital centers, which may represent more complex cases with a multimorbid patient group [10].

2. Methods

2.1. Data Source and Patient Selection

Data were collected between 2008 and 2020 from the American College of Surgeons National Surgical Quality Improvement Program (ACS-NSQIP) database. As a multi-institutional catalog, the ACS-NSQIP records over 150 pre-, peri-, and postoperative data points. Since the records analyzed did not contain patient-identifying information, the study was exempt from Institutional Review Board approval.

The ACS-NSQIP database was queried to identify all patients who underwent surgical treatment for obstructive sleep apnea (OSA). Specifically, 13 annual records between 2008 and 2020 were searched for ICD-9-CM 327.23 ("Obstructive sleep apnea") and ICD-10-CM G47.33 ("Obstructive sleep apnea") codes. In a second step, we screened this OSA cohort of 4781 cases and retrieved all cases in which bariatric surgical procedures were performed. We excluded a total of 119 cases of bariatric treatment to obtain a more homogeneous cohort undergoing head and neck surgery as the only therapeutic management for OSA. Thus, the analyzed cohort did not include any case of bariatric OSA treatment, either as the main procedure or as a concomitant procedure. Finally, the generated patient pool was manually cross-checked by two investigators (S.K. and A.C.P.), and the classification as head and neck OSA surgery was confirmed for each individual case. A third investigator (L.K.) was consulted in cases of discrepant assessments, with any unclear records being excluded from the analysis.

2.2. Variable Extraction

Pre-, peri-, and thirty-day postoperative variables were extracted for analysis.

(i) Preoperative data were evaluated as follows: (a) patient demographics (sex, age, race, height in inches, and weight in pounds), (b) comorbidities (history of chronic obstructive pulmonary disease (COPD) or congestive heart failure (CHF), active dialysis treatment, diabetes mellitus, hypertension, dyspnea, metastatic cancer, smoking status in the past year, steroid or immunosuppressive therapy use, weight loss greater than 10% of body weight, wound infections, ventilator dependency, and functional health status), (c) preoperative scores (wound classification (score of 1–4) and American Society of Anesthesiology (ASA) physical status classification (score of 1–5)), and (d) preoperative laboratory values, including serum sodium, blood urea nitrogen (BUN), serum creatinine, serum albumin, total bilirubin, serum glutamic-oxaloacetic transaminase (SGOT), alkaline phosphatase (ALP), white blood count (WBC), hematocrit, platelet count, partial thromboplastin time (PTT), international normalized ratio (INR), and prothrombin time (PT). In addition, we calculated the body mass index (BMI) for all patients using the following formula: weight (pounds)/height (inches)$^2 \times 703$. All extracted preoperative variables are shown in Table 1.

Table 1. Patient demographics and comorbidities. Reported as n (%), unless otherwise stated.

Characteristic	Patients (n = 4662)
Demographics	
Sex	
Female (n)	1273 (27)
Male (n)	3388 (73)
Age, mean ± SD	42 ± 13
BMI, mean ± SD	33 ± 7.3
Race	
American Indian or Alaskan Native	28 (0.6)
Asian	244 (5.2)
Native Hawaiian or Pacific Islander	51 (1.1)
Black or African American	544 (12)
White	2979 (64)
Other or unknown	804 (17)
Preoperative health and comorbidities	
Diabetes	469 (10)
Insulin-treated diabetes	137 (2.9)
COPD	60 (1.3)
CHF	5 (0.1)
Obesity	2909 (62)
Hypertension	1435 (31)
Dyspnea	229 (4.9)
Current smoker	742 (16)
Corticosteroid use	80 (1.7)
Wound infection	13 (0.3)
ASA physical status classification score	
1—No disturbance	217 (4.7)
2—Mild disturbance	2650 (57)
3—Severe disturbance	1744 (37)
4—Life-threatening	45 (1.0)
Wound class	
1—Clean	179 (3.8)
2—Clean/contaminated	4396 (94)
3—Contaminated	63 (1.4)
4—Dirty/infected	24 (0.5)
Functional Status	
Independent	4606 (99)
Partially or totally dependent	56 (1.2)

ASA, American Society of Anesthesiology.

(ii) In terms of perioperative data, we evaluated the type of anesthesia (general, monitored, epidural or spinal, local or regional, and other), surgical specialty (otolaryngology, general surgery, and other), setting (inpatient or outpatient), year of surgery within the 13-year period of 2008–2020, and total operative time in minutes. All perioperative data are shown in Tables 2 and 3.

Table 2. Surgical characteristics. Reported as n (%), unless otherwise stated.

Characteristic	Patients (n = 4662)
Surgical specialty	
General	39 (0.8)
ENT	4587 (98)
Other	36 (0.8)
Type of anesthesia	
General	4642 (100)
Local	3 (0.06)
Monitored anesthesia care	8 (0.2)
Epidural or spinal	6 (0.1)
Other or unknown	3 (0.06)
Setting	
Inpatient	1382 (30)
Outpatient	3280 (70)
Year of surgery	
2008	173 (3.7)
2009	202 (4.3)
2010	306 (6.6)
2011	120 (2.6)
2012	441 (9.5)
2013	429 (9.2)
2014	440 (9.4)
2015	455 (9.8)
2016	457 (9.8)
2017	516 (11)
2018	445 (9.5)
2019	376 (8.1)
2020	302 (6.5)

Table 3. (Sub)Types of surgery. Reported as n (%), unless otherwise stated.

Type of Surgery	N of Patients (%)
Isolated Uvulopalatopharyngoplasty (UPPP)	321 (6.9)
+ tonsillectomy	46 (1.0)
+ turbinate reduction	14 (0.3)
+ tongue radiofrequency ablation (RFA) + tonsillectomy	1 (0.02)
+ turbinate reduction + tongue RFA	3 (0.06)
+ tongue RFA	2 (0.04)
+ turbinate reduction + tonsillectomy	7 (0.2)
Isolated Palatopharyngoplasty (PPP)	1161 (25)
+ tonsillectomy	887 (19)
+ tonsillectomy + turbinate reduction	306 (6.6)
+ tonsillectomy + tongue RFA	70 (1.5)
+ tonsillectomy + turbinate reduction + tongue RFA	43 (0.9)
+ tonsillectomy + hyoid myotomy and suspension + turbinate reduction	5 (0.1)
+ turbinate reduction + sinus surgery	27 (0.6)
+ tongue RFA	76 (1.6)
+ turbinate reduction	409 (8.8)
+ sinus surgery	22 (0.5)
+ tonsillectomy + sinus surgery	9 (0.2)
+ turbinate reduction + tongue RFA	41 (0.9)
+ tonsillectomy + sinus surgery + turbinate reduction	9 (0.2)
+ tonsillectomy + turbinate reduction + sinus surgery + tongue RFA	2 (0.04)
+ turbinate reduction + sinus surgery + tongue RFA	1 (0.02)
+ sinus surgery + turbinate reduction + tonsillectomy	2 (0.04)

Table 3. Cont.

Type of Surgery	N of Patients (%)
+ sinus surgery + tongue RFA	1 (0.02)
+ sinus surgery + tonsillectomy + tongue RFA	1 (0.02)
Isolated Tonsillectomy	578 (12)
+ turbinate reduction	85 (1.8)
+ turbinate reduction + sinus surgery	7 (0.2)
+ uvulectomy	76 (1.6)
+ uvulectomy + sinus surgery	2 (0.04)
+ turbinate reduction + uvulectomy	18 (0.4)
+ uvulectomy + tongue RFA	3 (0.06)
+ turbinate reduction + tongue RFA	1 (0.02)
+ tongue RFA	3 (0.06)
+ sinus surgery	2 (0.04)
Isolated Uvulectomy	31 (0.7)
+ turbinate reduction	14 (0.3)
+ sinus surgery + turbinate reduction	2 (0.04)
+ sinus surgery	1 (0.02)
Isolated Partial Glossectomy	13 (0.3)
+ PPP	35 (0.8)
+ PPP + turbinate reduction	6 (0.1)
+ turbinate reduction	4 (0.09)
+ PPP + tonsillectomy	28 (0.6)
+ tonsillectomy + PPP + turbinate reduction	7 (0.2)
+ tonsillectomy + turbinate reduction	3 (0.06)
+ tonsillectomy	2 (0.04)
+ hyoid myotomy and suspension	1 (0.02)
Isolated Genioglossus Advancement	0 (0.0)
+ maxillomandibular advancement	15 (0.3)
+ PPP + turbinate reduction	1 (0.02)
+ PPP + tonsillectomy	3 (0.06)
+ maxillomandibular advancement + sinus surgery + turbinate reduction	1 (0.02)
+ maxillomandibular advancement + PPP	4 (0.09)
+ maxillomandibular advancement + PPP + tonsillectomy	2 (0.04)
+ maxillomandibular advancement + PPP + turbinate reduction	2 (0.04)
+ maxillomandibular advancement + turbinate reduction	1 (0.02)
+ turbinate reduction	1 (0.02)
+ PPP	1 (0.02)
Isolated Maxillomandibular Advancement	25 (0.5)
Isolated Hyoid Myotomy and Suspension	35 (0.8)
+ tonsillectomy	6 (0.1)
+ PPP	26 (0.6)
+ tongue RFA	3 (0.06)
+ PPP + turbinate reduction	10 (0.2)
+ PPP + partial glossectomy	1 (0.02)
+ tongue RFA + turbinate reduction	4 (0.09)
+ PPP + tonsillectomy	7 (0.2)
+ PPP + tongue RFA	2 (0.04)
+ turbinate reduction	1 (0.02)
Procedures Including Craniofacial Osteotomies	32 (0.7)
Procedures Including Epiglottidectomy	16 (0.3)
Procedures Including Tracheostomy	18 (0.4)
Other	57 (1.2)

For an in-depth evaluation, we manually analyzed all cases of head and neck OSA surgery and first classified them into one of the following types of surgery (based on the most invasive procedure or the entered main procedure): uvulopalatopharyngoplasty (UPPP), palatopharyngoplasty (PPP), tonsillectomy, uvulectomy, partial glossectomy, genioglossus advancement, maxillomandibular advancement, hyoid myotomy and suspension, cases including craniofacial osteotomy, cases including epiglottidectomy, cases including tracheostomy, and other. Next, we refined this classification system by specifying which concomitant (less invasive) procedures were entered in parallel.

When classifying and labeling the individual types of surgery, we closely adhered to the nomenclature recorded in the NSQIP database. Accordingly, the specification of the surgical types was based on the procedural description and the recorded Current Procedural Terminology (CPT) codes. Further, we followed the guidelines of the American Society of Anesthesiologists Task Force on the management of patients with OSA in assessing the invasiveness of the procedures [11]. In rare cases, for example, craniofacial osteotomies, a more precise specification was not possible due to limited case information. Surgical characteristics, including the classification pattern and the prevalence of each (sub)type of surgery, are summarized in Table 3 and Figure 1.

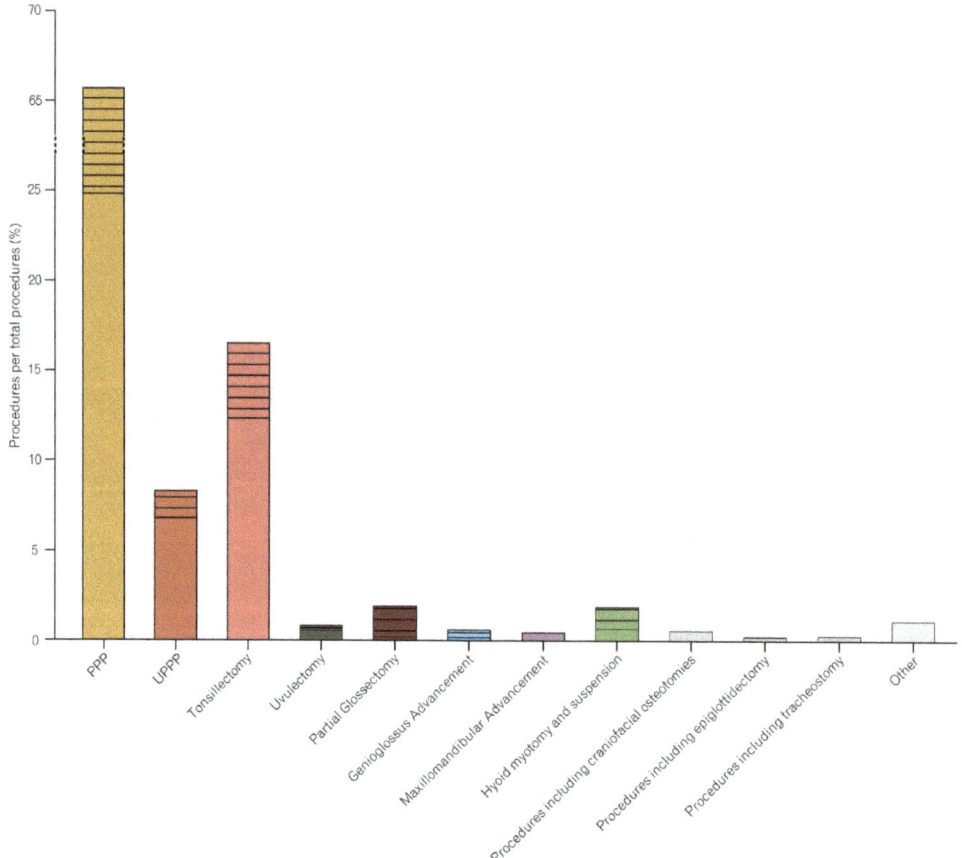

Figure 1. Procedure distribution. Procedures performed concomitantly with other procedures (combined procedures) are shown with a striped pattern. The majority of procedures (>65%) were PPPs, followed by tonsillectomies. The exact numbers are shown in Table 3. PPP, palatopharyngoplasty; UPPP, uvulopalatopharyngoplasty.

(iii) The gathered and analyzed 30-day postoperative outcomes included discharge destination (home, not home, and other or unknown) and length of hospital stay (LOS). LOS was counted as the difference in days between the date of admission and the date of discharge. Any complication was defined as the occurrence of any of the following: mortality, reoperation, readmission or unplanned readmission, and surgical or medical complications. For further analyses, all surgical complications reported in the ACS-NSQIP database (i.e., superficial and deep incision-site infections, organ-space infections, wound lacerations or dehiscences, and blood transfusions) that arose at least once were considered. Similarly, while evaluating all medical complications captured in the ACS-NSQIP catalog (i.e., pulmonary embolism, pneumonia, reintubation, ventilator use for more than 48 h, infection of the urinary tract, renal insufficiency, acute renal failure, deep-vein thrombosis or thrombophlebitis, cardiac arrest, cerebrovascular incident or stroke, myocardial infarction, sepsis, and septic shock), we focused on those for which at least one case was reported. Detailed information on postoperative outcomes after head and neck OSA surgery is listed in Tables 4–6.

Table 4. Operative and postoperative outcomes for all patients undergoing head and neck OSA surgery. Reported as n (%), unless otherwise stated.

Outcome	Patients (n = 4662)
Length of Hospital Stay, mean days ± SD	0.9 ± 2.0
Operative Time, mean minutes ± SD	66 ± 54
Any Complication	292 (6.3)
Mortality within 30 days	2 (0.04)
Reoperation	163 (3.5)
Readmission	100 (2.1)
Unplanned Readmission	99 (2.1)
Surgical Complication	48 (1.0)
Superficial Incisional Infection	26 (0.6)
Deep Incisional Infection	4 (0.09)
Organ-Space Infection	8 (0.2)
Dehiscence	10 (0.2)
Medical Complication	55 (1.2)
Pneumonia	21 (0.5)
Reintubation	17 (0.4)
Pulmonary Embolism	4 (0.09)
Ventilator > 48 h	10 (0.2)
Myocardial Infarction	1 (0.02)
Cardiac Arrest Requiring CPR	1 (0.02)
DVT or Thrombophlebitis	5 (0.1)
Urinary Tract Infection	11 (0.2)
Septic Shock	1 (0.02)
Sepsis	8 (0.2)
Discharge destination	
Home	3956 (85)
Not Home	16 (0.3)
Other or Unknown	8 (0.2)

Table 5. Distribution of procedures with the type-specific occurrence of any complication.

Type of Surgery	Total	Any Complication	Any Complication (Total %)
Uvulopalatopharyngoplasty (UPPP), of which:			
Isolated	321	13	4.0
+ tonsillectomy	46	3	6.5
+ turbinate reduction	14	1	7.1

Table 5. Cont.

Type of Surgery	Total	Any Complication	Any Complication (Total %)
+ tongue radiofrequency ablation (RFA)	2	0	0.0
+ turbinate reduction + tonsillectomy	7	0	0.0
+ turbinate reduction + tongue RFA	3	0	0.0
+ tongue RFA + tonsillectomy	1	0	0.0
Palatopharyngoplasty (PPP), of which:			
Isolated	1161	65	5.6
+ tonsillectomy	887	57	6.4
+ tonsillectomy + turbinate reduction	306	18	5.9
+ tonsillectomy + tongue RFA	70	9	13
+ tonsillectomy + turbinate reduction + tongue RFA	43	0	0.0
+ tonsillectomy + hyoid myotomy and suspension + turbinate reduction	5	1	20
+ turbinate reduction + sinus surgery	27	2	7.4
+ tongue RFA	76	5	6.6
+ turbinate reduction	409	18	4.4
+ sinus surgery	22	0	0.0
+ tonsillectomy + sinus surgery	9	2	22
+ turbinate reduction + tongue RFA	41	4	9.8
+ tonsillectomy + sinus surgery + turbinate reduction	9	1	11
+ tonsillectomy + turbinate reduction + sinus surgery + tongue RFA	2	0	0.0
+ turbinate reduction + sinus surgery + tongue RFA	1	0	0.0
+ sinus surgery + turbinate reduction + tonsillectomy	2	0	0.0
+ sinus surgery + tongue RFA	1	0	0.0
+ sinus surgery + tonsillectomy + tongue RFA	1	0	0.0
Tonsillectomy, of which:			
Isolated	578	50	8.7
+ turbinate reduction	85	4	4.7
+ turbinate reduction + sinus surgery	7	0	0.0
+ uvulectomy	76	4	5.4
+ uvulectomy + sinus surgery	2	0	0.0
+ turbinate reduction + uvulectomy	18	2	11
+ uvulectomy + tongue RFA	3	0	0.0
+ turbinate reduction + tongue RFA	1	0	0.0
+ tongue RFA	3	0	0.0
+ sinus surgery	2	0	0.0
Uvulectomy, of which:			
Isolated	31	0	0.0
+ turbinate reduction	14	2	14
+ sinus surgery + turbinate reduction	2	0	0.0
+ sinus surgery	1	0	0.0
Partial Glossectomy, of which:			
Isolated	13	0	0.0
+ PPP	35	2	5.7
+ PPP + turbinate reduction	6	1	17
+ turbinate reduction	4	0	0.0
+ PPP + tonsillectomy	28	3	11
+ tonsillectomy + PPP + turbinate reduction	7	0	0.0
+ tonsillectomy + turbinate reduction	3	0	0.0
+ tonsillectomy	2	0	0.0
+ hyoid myotomy and suspension	1	0	0.0
Genioglossus Advancement, of which:			
Isolated	0	0	0.0
+ maxillomandibular advancement	15	2	13
+ PPP + turbinate reduction	1	0	0.0

Table 5. *Cont.*

Type of Surgery	Total	Any Complication	Any Complication (Total %)
+ PPP + tonsillectomy	3	0	0.0
+ maxillomandibular advancement + sinus surgery + turbinate reduction	1	0	0.0
+ maxillomandibular advancement + PPP	4	0	0.0
+ maxillomandibular advancement + PPP + tonsillectomy	2	1	50
+ maxillomandibular advancement + PPP + turbinate reduction	2	1	50
+ maxillomandibular advancement + turbinate reduction	1	0	0.0
+ turbinate reduction	1	0	0.0
+ PPP	1	0	0.0
Isolated Maxillomandibular Advancement	25	2	8.0
Hyoid Myotomy and Suspension, of which:			
Isolated	35	3	8.6
+ tonsillectomy	6	0	0.0
+ PPP	26	3	12
+ tongue RFA	3	0	0.0
+ PPP + turbinate reduction	10	1	10
+ PPP + partial glossectomy	1	0	0.0
+ tongue RFA + turbinate reduction	4	1	25
+ PPP + tonsillectomy	7	0	0.0
+ PPP + tongue RFA	2	0	0.0
+ turbinate reduction	1	0	0.0
Procedures Including Craniofacial Osteotomies	32	2	6.3
Procedures Including Epiglottidectomy	16	0	0.0
Procedures Including Tracheostomy	18	4	22
Other	57	5	8.8

Of note, as the primary composite outcome, we defined the occurrence of any complication, i.e., mortality, reoperation, readmission, unplanned readmission, any surgical complication, or any medical complication. In this context, it is important to mention that we counted the total number of patient cases and not the sheer number of complications. In other words, if a patient both returned to the operating room and experienced a medical complication, this was recorded as any complication n = 1. Second, we analyzed all individual outcomes separately and determined the mean length of hospital stay. To this end, we evaluated the frequency of mortality, reoperation, (unplanned) readmission, any surgical, and any medical complication. The latter two included the occurrence of superficial or deep incisional infection, organ-space infection, dehiscence, pneumonia, reintubation, pulmonary embolism, ventilator use for more than 48 h, myocardial infarction, cardiac arrest, deep-vein thrombosis or thrombophlebitis, urinary tract infection, sepsis, and septic shock.

Table 6. Risk-associated factors for complications. Reported as n (%), unless otherwise stated. Statistically significant p-values are highlighted in bold.

Characteristic	Any Complication Yes (n = 292)	Any Complication No (n = 4370)	p-Value	Surgical Complication Yes (n = 48)	Surgical Complication No (n = 4614)	p-Value	Medical Complication Yes (n = 55)	Medical Complication No (n = 4607)	p-Value
Demographics									
Sex			0.03			0.20			0.36
Female (n)	64 (22)	1209 (28)		9 (19)	1264 (27)		18 (33)	1255 (27)	
Male (n)	228 (78)	3160 (72)		39 (81)	3349 (73)		37 (67)	3351 (73)	
Age, mean ± SD	41 ± 13	42 ± 13	0.44	46 ± 13	42 ± 13	**0.04**	45 ± 13	42 ± 13	**0.05**
BMI, mean ± SD	34 ± 8	33 ± 7	**0.01**	32 ± 6	33 ± 7	0.46	38 ± 9	33 ± 7	**<0.0001**
Race			0.30			**0.02**			0.66
American Indian or Alaskan Native	2 (0.7)	26 (0.6)		0 (0)	28 (0.1)		0 (0)	28 (0.6)	
Asian	23 (7.9)	221 (5.1)		2 (4.2)	242 (5.2)		3 (5.5)	241 (5.2)	
Native Hawaiian or Pacific Islander	4 (1.4)	47 (1.1)		1 (2.1)	50 (1.1)		0 (0)	51 (1.1)	
Black or African American	32 (11)	512 (12)		3 (6.3)	541 (12)		10 (18)	534 (12)	
White	173 (59)	2806 (64)		23 (48)	2956 (64)		32 (58)	2947 (64)	
Other or unknown	55 (19)	749 (17)		17 (35)	787 (17)		10 (18)	794 (17)	
Setting			**<0.0001**			**0.0002**			**<0.0001**
Outpatient	167 (57)	3113 (71)		22 (46)	3258 (71)		24 (44)	3256 (71)	
Inpatient	125 (43)	1257 (29)		26 (54)	1356 (29)		31 (56)	1351 (29)	
Preop health and comorbidities									
Diabetes	45 (15)	424 (9.7)	**0.002**	6 (13)	463 (10)	0.48	15 (27)	454 (9.9)	**<0.0001**
Insulin-treated diabetes	15 (5.1)	122 (2.8)	**0.02**	2 (4.2)	135 (2.9)	0.65	5 (9.1)	132 (2.9)	**0.02**
COPD	8 (2.7)	52 (1.2)	0.05	4 (8.3)	56 (1.2)	**0.003**	2 (3.6)	58 (1.3)	0.16
CHF	1 (0.3)	4 (0.09)	0.28	0 (0)	5 (0.1)	>0.99	1 (1.8)	4 (0.09)	0.06
Obesity	195 (67)	2714 (62)	0.11	29 (60)	2880 (62)	0.78	45 (82)	2864 (62)	**0.003**
Hypertension	106 (36)	1329 (30)	**0.03**	18 (38)	1417 (31)	0.31	21 (38)	1414 (31)	0.23
Dyspnea	21 (7.2)	208 (4.8)	0.06	6 (13)	223 (4.8)	**0.03**	6 (11)	223 (4.8)	0.05
Current smoker	52 (18)	690 (16)	0.36	7 (15)	735 (16)	>0.99	10 (18)	732 (16)	0.64
Corticosteroid use	7 (2.4)	73 (1.7)	0.35	2 (4.2)	78 (1.7)	0.20	4 (7.3)	76 (1.6)	**0.01**
Wound infection	2 (0.7)	11 (0.3)	1.19	0 (0)	13 (0.3)	>0.99	1 (1.8)	12 (0.3)	0.14
ASA physical status classification score			**<0.0001**			0.48			**0.0006**
1—No disturbance	13 (4.5)	204 (4.7)		4 (8.3)	213 (4.6)		1 (1.8)	216 (4.7)	
2—Mild disturbance	149 (51)	2501 (57)		24 (50)	2626 (57)		19 (35)	2631 (57)	

Table 6. Cont.

Characteristic	Any Complication			Surgical Complication			Medical Complication		
	Yes (n = 292)	No (n = 4370)	p-Value	Yes (n = 48)	No (n = 4614)	p-Value	Yes (n = 55)	No (n = 4607)	p-Value
3—Severe disturbance	119 (41)	1625 (37)		19 (40)	1725 (37)		33 (60)	1711 (37)	
4—Life-threatening	10 (3.4)	35 (0.8)		1 (2.1)	44 (1.0)		2 (3.6)	43 (0.9)	
Wound class			0.81			0.82			0.22
1—Clean	14 (4.8)	165 (3.8)		2 (4.2)	177 (3.8)		4 (7.3)	175 (3.8)	
2—Clean/Contaminated	272 (93)	4124 (94)		46 (96)	4350 (94)		50 (91)	4346 (94)	
3—Contaminated	4 (1.4)	59 (1.4)		0 (0)	63 (1.4)		0 (0)	63 (1.4)	
4—Dirty/Infected	2 (0.7)	22 (0.5)		0 (0)	24 (0.5)		1 (1.8)	23 (0.5)	
Functional Status			0.08			0.44			0.03
Independent	285 (98)	4321 (99)		47 (98)	4559 (99)		52 (95)	4554 (99)	
Partially or totally dependent	7 (2.4)	49 (1.1)		1 (2.1)	55 (1.2)		3 (5.5)	53 (1.2)	

ASA, American Society of Anesthesiology.

2.3. Statistical Analysis

Data were collected and stored in an electronic laboratory notebook (LabArchives, LLC, San Marcos, CA, USA) and evaluated with GraphPad Prism (V9.00 for MacOS, GraphPad Software, La Jolla, CA, USA). Continuous variables (i.e., age and BMI) were analyzed with independent *t*-tests and reported as means with standard deviations. Pearson's chi-squared test was used to measure differences in categorical variables. In cases with fewer than 10 events, Fisher's exact test was applied. Statistical significance was measured at $p < 0.05$. a univariable subgroup analysis was performed to accomplish risk-associated factors for complications by separating the cohort into three groups depending on the occurrence of any, surgical, or medical complications. An in-depth statistical analysis was conducted using ordinary least squares (OLS) based on a multivariate logistic regression analysis. OLS regression is a statistical-mathematical method calculating the association between one or more independent variables and a dependent variable. Multivariate regression is considered an advanced version of normal OLS regression. These models were performed to control for confounding by including all variables found to be significant risk-associated factors for the occurrence of any, surgical, or medical complications. More specifically, this analysis was adjusted for gender, BMI, setting, diabetes, hypertension, and ASA physical status classification (any complications); for age, race, setting, COPD, and dyspnea (surgical complications); and for BMI, setting, diabetes, obesity, corticosteroid use, ASA physical status classification, and functional status (medical complications).

3. Results

3.1. Patient Demographics

The study population included 4662 patients who underwent OSA surgery over a 13-year review period (2008–2020). The average patient age was 42 ± 13, while male (n = 3388; 73%) and white (n = 2979; 64) patients with class-1 or -2 obesity (BMI: 33 ± 7.7) accounted for the majority of OSA surgery candidates. Obesity (n = 2909; 63%) and hypertension (n = 1435; 31%) were the most frequent comorbidities. In our study population, 16% (n = 742) declared to be current smokers. Detailed demographic data and comorbidities of the entire study population are described in Table 1. Supplementary Table S1 focuses on patients who underwent isolated uvulopalatopharyngoplasty, palatopharyngoplasty, and tonsillectomy procedures and provides a breakdown of their characteristics.

3.2. Surgical Characteristics

Isolated palatopharyngoplasty (PPP) (n = 1161; 25%) was the most frequently performed surgery, with tonsillectomy (PPP with tonsillectomy) (n = 887; 19%) and turbinate reduction (PPP with turbinate reduction) (n = 409; 8.8%) as most common multilevel procedures. Most procedures were performed in an outpatient setting (n = 3280; 70%). Tables 2 and 3 display surgical characteristics in detail.

3.3. Perioperative Outcomes

The mean operation time was 66 ± 54 min. After a postoperative LOS of 0.9 ± 2.0 days on average, 84% (n = 3956) of patients were discharged home (Table 4).

3.4. Postoperative Surgical and Medical Outcomes

The occurrence of any complication (i.e., mortality, reoperation, readmission, unplanned readmission, any surgical complication, or any medical complication) was recorded in 292 patient cases (6.3%) (Table 4). While two (0.04%) deaths were reported within the 30-day postoperative period, the reoperation rate amounted to 3.5% (n = 163). The surgical complication rate was 1.0% (n = 48), with superficial incisional infection (n = 26; 0.6%) as the most frequently reported adverse surgical event. Medical complications occurred in 55 (1.2%) cases, of which pneumonia constituted 21 (0.5%) cases. Male sex ($p = 0.03$), increased BMI ($p = 0.01$), inpatient setting ($p < 0.0001$), history of diabetes ($p = 0.002$), hypertension requiring treatment ($p = 0.03$), and ASA scores ≥ 4 ($p < 0.0001$) were identified as risk-associated factors for the occurrence of any postoperative complications. Advanced age ($p = 0.04$), inpatient setting ($p = 0.0002$), history of COPD ($p = 0.003$), and dyspnea ($p = 0.03$) were identified as risk-associated factors for the occurrence of any surgical complication. In terms of medical complications, increased BMI ($p < 0.0001$), inpatient setting ($p < 0.0001$), history of diabetes ($p < 0.0001$), corticosteroid use ($p = 0.01$), and ASA scores ≥ 4 ($p = 0.0006$) were identified as risk-associated factors. A multivariable analysis confirmed that ASA score and diabetes were independent risk-associated factors for the occurrence of any complication ($p = 0.03$ and $p = 0.001$, respectively; Table 7). Further details about the multivariable assessments of any, surgical, and medical complications are described in Tables 7 and 8. Increased alkaline phosphatase (ALP) was identified as a risk-associated factor for the occurrence of any complication ($p = 0.02$) and medical complications ($p = 0.001$). Detailed preoperative lab value data are described in Table 9.

Table 7. Multivariable assessment of any, surgical, and medical complication occurrences for all patients undergoing head and neck OSA surgery.

Risk-Associated Factors	OR	95% CI	p-Value
Any complications			
Sex (female)	−0.02	−0.04−−0.01	0.003
Diabetes	0.03	0.00–0.05	0.03
ASA physical status classification score ($\geq$4)	0.12	0.05–0.20	0.001
Surgical complications			
Race (White)	−0.02	−0.02−−0.01	<0.0001
Race (Black or African American)	−0.02	−0.03−−0.01	0.004
COPD	0.05	0.02–0.07	0.0006
Medical complications			
Diabetes	0.02	0.01–0.03	0.003
History of CHF	0.15	0.05–0.24	0.004
Corticosteroid use	0.03	0.01–0.06	0.006
Underweight; BMI < 18.5	0.08	0.01–0.14	0.02
Extreme Obesity Class 3; BMI > 40	0.01	0.00–0.02	0.02

ASA, American Society of Anesthesiology.

Table 8. Multivariable assessment of any, surgical, and medical complication occurrences with regard to different types of surgeries.

Risk-Associated Factors	OR	95% CI	p-Value
Any complications			
Isolated tonsillectomy	0.05	0.02–0.09	0.003
Procedures including tracheostomy	0.12	0.00–0.25	0.04
PPP + tonsillectomy + tongue RFA	0.09	0.02–0.15	0.007
PPP + tonsillectomy + sinus surgery	0.17	0.01–0.33	0.03
Genioglossus advancement + maxillomandibular advancement + PPP + tonsillectomy	0.45	0.11–0.78	0.009
Genioglossus advancement + maxillomandibular advancement + turbinate reduction	0.96	0.48–1.43	<0.0001
Surgical complications			
Genioglossus advancement + maxillomandibular advancement	0.06	0.01–0.11	0.03
Genioglossus advancement + maxillomandibular advancement + turbinate reduction	0.99	0.79–1.18	<0.0001
Hyoid myotomy and suspension	0.07	0.04–0.11	<0.0001
Hyoid myotomy and suspension + PPP	0.06	0.02–0.10	0.001
Hyoid myotomy and suspension + tongue RFA + turbinate reduction	0.24	0.15–0.34	<0.0001
Medical complications			
Procedures including tracheostomy	0.06	0.00–0.11	0.04
Genioglossus advancement + maxillomandibular advancement	0.06	0.00–0.11	0.04

Table 8. Cont.

Risk-Associated Factors	OR	95% CI	p-Value
PPP + tonsillectomy + tongue RFA	0.03	0.00–0.06	0.04
PPP + tonsillectomy + sinus surgery	0.09	0.02–0.17	0.01
PPP + tonsillectomy + sinus surgery + turbinate reduction	0.11	0.03–0.18	0.004
Hyoid myotomy and suspension + PPP + turbinate reduction	0.09	0.02–0.16	0.01
UPPP + turbinate reduction	0.07	0.01–0.13	0.02

PPP: palatopharyngoplasty; RFA: radiofrequency ablation; UPPP, uvulopalatopharyngoplasty.

To delineate a correlation pattern between the type of procedure performed and the occurrence of adverse events, we first reviewed the total number of complications. We found that most complications occurred in patients who underwent palatopharynoplasty (PPP), (n = 65) followed by patients receiving tonsillectomy (n = 50) (Table 5). This was not surprising considering that these two surgical procedures also numerically accounted for the largest proportion of the cohort (Figure 1). We, therefore, calculated a complication rate (defined as the number of complications within a surgery type relative to the total number of patients who underwent that specific procedure; Table 5). A comparison of complication rates among the different (sub)types of surgery revealed that there were no statistically significant differences between isolated procedures and multilevel surgeries (Supplementary Table S2). When focusing exclusively on isolated procedures, we found isolated tonsillectomy to be associated with a significantly higher risk than isolated uvulopalatopharyngoplasty ($p = 0.009$) and isolated palatopharyngoplasty ($p = 0.02$; Supplementary Table S3). Further, tracheostomy showed significantly higher complication rates than isolated uvulopalatopharyngoplasty ($p = 0.009$), isolated palatopharyngoplasty ($p = 0.02$), and isolated uvulectomy ($p = 0.01$; Figure 2 and Supplementary Table S3). Comparable trends were also noticeable in the multivariable assessment of complication occurrences among the different (sub)types of surgery. While isolated tonsillectomy was found to be statistically significantly associated with any complications ($p = 0.003$), tracheostomy surgery was associated with significantly higher risks for any ($p = 0.04$) and medical complications ($p = 0.04$; Table 8). The multivariable analysis suggested two surgical combinations as high-risk conditions for the occurrence of postoperative complications. Namely, combined genioglossus advancement and maxillomandibular advancement, as well as combined palatopharyngoplasty and tonsillectomy, were frequent among the risk-associated types of surgery (Table 8).

Table 9. Preoperative lab values for complications. Statistically significant p-values are highlighted in bold.

Characteristic	Any Complication			Surgical Complication			Medical Complication			Reference Range
	Yes (n = 292)	No (n = 4370)	p-Value	Yes (n = 48)	No (n = 4614)	p-Value	Yes (n = 55)	No (n = 4607)	p-Value	
Serum sodium (mmol/L)	139.5 (2.7)	139.4 (2.5)	0.45	139.0 (3.2)	139.4 (2.5)	0.51	139.6 (2.3)	139.4 (2.5)	0.57	135–145 mmol/L
BUN (mg/dL)	15.3 (8.3)	15.1 (5.4)	0.64	16.2 (4.8)	15.1 (5.6)	0.43	16.5 (12.0)	15.1 (5.4)	0.14	8–25 mg/dL
Creatinine (g/D)	0.9 (0.5)	1.0 (0.5)	0.65	1.0 (0.3)	1.0 (0.5)	0.79	1.0 (0.5)	1.0 (0.5)	0.61	F 0.6–1.8, M 0.8–2.4 g/D
Serum albumin (g/dL)	4.2 (0.5)	4.3 (0.4)	0.38	4.3 (0.5)	4.2 (0.4)	0.78	4.1 (0.4)	4.3 (0.4)	0.16	3.1–4.3 g/dL
Total bilirubin (mg/dL)	0.7 (0.9)	0.6 (0.5)	0.07	0.6 (0.3)	0.6 (0.6)	0.91	0.7 (0.5)	0.6 (0.6)	0.40	0–1 mg/dL
SGOT (U/L)	28.4 (15.4)	27.1 (25.5)	0.68	20.0 (4.7)	27.3 (25.0)	0.35	25.3 (10.2)	27.3 (25.1)	0.74	F 9–25, M 10–40 U/L
Alkaline phosphatase (U/L)	81.5 (32.8)	74.4 (23.5)	**0.02**	70.3 (18.9)	75.0 (24.3)	0.57	94.1 (43.5)	74.6 (23.7)	**0.001**	F 30–100 U/L
WBC × 10^3/mm^3	7.8 (2.6)	7.4 (2.8)	0.09	7.2 (2.1)	7.5 (2.8)	0.66	8.1 (2.2)	7.4 (2.8)	0.15	4.5–11 × 10^3/mm^3
Hematocrit (% of RBCs)	43.0 (4.9)	42.8 (4.2)	0.64	43.8 (3.9)	42.8 (4.2)	0.26	42.4 (4.5)	42.8 (4.2)	0.58	F 36.0–46.0%, M 37.0–49.0% of RBCs
Platelet count × 10^3/μL	248.2 (62.9)	250.4 (64.3)	0.68	240.7 (46.1)	250.4 (64.4)	0.48	242.3 (55.3)	250.4 (64.4)	0.47	130–400 × 10^3/μL
PTT (s)	30.2 (3.7)	29.3 (5.2)	0.20	31.7 (4.7)	29.4 (5.1)	0.19	29.8 (4.7)	29.4 (5.1)	0.77	25–35 s
INR of PT values	1.0 (0.1)	1.0 (0.3)	0.86	1.0 (0.1)	1.0 (0.3)	0.89	1.0 (0.1)	1.0 (0.3)	0.95	<1.1

BUN, blood urea nitrogen; SGOT, serum glutamic-oxaloacetic transaminase; WBC, white blood cell; PTT, partial thromboplastin time; INR, international normalized ratio; PT, prothrombin time; s, seconds; SD, standard deviation; RBC, red blood cell.

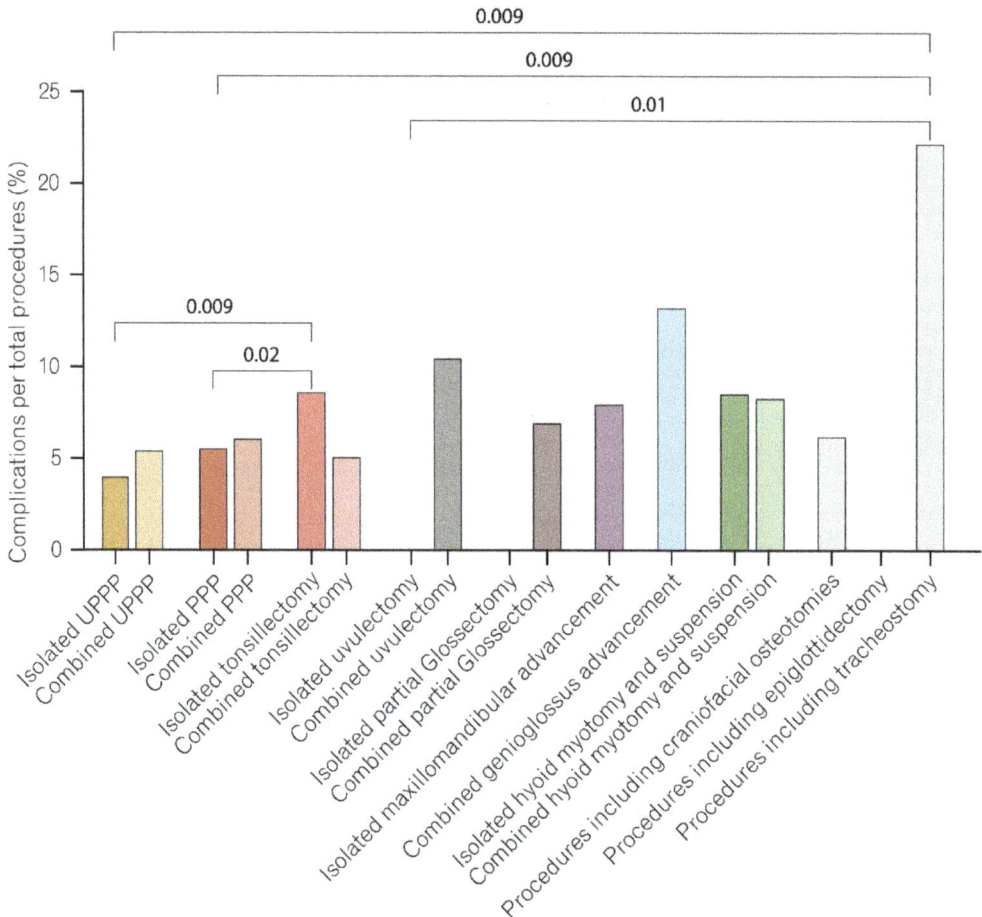

Figure 2. Complications rates for different procedures. Isolated and combined procedures did not significantly differ in terms of complication rates. Tonsillectomy, when performed as an isolated procedure, had a significantly higher rate of complications than isolated UPPP or isolated PPP. Tracheostomy procedures had the highest rate of complications, significantly higher than isolated UPPP, isolated PPP, and isolated uvulectomy. The exact numbers are shown in Supplementary Tables S2 and S3.

4. Discussion

Big databases represent a powerful tool for tracking surgical outcomes and improving patient care. For OSA patients, as a vulnerable patient group per se, it is important for surgeons to thoroughly determine a patient's risk profile prior to undergoing surgery [12]. We queried the ACS-NSQIP database to investigate medical and surgical complications and risk-associated factors, as well as 30-day postoperative outcomes, in 4662 OSA surgery cases.

For the purpose of a homogeneous patient cohort (and, thus, for better interindividual comparability), we excluded all cases of bariatric surgery as a therapeutic approach for OSA. Nonetheless, in our study population undergoing head and neck surgery, middle-aged (42 ± 13 years of age) males with class-1 obesity (BMI: 33 ± 7.3 kg/m^2) still represented the most common OSA patient. This finding aligns with recent studies by Du et al. and Zaghi et al. who each investigated demographic patterns in OSA surgery [13,14]. Further, we found that 62% of patients undergoing upper airway surgery suffered from obesity and 31% from hypertension, while 16% of patients were current smokers. The high prevalence of comorbidities, such as obesity, was also reported in a 2014 Korean population study of 348 patients, as well as in a 2015 study by Heinzer et al. including 2121 OSA patients [15,16]. The high prevalence of nicotine abuse in OSA patients has also been described in the scientific literature [17,18]. Our findings, therefore, underscore the vulnerability of this specific patient group (i.e., middle-aged, male, and obese patients with a medical record of nicotine abuse) to OSA. With the background of increasing worldwide obesity rates and persistently high smoking prevalence, joint efforts are needed to sensitize and target risk patients, such as overweight adolescents or current smokers, before the clinical manifestation of OSA symptoms [19–21].

Surgical OSA therapy is a case-to-case decision based upon individual anatomical findings with the possible combination of different surgical techniques in multilevel surgeries [2,22]. Of note, UPPP, which was considered the standard OSA surgery prior, has been successively replaced by multilevel surgery to simultaneously address variables that predispose patients to UPPP-resistant OSA (e.g., narrowing or collapse at sites other than the retropalate) [23]. The multilevel approach renders perioperative risk evaluation more challenging and necessitates procedure-adjusted complication assessment. In our study, isolated UPPP accounted for 6.9% of the cases, while palatopharyngoplasty combined with different concurrent procedures accounted for 40% of the patients (Figure 1). This distribution pattern corroborates the ongoing shift toward concomitant surgeries in OSA patients.

Regarding complication rates, different studies have shown overall perioperative complication rates in OSA surgery ranging between 1.0% and 15% [22,24]. More recent reports have indicated relatively low complication rates for OSA surgery: while van Daele et al. documented reoperation rates and surgical site infections in 4.8% and 0.9% of all cases, respectively, Rosero et al. found postoperative complications occurring in 6.4% of surgical OSA patients [25,26]. Both authors reported surgery-related mortality rates of less than 0.1%. Overall, these numbers are comparable to our analysis, where we found 2 cases of death (0.4%), 292 (6.3%) cases of any complications, and 163 reoperations (3.5%) due to complications.

Interestingly, in our study, no significant differences in the occurrences of complications and the incidences of readmissions and reoperations were found between multilevel surgeries and isolated procedures (Supplementary Table S2). The stacking of concomitant procedures for customized patient therapy was not associated with a significantly increased risk. This finding is in line with recent studies that have highlighted the safety profile of multilevel OSA surgery [27–31]. More specifically, the SAMS randomized clinical trial involved 51 patients undergoing multilevel OSA surgery (i.e., uvulopalatopharyngoplasty and minimally invasive tongue volume reduction), with only two participants (4%) experiencing postoperative adverse events [30]. Similarly, Bosco et al. reported the absence of any unexpected complications during the postoperative follow-up of 24 patients receiving one-stage multilevel OSA surgery (pharyngoplasty, tongue base reduction, or partial epiglottectomy) [31]. In 2021, a meta-analysis evaluated 37 studies and a total of 1639 patients undergoing multilevel OSA surgery. With major complications being reported in only 1.1% of all cases, this analysis further validated the procedures' safety [29]. Thus, our study substantiates the current trend towards multilevel OSA surgery also from a risk-associated standpoint. However, we identified two surgical combinations (i) genioglossus advancement plus concomitant maxillomandibular advancement and ii) palatopharyngoplasty plus parallel tonsillectomy) as high-risk procedures. Therefore, although this study may encourage surgeons to consider concomitant procedures for more tailored surgical management of OSA patients, surgeons should pay particular attention to these two combinations during preoperative planning and critically evaluate patients' eligibility. In this context, we advocate an individualized case-by-case decision that takes into account both the patient characteristics and the relevant circumstances (such as psychosocial support, monetary burden, and available (mid- and long-term) nursing). The proposed predictive factors, including patient gender, body weight, comorbidities, and laboratory values, may aid in achieving an evidence-based risk assessment.

Of note, tracheostomy was also identified as a risk-associated factor for both any and medical complications, regardless of the main surgical procedure. In general, tracheostomy has been shown to be a safe airway management technique in most cases, as well as a potential, yet uncommon, therapeutic alternative for patients with severe OSA [32–36]. Still, tracheostomy is an invasive procedure that carries a risk of high morbidity. The spectrum of potential adverse events is broad, ranging from postoperative bleeding and infection to tracheal wall injury and tube obstruction. Further tracheostomy-related complications (such as stenosis, malacia, and fistula formation) may also be life-threatening by affecting airway passability, ultimately rendering this procedure one of the most morbid in the wide field of OSA therapy [37–39]. Koitschev et al. showed that the surgical technique used for tracheotomy influenced the risk for tracheostomy-related complications. They found that surgical approaches resulting in an epithelialized tracheostoma minimized the risk for tracheostomy-related complications [40]. To our knowledge, this is the first study to outline the increased risk of tracheostomy in OSA surgery. Therefore, surgeons may critically weigh the potential benefits of tracheostomy, such as enhanced nursing care, against the additional complication risk in OSA patients. However, this finding should be corroborated on larger scales.

OSA patients represent a vulnerable patient group in surgical risk management [12,41]. Therefore, the identification of risk-associated factors plays a pivotal role in enhancing patient care. In our analysis, we found male gender, diabetes mellitus, and ASA scores ≥ 4 to be predictive of any complications. While these factors have been described as risk-associated factors in other fields of surgery, this is the first study to reveal an increased risk for this patient profile when undergoing OSA surgery [42–48]. For medical complications, we not only found extreme obesity (i.e., BMI > 40 kg/m^2) but also underweight status (i.e., BMI < 18.5 kg/m^2) to be significant risk-associated factors (Table 7; Supplementary Figure S1). While Du et al. found the same for OSA surgery patients in obesity classes 2 and 3 when analyzing 1923 OSA surgery cases, this is the first study to reveal an increased risk of medical complications in underweight patients who underwent OSA surgery. Further, we identified elevated alkaline phosphatase (ALP) values to be predictive of medical and surgical complications following OSA surgery. Increased ALP levels can be due to hepatic and biliary diseases, as well as bone disorders [49,50]. Increased ALP values have been implicated with elevated complication rates in other types of surgery, but the exact pathomechanism by which ALP influences perioperative patient health remains to be determined [51,52]. Based on our analysis, we propose that particular attention be paid to patients with ALP levels lower than 81.5 U/L given the association with postoperative complications.

Although the experience, dexterity, and expertise of the surgeon can have a substantial impact on therapeutic success, a series of pre- and perioperative measures can help optimize patient safety. Care providers may, therefore, wish to implement the identified risk-associated factors into their clinical workflow to optimize (i) patient counseling, (ii) high-risk patient group identification, (iii) preoperative patient-tailored planning, (iv) perioperative multimodal monitoring, and (v) postoperative (long-term) follow-up. Thus, by updating and upgrading the risk assessment armamentarium, an individual surgeon can contribute to further honing surgical OSA management.

Limitations

To the best of our knowledge, the study is the first to analyze risks, complications, and outcomes after different kinds of surgical treatment in OSA patients based on multicenter data collected over more than a decade. However, interpretation of the findings considering the study's limitations is mandatory. First, we would like to emphasize that we analyzed correlations and not causalities with the statistical calculations. We identified factors that were associated with higher perioperative risk. However, the underlying causal mechanisms remain to be elucidated. In general, the NSQIP database only provides a limited postoperative follow-up for a 30-day period, meaning that long-term complications, e.g., disease recurrence, remain uncovered [53]. Further, this study entails the risk of unconsidered bias and confounding factors due to its conceptualization as a retrospective data analysis. Due to subjectivity and the unequal expertise of professional database documentation, intra- and interinstitutional differences in the precision and completeness of data collection represent additional limitations in data comparison [54]. However, the robustness, quality, and validity of the entered information are warranted by spot audits and peer controls [55,56]. In fact, according to Shiloach et al., the NSQIP database established low variance in heterogeneity by means of trained data collectors and ongoing audits of data reliability [57].

The range of OSA therapy is far-reaching. The ACS-NSQIP does not cover all of the available treatment modalities [25]. As such, e.g., the implantation and use of a hypoglossal nerve stimulator device ("upper airway stimulation system") is not included in this study. Protocols and therapeutic approaches in the surgical management of OSA vary across the globe [58–61]. Since the NSQIP is a national US database, the transferability of our findings is limited to the American healthcare system [62]. Lacking information about significant subgroup variables, including OSA severity and primary OSA treatment, may lead to deviating outcomes in patient cases. Not considering the initial severity of OSA and the corresponding degree of invasiveness of the surgical procedure, complication rates constitute a kind of average value without the possibility of exact procedure identification. The NSQIP database does not provide information regarding the improvement of OSA symptoms after surgery; thus, no conclusions regarding the impact of risk-associated factors on surgical success rates could be drawn. Furthermore, the ACS-NSQIP database does not specify the criteria upon which an OSA diagnosis is generated and validated. Thus, it cannot be ascertained whether overnight polysomnography was used as a diagnostic procedure. Nevertheless, despite the aforementioned limitations, we are convinced of the study's significance, validity, and value. The described findings may help further refine the perioperative protocols of OSA surgery and, ultimately, optimize patient care.

5. Conclusions

Utilizing the NSQIP-ACS big database, we analyzed 4662 patients undergoing OSA surgery over a 13-year period. We identified that elevated ALP levels (≥ 81.5 U/L), male gender, diabetes mellitus, values at extreme ends of the BMI scale (BMI < 18.5 kg/m^2 and >40 kg/m^2), and ASA scores ≥ 4 were predictive factors for postoperative complications. Awareness of these risk-associated factors may help surgeons carefully balance a patient's eligibility and refine their perioperative management. More specifically, by accounting for these factors during the preoperative planning stage, high-risk patients can be preemptively identified and closely monitored. Moreover, we noted no significant differences in the safety profiles between multilevel surgeries and isolated interventions. While these findings generally imply a step toward treatment individualization, we revealed two (relatively) high-risk surgical combinations (i.e., genioglossus advancement plus concomitant maxillomandibular advancement and palatopharyngoplasty plus parallel tonsillectomy). In addition, cases involving tracheostomy were found to be associated with an increased incidence of adverse events. OSA surgeons should be mindful of these correlations when planning individual treatments and counseling patients.

Supplementary Materials: The following supporting information can be downloaded at: https://www.mdpi.com/article/10.3390/jcm11247371/s1. Table S1: Demographics and comorbidities of all patients who underwent isolated uvulopalatopharyngoplasty (UPPP), palatopharyngoplasty (PPP), and tonsillectomy. Table S2: Comparison of complication rates in the different procedures when the procedures were performed as isolated procedures and when they were performed in combination with other procedures. Table S3: Comparison of complication rates in the different procedures when the procedures were performed as isolated procedures. Figure S1: Frequency of complications stratified by BMI classes.

Author Contributions: Conceptualization, S.K., L.K. and A.C.P.; Methodology, S.K., L.K., H.B. and A.C.P.; Formal analysis, S.K., L.K., M.K.-N. and A.C.P.; Investigation, S.K. and L.K.; Data curation, M.K.-N.; Writing—original draft, S.K., L.K. and A.C.P.; Writing—review & editing, H.B., M.K.-N., D.O., C.C.H., Y.F.D., P.S.V., U.H., U.K. and A.C.P.; Visualization, D.O., C.C.H. and A.C.P.; Supervision, U.K. and A.C.P.; Project administration, M.K-N. All authors have read and agreed to the published version of the manuscript.

Funding: This research received no external funding.

Informed Consent Statement: Not applicable.

Data Availability Statement: Restrictions apply to the availability of these data. Data were obtained from the American College of Surgeons—National Surgical Quality Improvement Program. The application can be submitted at https://accreditation.facs.org/programs/nsqip.

Conflicts of Interest: None of the authors have financial interest in any of the products, devices, or drugs mentioned in this manuscript.

References

1. Epstein, L.J.; Kristo, D.; Strollo, P.J., Jr.; Friedman, N.; Malhotra, A.; Patil, S.P.; Ramar, K.; Rogers, R.; Schwab, R.J.; Weaver, E.M.; et al. Clinical guideline for the evaluation, management and long-term care of obstructive sleep apnea in adults. *J. Clin. Sleep Med.* **2009**, *5*, 263–276.
2. Jordan, A.S.; White, D.P. Pharyngeal motor control and the pathogenesis of obstructive sleep apnea. *Respir. Physiol. Neurobiol.* **2008**, *160*, 1–7. [CrossRef]
3. Gottlieb, D.J.; Punjabi, N.M. Diagnosis and Management of Obstructive Sleep Apnea: A Review. *JAMA* **2020**, *323*, 1389–1400. [CrossRef]
4. Mehra, R. Sleep apnea and the heart. *Cleve Clin. J. Med.* **2019**, *86*, 10–18. [CrossRef]
5. Sabil, A.; Bignard, R.; Gerves-Pinquie, C.; Philip, P.; Le Vaillant, M.; Trzepizur, W.; Meslier, N.; Gagnadoux, F. Risk Factors for Sleepiness at the Wheel and Sleep-Related Car Accidents Among Patients with Obstructive Sleep Apnea: Data from the French Pays de la Loire Sleep Cohort. *Nat. Sci. Sleep* **2021**, *13*, 1737–1746. [CrossRef]
6. Hirsch Allen, A.J.M.; Bansback, N.; Ayas, N.T. The effect of OSA on work disability and work-related injuries. *Chest* **2015**, *147*, 1422–1428. [CrossRef]
7. Patil, S.P.; Ayappa, I.A.; Caples, S.M.; Kimoff, R.J.; Patel, S.R.; Harrod, C.G. Treatment of Adult Obstructive Sleep Apnea With Positive Airway Pressure: An American Academy of Sleep Medicine Systematic Review, Meta-Analysis, and GRADE Assessment. *J. Clin. Sleep Med.* **2019**, *15*, 301–334. [CrossRef]
8. Kezirian, E.J.; Maselli, J.; Vittinghoff, E.; Goldberg, A.N.; Auerbach, A.D. Obstructive sleep apnea surgery practice patterns in the United States: 2000 to 2006. *Otolaryngol. Head Neck Surg.* **2010**, *143*, 441–447. [CrossRef]
9. Liao, P.; Yegneswaran, B.; Vairavanathan, S.; Zilberman, P.; Chung, F. Postoperative complications in patients with obstructive sleep apnea: A retrospective matched cohort study. *Can. J. Anesth./J. Can. D'anesthésie* **2009**, *56*, 819. [CrossRef]
10. Kezirian, E.J.; Weaver, E.M.; Yueh, B.; Deyo, R.A.; Khuri, S.F.; Daley, J.; Henderson, W. Incidence of serious complications after uvulopalatopharyngoplasty. *Laryngoscope* **2004**, *114*, 450–453. [CrossRef]
11. Practice guidelines for the perioperative management of patients with obstructive sleep apnea: An updated report by the American Society of Anesthesiologists Task Force on Perioperative Management of patients with obstructive sleep apnea. *Anesthesiology* **2014**, *120*, 268–286. [CrossRef]
12. Kaw, R.; Pasupuleti, V.; Walker, E.; Ramaswamy, A.; Foldvary-Schafer, N. Postoperative complications in patients with obstructive sleep apnea. *Chest* **2012**, *141*, 436–441. [CrossRef]
13. Zaghi, S.; Holty, J.E.; Certal, V.; Abdullatif, J.; Guilleminault, C.; Powell, N.B.; Riley, R.W.; Camacho, M. Maxillomandibular Advancement for Treatment of Obstructive Sleep Apnea: A Meta-analysis. *JAMA Otolaryngol. Head Neck Surg.* **2016**, *142*, 58–66. [CrossRef]
14. Du, A.L.; Tully, J.L.; Curran, B.P.; Gabriel, R.A. Obesity and outcomes in patients undergoing upper airway surgery for obstructive sleep apnea. *PLoS ONE* **2022**, *17*, e0272331. [CrossRef]

15. Heinzer, R.; Vat, S.; Marques-Vidal, P.; Marti-Soler, H.; Andries, D.; Tobback, N.; Mooser, V.; Preisig, M.; Malhotra, A.; Waeber, G.; et al. Prevalence of sleep-disordered breathing in the general population: The HypnoLaus study. *Lancet Respir. Med.* **2015**, *3*, 310–318. [CrossRef]
16. Lee, S.D.; Kang, S.H.; Ju, G.; Han, J.W.; Kim, T.H.; Lee, C.S.; Kim, T.; Kim, K.W.; Yoon, I.Y. The prevalence of and risk factors for sleep-disordered breathing in an elderly Korean population. *Respiration* **2014**, *87*, 372–378. [CrossRef]
17. Bednarek, M.; Plywaczewski, R.; Jonczak, L.; Zielinski, J. There is no relationship between chronic obstructive pulmonary disease and obstructive sleep apnea syndrome: A population study. *Respiration* **2005**, *72*, 142–149. [CrossRef]
18. Choi, K.M.; Thomas, R.J.; Kim, J.; Lee, S.K.; Yoon, D.W.; Shin, C. Overlap syndrome of COPD and OSA in Koreans. *Medicine* **2017**, *96*, e7241. [CrossRef]
19. Reitsma, M.B.; Kendrick, P.J.; Ababneh, E.; Abbafati, C.; Abbasi-Kangevari, M.; Abdoli, A.; Abedi, A.; Abhilash, E.S.; Abila, D.B.; Aboyans, V.; et al. Spatial, temporal, and demographic patterns in prevalence of smoking tobacco use and attributable disease burden in 204 countries and territories, 1990–2019: A systematic analysis from the Global Burden of Disease Study 2019. *Lancet* **2021**, *397*, 2337–2360. [CrossRef]
20. Chooi, Y.C.; Ding, C.; Magkos, F. The epidemiology of obesity. *Metabolism* **2019**, *92*, 6–10. [CrossRef]
21. Islami, F.; Torre, L.A.; Jemal, A. Global trends of lung cancer mortality and smoking prevalence. *Transl. Lung Cancer Res.* **2015**, *4*, 327–338. [CrossRef]
22. Lin, H.C.; Weaver, E.M.; Lin, H.S.; Friedman, M. Multilevel Obstructive Sleep Apnea Surgery. *Adv. Otorhinolaryngol.* **2017**, *80*, 109–115. [CrossRef]
23. Friedman, J.J.; Salapatas, A.M.; Bonzelaar, L.B.; Hwang, M.S.; Friedman, M. Changing Rates of Morbidity and Mortality in Obstructive Sleep Apnea Surgery. *Otolaryngol. Head Neck Surg.* **2017**, *157*, 123–127. [CrossRef]
24. Barrera, J.E. Skeletal Surgery for Obstructive Sleep Apnea. *Otolaryngol. Clin. N. Am.* **2016**, *49*, 1433–1447. [CrossRef]
25. Van Daele, D.J.; Cromwell, J.W.; Hsia, J.K.; Nord, R.S. Post-operative Complication Rate Comparison Between Airway Surgery and Upper Airway Stimulation Using NSQIP and ADHERE. *OTO Open* **2021**, *5*, 2473974X211051313. [CrossRef]
26. Rosero, E.B.; Joshi, G.P. Outcomes of Sleep Apnea Surgery in Outpatient and Inpatient Settings. *Anesth. Analg.* **2021**, *132*, 1215–1222. [CrossRef]
27. Saenwandee, P.; Neruntarat, C.; Saengthong, P.; Wiriyaamornchai, P.; Khuancharee, K.; Sirisomboonwech, S.; Chuoykwamdee, N. Barbed pharyngoplasty for obstructive sleep apnea: A meta-analysis. *Am. J. Otolaryngol.* **2022**, *43*, 103306. [CrossRef]
28. Gafar, H.A.-L.; Abdulla, A.E.-D.A.; Ghanem, Y.Y.; Bahgat, A.Y. Comparative study between single-stage multilevel surgery and staged surgery for management of snoring and/or obstructive sleep apnea. *Egypt. J. Otolaryngol.* **2022**, *38*, 90. [CrossRef]
29. Zhou, N.; Ho, J.T.F.; Huang, Z.; Spijker, R.; de Vries, N.; Aarab, G.; Lobbezoo, F.; Ravesloot, M.J.L.; de Lange, J. Maxillomandibular advancement versus multilevel surgery for treatment of obstructive sleep apnea: A systematic review and meta-analysis. *Sleep Med. Rev.* **2021**, *57*, 101471. [CrossRef]
30. MacKay, S.; Carney, A.S.; Catcheside, P.G.; Chai-Coetzer, C.L.; Chia, M.; Cistulli, P.A.; Hodge, J.-C.; Jones, A.; Kaambwa, B.; Lewis, R.; et al. Effect of Multilevel Upper Airway Surgery vs Medical Management on the Apnea-Hypopnea Index and Patient-Reported Daytime Sleepiness Among Patients With Moderate or Severe Obstructive Sleep Apnea: The SAMS Randomized Clinical Trial. *JAMA* **2020**, *324*, 1168–1179. [CrossRef]
31. Bosco, G.; Morato, M.; Pérez-Martín, N.; Navarro, A.; Racionero, M.A.; O'Connor-Reina, C.; Baptista, P.; Plaza, G. One-Stage Multilevel Surgery for Treatment of Obstructive Sleep Apnea Syndrome. *J. Clin. Med.* **2021**, *10*, 4822. [CrossRef] [PubMed]
32. Browaldh, N.; Markström, A.; Friberg, D. Elective tracheostomy is an alternative treatment in patients with severe obstructive sleep apnoea syndrome and CPAP failure. *Acta Otolaryngol.* **2009**, *129*, 1121–1126. [CrossRef]
33. Camacho, M.; Zaghi, S.; Chang, E.T.; Song, S.A.; Szelestey, B.; Certal, V. Mini Tracheostomy for Obstructive Sleep Apnea: An Evidence Based Proposal. *Int. J. Otolaryngol.* **2016**, *2016*, 7195349. [CrossRef]
34. Rizzi, C.J.; Amin, J.D.; Isaiah, A.; Valdez, T.A.; Jeyakumar, A.; Smart, S.E.; Pereira, K.D. Tracheostomy for Severe Pediatric Obstructive Sleep Apnea: Indications and Outcomes. *Otolaryngol. Head Neck Surg.* **2017**, *157*, 309–313. [CrossRef]
35. Camacho, M.; Certal, V.; Brietzke, S.E.; Holty, J.E.; Guilleminault, C.; Capasso, R. Tracheostomy as treatment for adult obstructive sleep apnea: A systematic review and meta-analysis. *Laryngoscope* **2014**, *124*, 803–811. [CrossRef]
36. Thatcher, G.W.; Maisel, R.H. The long-term evaluation of tracheostomy in the management of severe obstructive sleep apnea. *Laryngoscope* **2003**, *113*, 201–204. [CrossRef]
37. Fernandez-Bussy, S.; Mahajan, B.; Folch, E.; Caviedes, I.; Guerrero, J.; Majid, A. Tracheostomy Tube Placement: Early and Late Complications. *J. Bronchol. Interv. Pulmonol.* **2015**, *22*, 357–364. [CrossRef]
38. Rosero, E.B.; Corbett, J.; Mau, T.; Joshi, G.P. Intraoperative Airway Management Considerations for Adult Patients Presenting With Tracheostomy: A Narrative Review. *Anesth. Analg.* **2021**, *132*, 1003–1011. [CrossRef]
39. Cipriano, A.; Mao, M.L.; Hon, H.H.; Vazquez, D.; Stawicki, S.P.; Sharpe, R.P.; Evans, D.C. An overview of complications associated with open and percutaneous tracheostomy procedures. *Int. J. Crit. Illn. Inj. Sci.* **2015**, *5*, 179–188. [CrossRef]
40. Koitschev, A.; Simon, C.; Blumenstock, G.; Mach, H.; Graumueller, S. Surgical technique affects the risk for tracheostoma-related complications in post-ICU patients. *Acta Otolaryngol.* **2006**, *126*, 1303–1308. [CrossRef]
41. Kaw, R.; Gali, B.; Collop, N.A. Perioperative care of patients with obstructive sleep apnea. *Curr. Treat. Options Neurol.* **2011**, *13*, 496–507. [CrossRef] [PubMed]

42. Bamba, R.; Gupta, V.; Shack, R.B.; Grotting, J.C.; Higdon, K.K. Evaluation of Diabetes Mellitus as a Risk Factor for Major Complications in Patients Undergoing Aesthetic Surgery. *Aesthet. Surg. J.* **2016**, *36*, 598–608. [CrossRef] [PubMed]
43. Dulai, M.; Tawfick, W.; Hynes, N.; Sultan, S. Female Gender as a Risk Factor for Adverse Outcomes After Carotid Revascularization. *Ann. Vasc. Surg.* **2019**, *60*, 254–263. [CrossRef] [PubMed]
44. Fitz-Henry, J. The ASA classification and peri-operative risk. *Ann. R. Coll. Surg. Engl.* **2011**, *93*, 185–187. [CrossRef] [PubMed]
45. Negus, O.J.; Watts, D.; Loveday, D.T. Diabetes: A major risk factor in trauma and orthopaedic surgery. *Br. J. Hosp. Med.* **2021**, *82*, 1–5. [CrossRef]
46. Hackett, N.J.; De Oliveira, G.S.; Jain, U.K.; Kim, J.Y. ASA class is a reliable independent predictor of medical complications and mortality following surgery. *Int. J. Surg.* **2015**, *18*, 184–190. [CrossRef]
47. Davenport, D.L.; Bowe, E.A.; Henderson, W.G.; Khuri, S.F.; Mentzer, R.M., Jr. National Surgical Quality Improvement Program (NSQIP) risk factors can be used to validate American Society of Anesthesiologists Physical Status Classification (ASA PS) levels. *Ann. Surg.* **2006**, *243*, 636–641; discussion 641–634. [CrossRef]
48. Kandasamy, T.; Wright, E.D.; Fuller, J.; Rotenberg, B.W. The incidence of early post-operative complications following uvulopalatopharyngoplasty: Identification of predictive risk factors. *J. Otolaryngol. Head Neck Surg.* **2013**, *42*, 15. [CrossRef]
49. Maldonado, O.; Demasi, R.; Maldonado, Y.; Taylor, M.; Troncale, F.; Vender, R. Extremely high levels of alkaline phosphatase in hospitalized patients. *J. Clin. Gastroenterol.* **1998**, *27*, 342–345. [CrossRef]
50. Moss, D.W. Alkaline phosphatase isoenzymes. *Clin. Chem.* **1982**, *28*, 2007–2016. [CrossRef]
51. Karhade, A.V.; Thio, Q.; Ogink, P.T.; Schwab, J.H. Serum alkaline phosphatase and 30-day mortality after surgery for spinal metastatic disease. *J. Neurooncol.* **2018**, *140*, 165–171. [CrossRef] [PubMed]
52. Kudsk, K.A.; Tolley, E.A.; DeWitt, R.C.; Janu, P.G.; Blackwell, A.P.; Yeary, S.; King, B.K. Preoperative albumin and surgical site identify surgical risk for major postoperative complications. *JPEN J. Parenter. Enter. Nutr.* **2003**, *27*, 1–9. [CrossRef] [PubMed]
53. Panayi, A.C.; Haug, V.; Kauke-Navarro, M.; Foroutanjazi, S.; Diehm, Y.F.; Pomahac, B. The modified 5-item frailty index is a predictor of perioperative risk in head and neck microvascular reconstruction: An analysis of 3795 cases. *Am. J. Otolaryngol.* **2021**, *42*, 103121. [CrossRef] [PubMed]
54. Nørgaard, M.; Ehrenstein, V.; Vandenbroucke, J.P. Confounding in observational studies based on large health care databases: Problems and potential solutions—A primer for the clinician. *Clin. Epidemiol.* **2017**, *9*, 185–193. [CrossRef]
55. American College of Surgeons. Quality Programs. *Frequently Asked Questions.* Available online: https://www.facs.org/quality-programs/data-and-registries/acs-nsqip/faq/ (accessed on 18 November 2022).
56. American College of Surgeons. User Guide for the 2016 ACS NSQIP Participant Use Data File (PUF). Available online: https://www.facs.org/media/kthpmx3h/nsqip_puf_userguide_2016.pdf (accessed on 18 November 2022).
57. Shiloach, M.; Frencher, S.K., Jr.; Steeger, J.E.; Rowell, K.S.; Bartzokis, K.; Tomeh, M.G.; Richards, K.E.; Ko, C.Y.; Hall, B.L. Toward robust information: Data quality and inter-rater reliability in the American College of Surgeons National Surgical Quality Improvement Program. *J. Am. Coll. Surg.* **2010**, *210*, 6–16. [CrossRef]
58. MacKay, S.G.; Lewis, R.; McEvoy, D.; Joosten, S.; Holt, N.R. Surgical management of obstructive sleep apnoea: A position statement of the Australasian Sleep Association. *Respirology* **2020**, *25*, 1292–1308. [CrossRef]
59. Tan, J.W.C.; Leow, L.C.; Wong, S.; Khoo, S.M.; Kasai, T.; Kojodjojo, P.; Sy, D.Q.; Lee, C.P.; Chirakalwasan, N.; Li, H.Y.; et al. Asian Pacific Society of Cardiology Consensus Statements on the Diagnosis and Management of Obstructive Sleep Apnoea in Patients with Cardiovascular Disease. *Eur. Cardiol.* **2022**, *17*, e16. [CrossRef]
60. Rösslein, M.; Bürkle, H.; Walther, A.; Stuck, B.A.; Verse, T. Positionspapier zum perioperativen Management von erwachsenen Patienten mit obstruktiver Schlafapnoe bei HNO-ärztlichen Eingriffen. [Position Paper: Perioperative Management of Adult Patients with Obstructive Sleep Apnea in ENT Surgery]. *Laryngorhinootologie* **2015**, *94*, 516–523. [CrossRef]
61. Chang, J.L.; Goldberg, A.N.; Alt, J.A.; Ashbrook, L.; Auckley, D.; Ayappa, I.; Bakhtiar, H.; Barrera, J.E.; Bartley, B.L.; Billings, M.E.; et al. International consensus statement on obstructive sleep apnea. *Int. Forum Allergy Rhinol.* **2022**. [CrossRef]
62. Haug, V.; Kadakia, N.; Wang, A.T.; Dorante, M.I.; Panayi, A.C.; Kauke-Navarro, M.; Hundeshagen, G.; Diehm, Y.F.; Fischer, S.; Hirche, C.; et al. Racial disparities in short-term outcomes after breast reduction surgery-A National Surgical Quality Improvement Project Analysis with 23,268 patients using Propensity Score Matching. *J. Plast Reconstr. Aesthet. Surg.* **2022**, *75*, 1849–1857. [CrossRef]

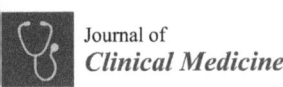

Article

Provider Perspectives on Sleep Apnea from Appalachia: A Mixed Methods Study

Robert Stansbury [1,2,*], Toni Rudisill [3], Rachel Salyer [4], Brenna Kirk [3], Caterina De Fazio [3], Adam Baus [3], Shubekchha Aryal [1], Patrick J. Strollo [2,5], Sunil Sharma [1] and Judith Feinberg [4]

[1] Section of Pulmonary, Critical Care, and Sleep Medicine, West Virginia University, Morgantown, WV 26506, USA; shubekchha.aryal@hsc.wvu.edu (S.A.); sunil.sharma@hsc.wvu.edu (S.S.)
[2] Department of Medicine, University of Pittsburgh, Pittsburgh, PA 15213, USA; strollopj@upmc.edu
[3] School of Public Health, West Virginia University, Morgantown, WV 26501, USA; trudisill@hsc.wvu.edu (T.R.); bok0001@hsc.wvu.edu (B.K.); caterina.defazio@hsc.wvu.edu (C.D.F.); abaus@hsc.wvu.edu (A.B.)
[4] Department of Medicine, West Virginia University, Morgantown, WV 26506, USA; rachel.salyer@hsc.wvu.edu (R.S.); judith.feinberg@hsc.wvu.edu (J.F.)
[5] Department of Medicine, Veterans Affairs Pittsburgh, Pittsburgh, PA 15240, USA
* Correspondence: rstansbury@hsc.wvu.edu

Citation: Stansbury, R.; Rudisill, T.; Salyer, R.; Kirk, B.; De Fazio, C; Baus, A.; Aryal, S.; Strollo, P.J.; Sharma, S.; Feinberg, J. Provider Perspectives on Sleep Apnea from Appalachia: A Mixed Methods Study. *J. Clin. Med.* **2022**, *11*, 4449. https://doi.org/10.3390/jcm11154449

Academic Editor: Yuksel Peker

Received: 15 June 2022
Accepted: 27 July 2022
Published: 30 July 2022

Publisher's Note: MDPI stays neutral with regard to jurisdictional claims in published maps and institutional affiliations.

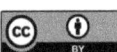

Copyright: © 2022 by the authors. Licensee MDPI, Basel, Switzerland. This article is an open access article distributed under the terms and conditions of the Creative Commons Attribution (CC BY) license (https://creativecommons.org/licenses/by/4.0/).

Abstract: Abstract: BackgroundWest Virginia (WV) has the highest rates of obesity and cardiopulmonary disease in the United States (U.S.). Recent work has identified a significant care gap in WV for obstructive sleep apnea (OSA). This OSA care gap likely has significant health implications for the region given the high rates of obesity and cardiopulmonary disease. The purpose of this mix methods study was to identify barriers that contribute to the rural OSA care disparity previously identified in WV. **Methods:** This study used mixed methods to evaluate the barriers and facilitators to management of OSA at Federally Qualified Health Centers serving communities in southern WV. Focus groups were conducted at federally qualified health centers with providers serving Appalachian communities. Participants also completed the validated Obstructive Sleep Apnea Knowledge and Attitudes (OSAKA) questionnaire to gain insight into provider knowledge and beliefs regarding OSA. EMR analysis using diagnostic codes was completed at the sites to assess OSA prevalence rates. The same individual served as the interviewer in all focus group sessions to minimize interviewer variability/bias. Our team checked to ensure that the professional transcriptions were correct and matched the audio via spot checks. **Results:** Themes identified from the focus groups fell into three broad categories: (1) barriers to OSA care delivery, (2) facilitators to OSA care delivery, and (3) community-based care needs to optimize management of OSA in the targeted rural areas. Questionnaire data demonstrated rural providers feel OSA is an important condition to identify but lack confidence to identify and treat OSA. Evaluation of the electronic medical record demonstrates an even larger OSA care gap in these rural communities than previously described. **Conclusion:** This study found a lack of provider confidence in the ability to diagnose and treat OSA effectively and identified specific themes that limit OSA care in the communities studied. Training directed toward the identified knowledge gaps and on new technologies would likely give rural primary care providers the confidence to take a more active role in OSA diagnosis and management. An integrated model of care that incorporates primary care providers, specialists and effective use of modern technologies will be essential to address the identified OSA care disparities in rural WV and similar communities across the U.S. Community engaged research such as the current study will be essential to the creation of feasible, practical, relevant and culturally competent care pathways for providers serving rural communities with OSA and other respiratory disease to achieve health equity.

Keywords: respiratory health disparity; rural health; obstructive sleep apnea; mixed methods; community engaged research

1. Introduction

Appalachia—especially West Virginia (WV)—persistently has the highest rates of obesity, cardiovascular disease, and smoking-related pulmonary illness in the United States [1–3]. Despite federal support and other programs aimed at improving care in rural communities, these health disparities persist [4]. Among those with cardiopulmonary disease, research suggests significant improvements in health outcomes with treatment of obstructive sleep apnea (OSA) [5–9]. Given these highly prevalent comorbid conditions, identification and treatment of OSA is of particular importance in improving health outcomes in disadvantaged rural communities.

OSA prevalence in adults is increasing and recent work demonstrates nearly a billion people worldwide have undiagnosed sleep apnea suggesting a prevalence of 13% [10,11]. However, there is significant geographical variation in OSA prevalence, with some countries having a prevalence rate that exceeds 50% in the adult population [11]. This rise in OSA prevalence has been attributed in part to the increased prevalence of obesity, a key risk factor for OSA, and no region in the U.S. has been more affected by the obesity epidemic than Appalachia [12]. According to the CDC's Behavioral Risk Factor Surveillance System (BRFSS), WV has the highest obesity prevalence rate at almost 40% [1]. Previous work suggests that OSA is under-recognized and ineffectively managed in rural WV communities [13,14]. A large study analyzed the WV Medicaid database covering approximately 1/3 of the state's adult population and found that only 8% carried a diagnosis code for OSA compared to an expected prevalence in this population of 25% [15]. This OSA care gap in WV is likely related to healthcare disparities in rural Appalachian communities that lack access to specialty care.

Like many rural areas, WV has a dearth of specialty providers, and management of chronic respiratory conditions such as OSA typically falls to primary care providers. For this study, we conducted: (1) a community-engaged research project to assess the knowledge and beliefs of primary care providers with regard to OSA and how these may impact their decision to screen and treat OSA, (2) quantitative analysis of diagnostic patterns at the targeted Federally Qualified Health Centers (FQHCs). These community-based health care providers receive funds from the Health Resources and Services Administration to provide primary care services in underserved areas [16]. We hypothesized that unidentified barriers to care for OSA contribute to the rural OSA care disparity previously identified in WV.

2. Materials and Methods

This study used mixed methods to evaluate the barriers and facilitators to provider management of OSA at FQHCs serving communities in southern WV, an area with some of the poorest healthcare outcomes and healthcare disparities in the U.S. [4]. West Virginia has a population of ~1.7 million inhabitants [17]. Ninety-three percent of the population is Caucasian [17]. Unfortunately, 15.8% live in poverty and 8.3% do not have health insurance. Approximately 1/3 of the state's population has Medicaid insurance coverage [15]. On a per capita basis, there are about 69 PCPs per 100,000 persons in West Virginia. The specific FQHCs in this study were targeted for multiple reasons, including: (a) providing care for a rural population with significant healthcare disparities, (b) having providers who expressed interest in the study during preliminary discussions with our team, and (c) having support from the FQHC's executive leadership to pursue clinical research to improve care for the community served. Data sources included qualitative data from focus groups, questionnaires, and analysis of the FQHCs' electronic medical record. This study was reviewed by the West Virginia University IRB (Exempt Protocol 2009107631) and supported by funding through the West Virginia Clinical and Translational Sciences Institute (NIH/NIGMS 5U54GM104942-03).

2.1. Qualitative Methods

Targeted providers included primary care physicians and advanced practice providers who were recruited for participation through the support of the West Virginia Practice Based

Research Network (WVPBRN). The WVPBRN is a group of primary care clinicians and practices partnered with research centers (such as West Virginia University, the WV School of Osteopathic Medicine, and Charleston Area Medical Center) who work together to answer community-based healthcare questions and translate research findings into meaningful everyday practice. The WVPBRN contacted executive leadership and the chief medical officer at each FQHC, who subsequently offered participation to all providers. Provider focus groups were scheduled with the support of the WVPBRN and local collaborators championing our efforts at each of two clinical sites at two FQHCs, for a total of four sites.

All providers at the targeted clinic sites were included in the study (except one provider who was on vacation at the time of the focus group). No subspecialists participated in these focus groups; there were no exclusion criteria. Participants received USD 100 for their time and effort.

Each focus group had 3-to-5 participants (n = 14). A semi-structured interview guide was developed to assess understanding of provider knowledge and comfort level with OSA management as well as to explore their perspectives on the barriers and facilitators to OSA care in their rural communities (Table 1). Questions were developed based on input from rural practitioners and previous research [13–15]. Focus group sessions lasted approximately 45 min, were audio recorded and professionally transcribed. Professional transcription was completed with NVivo (QRS International Data^C, Ruggell, Liechtenstein). Saturation was achieved by the fourth focus group, where no new themes emerged. The same individual served as the interviewer in all focus group sessions to minimize interviewer variability/bias. Our team checked to ensure that the professional transcriptions were correct and matched the audio via spot checks.

Table 1. Focus Group Guide for Rural Practitioners.

Provider Knowledge and Beliefs of Sleep Apnea

1. Tell me what you know about sleep apnea.
2. Do you regularly screen patients for sleep apnea.
   a. Why or why not?
3. Are you comfortable managing obstructive sleep apnea?
   a. Are you comfortable reviewing sleep study results?
   b. If you decide to treat sleep apnea what therapies do you offer And why?
   c. Are you comfortable managing CPAP therapy for sleep apnea?

Provider Percieved Barriers to Osa Management in Rural Commmunities

1. If you have concerns of sleep apnea, what steps do you take to confirm the diagnosis?
   a. Are there barriers to successfully diagnose patients with sleep apnea. If so what are they?
   b. Is there anything that helps you successfully diagnose patients with sleep apnea?
2. Do you feel your patients are receptive or would be receptive to discussions on sleep apnea?
3. If you were to develop a special program to help improve screening and treatment of sleep apnea in your community:
   a. What would that program look like?
   b. What things would you include?

2.2. Quantitative Methods

Three data sources were utilized: demographic questionnaires, the validated Obstructive Sleep Apnea Knowledge and Attitudes (OSAKA) questionnaire [18], and the site electronic medical record (EMR). All focus group participants completed demographic questionnaires that captured gender, age, race, professional certification, board certification (if applicable), years in practice, and years in practice at the current FQHC. The OSAKA questionnaire was used to determine providers' OSA knowledge, using 18 true-false statements with a third option of "don't know." This portion is scored for correctness, with a higher score indicating greater OSA knowledge. Then, using a five-point Likert scale, providers rate their level of agreement with five statements. The first two statements are about the importance of OSA (1 = not important, 5 = extremely important) and next three statements are about their confidence in identifying and managing OSA (1 = strongly disagree, 5 = strongly agree). Higher scores for these two portions indicate greater rating of the importance of OSA and provider confidence in diagnosing and managing OSA. Questionnaires were completed in paper format. The data were then de-identified and stored in a HIPAA-compliant, secure Research Electronic Data Capture (REDCap) database (hosted at WVCTSI). Finally, we assessed OSA diagnosis rates at one of the targeted FQHCs through EMR interrogation for the period between 1 July 2019 and 19 October 2021. We queried adult patients with an ICD-10 code for sleep apnea during the reporting period [ICD-10 codes G4731 Primary Central Sleep Apnea; G4733 Obstructive Sleep Apnea (adult) (pediatric); G4739 Other Sleep Apnea].

2.3. Statistical Analysis

2.3.1. Qualitative Analysis: Focus Groups

Focus group transcripts were analyzed using content analysis to identify themes relating to facilitators and barriers of sleep apnea management. Two coders thoroughly read and reread the transcripts, and each coder independently developed code words/phrases to label thoughts or concepts that emerged. The research team met with the coders to compare their initial coding schemes and reached consensus on how to code thoughts and concepts. These codes were then operationally defined and documented in a data dictionary within the NVivo software. After all transcripts were coded, our team sorted and collapsed the operationally defined codes into broader, more encompassing themes or subthemes. Inter-rater reliability was evaluated using Cohen's kappa statistic. It was determined a priori that if a minimum kappa of 0.8 was not met, the coding process would occur iteratively until that value was reached. After core themes were determined, the transcripts were reread to ensure that these themes accurately depicted the data. Data management, including searching, coding and categorization of the text from transcripts, was completed with NVivo (V.12).

2.3.2. Quantitative Analysis

Questionnaires: Demographic data were analyzed descriptively as frequencies and percentages. Continuously scaled measures were summarized by means, standard deviations, medians, and ranges. The OSAKA questionnaire was used to determine providers' OSA knowledge, importance, and confidence. Provider responses to OSA knowledge items were analyzed for correctness. This dataset was analyzed with SPSS Windows version 28 (SPSS Inc., Chicago, IL, USA).

Electronic Medical Record: This analysis was completed in collaboration with West Virginia University Office of Health Affairs who have an agreement with the FQHCs to use the EMR data source for approved research projects. This partnership provides WVU faculty access to anonymized data. Record-level claims data from 2021 were aggregated at the individual level to assess the overall prevalence of sleep apnea among adult patients at the FQHC. We calculated the prevalence of OSA diagnoses by dividing the number of patients with a sleep apnea ICD-10 code by the number of unique patient encounters during the study timeframe. Descriptive statistics provided details on age, sex, race, and ethnicity for patients with an OSA diagnosis. JMP Statistical Discovery Software version 15 was used for this analysis (SAS Inc, Cary, NC, USA).

3. Results

3.1. Questionnaire Results

A total of 14 providers participated in the focus group sessions. Participants' demographic characteristics are shown in Table 2. Eight participants were advanced practice providers and six were physicians

Table 2. Characteristics of Providers Participating in Focus Groups.

AGE Mean (SD)	
Mean	53.0 years (12.5) [Range 31 years–75 years]
Gender, N (Percent)	
Male	3 (21.4%)
Female	11 (78.6%)
Race, N (Percent)	
Caucasian	14 (100%)
Practice Type, N (Percent)	
Advanced Practice Provider	8 (57.1%)
Physician	6 (42.9%)
Practice Tenure, Mean (SD) [Range]	
Total Years in Practice	16.2 (15.0) [less than one month to 43 years]
Total Years in Practice at FQHC	8.7 (13.5) [less than one month to 43 years]
Degree N (Percent)	
MD	5 (35.7%)
DO	1 (7.1%)
NP	6 (42.8%)
PA	2 (14.3%)

They had 16.2 mean years in practice overall and 8.7 mean years in practice at the FQHC; however, there was a wide range of years in practice. The majority of participants were female. All physicians were board- certified in Family Medicine.

Regarding the OSAKA questionnaire, the mean OSA importance rating was 9.1 for all providers with a highest possible score of 10 from the two Likert questions on the OSAKA regarding disease importance. The average OSA confidence rating was 9.6 with a highest possible score of 15 from the three Likert questions on the OSAKA regarding disease confidence in disease management. Knowledge scores ranged from 11 to 16 correct answers out of 18. The average number of correct answers for all providers was 14 (SD 1.6). Table 3 shows correct participant responses to each individual item. No provider answered all the knowledge questions correctly. The most common items answered incorrectly were item 3- OSA epidemiology (28.6% respondents answered correctly), Item 4- OSA symptoms (57.1% respondents answered correctly), and item 8- OSA treatment (28.6% respondents answered correct).

Table 3. Participants Answering OSAKA Knowledge Items Correctly ($n = 14$).

Item Number	Number and Percent Answer Correctly	Item Number	Number and Percent Answer Correctly
Item 1	14 (100%)	Item 10	13 (92.69%)
Item 2	10 (71.4%)	Item 11	14 (100%)
Item 3	4 (28.6%)	Item 12	14 (100%)

Table 3. *Cont.*

Item Number	Number and Percent Answer Correctly	Item Number	Number and Percent Answer Correctly
Item 4	8 (57.1%)	Item 13	11 (78.6%)
Item 5	12 (85.7%)	Item 14	14 (100%)
Item 6	13 (92.6%)	Item 15	11 (78.6%)
Item 7	12 (85.7%)	Item 16	12 (85.7%)
Item 8	4 (28.6%)	Item 17	9 (64.3%)
Item 9	12 (85.6%)	Item 18	14 (100%)

3.2. Focus Group Themes

Themes identified from the focus groups fell into 3 broad categories (Table 4): (1) barriers to OSA care delivery, (2) facilitators to OSA care delivery, and (3) community-based care needs to optimize management of OSA in the targeted rural areas.

Table 4. Categorization of Themes and Subthemes with Representative Quotes.

Theme	Subtheme	Representative Quotes
Barriers to OSA Care Delivery (N = 94)	OSA Care Access	"And lack of transportation."
	Provider Knowledge/Beliefs OSA	"I, uh, learned a little bit more about sleep apnea in the past several years from continuing education class. But I think there's a lot I don't know."
	Cost of OSA Care	"I noticed even before I started doing those physicals that some insurers prefer to just do the overnight sleep study without, uh, referral to a specialist, and so then I was left holding the results and was not real happy about that. So, so to me, the barrier, the biggest barrier is cost and coverage."
Facilitators to OSA care Delivery (N = 33)	Specialty Referral Access	They [specialist and DME] pretty much take care of all that stuff. As long as they do all that, then I'm pretty comfortable with that."
	Patient Characteristics	"I've never had any patient that closed the door on that discussion [regarding OSA] with me in my practice."
Community Based Care needs to improve OSA management in targeted rural areas (N = 19)	Community Programming	"A lot of them [patients] are these big burly gentlemen that are very manly, and they don't want to say that, 'Yeah. Well, maybe something's not right. I'm not tired'. But yet they can't lift five pounds, because they are so tired. So, you have this, no disrespect, but this 'man mentality' to some of these guys."
	Provider Preferences	"I mean, it's my responsibility, but since you're conducting this study, I would be interested in more education on it [OSA and CPAP]".
	Educational Needs	"I probably would consider learning how to manage it [OSA] more myself and prescribe CPAP."

3.2.1. Theme 1: Barriers to OSA Care Delivery

OSA Care Access: A major concern for providers was whether their patients could access care for OSA. Providers reported making referrals for OSA testing or specialist evaluation, but patients often did not follow-up. Reasons for lack of follow-up include lack of transportation or cost of transportation, scheduling difficulties, not wanting to stay overnight for a sleep study, patients not "trusting" other providers and only wanting to be treated by their primary care provider, and important aspects of the social determinants of health for the community including poverty, low health literacy and low educational levels. Even when patients followed through with referrals, it was difficult for the providers and patients to get feedback from the appointments and/or test results. Providers described the issues with patients' access to care:

"And lack of transportation. Most of the patients I see, they want to go close to here and there's only one facility here [sleep specialist] and sometimes scheduling is a nightmare just because you cannot get ahold of anybody there."

"[T]here's nothing here locally; they have to go Charleston or a lot of the other what have you and a lot of these people do not have cars or can't pay four zillion dollars, if they can't afford for somebody to transport them, then that's the problem."

"The constraints that I've seen though, nobody wants to do an overnight sleep study and some of the insurances don't want to pay for the home sleep studies, they only want them to go to a site and nobody wants to do that ... "

Treatment for OSA is also described as a challenge. Many patients will not accept continuous positive airway pressure therapy (CPAP). Those who do undergo a trial of CPAP therapy may encounter problems, but there is not good local support from durable medical equipment (DME) companies to address these issues. Patients don't communicate if they are having problems, and then just stop using CPAP. As providers explained:

"I don't know if it's related to the [DME] company versus a patient, but they [the patient] will usually come to you first and say, 'Oh, I couldn't get that last thing to work or whatever'. So, I don't know if it's because on that end they're [the DME company] hard to get in contact with or they [the patient] dropped the ball."

"[T]here's certainly some patients who don't do well with CPAP and they probably don't tell anybody and just don't get treatment."

"They [patients] don't tell you if it's actually not working I think."

"The patients are not very successful with trying to contact the companies once they've dropped the equipment .... It'll be stuck on us to try to get back in contact with the third [party] company."

Variable Provider Knowledge/Beliefs About OSA: In general, providers reported that screening patients for OSA was a low priority, but did note that there seems to be increasing awareness in the local medical community. Symptoms that may trigger OSA screening included fatigue/sleepiness, choking/coughing at night, spouse complaints of snoring, and chronic headaches. Hypertension was the mostly commonly reported disease that prompted OSA screening, although there was significant variability in reported conditions that led to OSA evaluation. Most providers will not evaluate patients with these conditions unless the patient has sleep-related complaints. As providers explained:

"Everybody in my practice complains of fatigue. And almost everybody complains of fatigue and fatigue is such a broad diagnosis. A lot of them you'll ask them, 'Do you snore'? 'Well, I don't know if I do or not'. They'll giggle and say, 'I don't listen to myself sleep'".

"I have to say in all honesty I think over my career I've probably done a lousy job of screening for sleep apnea. And I've probably only referred people for testing when they said they were sleepy. And, um, and even then, I think it was low down on my list of things to consider to do a sleep study and to think about sleep apnea."

"I don't think I'm screening and I don't think I'm doing follow up, um, uh, gosh, questions related to it. It's really not on, on my radar."

"I, uh, learned a little bit more about sleep apnea in the past several years from continuing education class. But I think there's a lot I don't know."

"If you mean do I have a questionnaire that I ask my patients or have them complete, the answer is no. But if you ask me if I screen the patient, I do. If you're obese and hypertensive, if you're obese and complain of not being able to sleep well at night, or that you wake up coughing or choking along with GERD symptoms, I mean, I screen that way."

Providers did not feel comfortable reviewing and interpreting sleep study data and "don't trust" the results of a negative home sleep test. Providers did not feel comfortable managing CPAP machines including trouble-shooting common issues and reviewing data downloaded from the device. Providers will order a portable sleep test, but will leave treatment decisions up to a specialist. Some providers were willing to refill prescriptions for CPAP supplies if a patient is doing well, but were not comfortable making any adjustments to the CPAP device. In general, there was limited knowledge about CPAP alternatives. As one provider explained:

"I was going to say I can read it [the results] and understand some. The last one I had, I thought it was kind of difficult to interpret the gist of the wording and stuff on the report."

"No, I feel more comfortable when I get the results and seeing its positive to send them [patients] somebody that can do that, not that I wouldn't, if I had the training, feel like I could do it. I've just never had the training."

"I just don't know like, you know, change in settings, you know, how many . . . if they're [patients] still having episodes of apnea, you know, all of the adjustments you have to make on the machines, I really don't even know where to start."

"I just refer and let them [specialists] manage it. I mean, if uh . . . Even in the dental appliances, I would not know where to . . . who to approach to about this fitting mouthpieces and things that they do, so I just, I just assume the uh, sleep center knows all that."

"I only ask them [patients] the last time that their equipment was replaced, like their face mask and that type of stuff, but outside of that I would have no clue."

Cost of OSA Care: High cost and variable insurance coverage are other sub-themes impacting OSA care in the targeted rural communities. Some insurances will not cover specialty referral and require a home sleep test through the primary care provider leaving the provider with results they do not understand. Some specialty providers will not accept patient insurance due to low reimbursement. Testing and equipment for OSA treatment are often denied by insurance. Insurance requirement for yearly OSA follow-up was also a noted barrier for many patients who cannot afford travel to specialty clinics or do not have access to transportation. As providers discussed:

"14% of people are uninsured and then you heard people comment that some of the insurances don't cover this specific test, or that specific, so definitely healthcare coverage is also a barrier."

"People's ability to get a test. And, and sometimes, um, they can't afford it. I, I do, um, patient physicals and the, the DOT [Department of Transportation] requires that everybody who uses a CPAP get a, an annual sleep study. And, um, we really run into a problem that a lot of these guys can't, or ladies, can't afford the follow-up sleep study or the follow-up visit. I'm not sure why it's not well covered by insurance."

"[T]he other thing is I noticed even before I started doing those physicals that some insurers prefer to just do the overnight sleep study without, uh, referral to a specialist, and so then I was left holding the results and was not real happy about that. So, so to me, the barrier, the biggest barrier is cost and coverage."

"And then they [dental professional] want some ridiculous amount for the, the [oral] appliance. People don't have the money."

"And, and, and besides those that pay for it, it's a question of does the specialist accept that kind of insurance? . . . . Because if the reimbursement is low, and I think that's an issue with our person in XXX."

3.2.2. Theme 2: Facilitators to OSA Care Delivery

Providers were able to identify certain characteristics that improved the likelihood of a patient successfully navigating the local OSA care pathway leading to diagnosis and effective treatment.

Specialty Referral Access: Rural providers with good access to specialty care clinics and DMEs felt more comfortable with OSA management although they still referred patients to specialists. In general, these providers were comfortable ordering sleep tests and CPAP supplies and would refer patients to DMEs for CPAP trouble-shooting. Proximity to specialty centers mitigated transportation issues for some patients. Increased access to and Medicaid coverage of home sleep testing also facilitated OSA care delivery. One provider explained the relationship with a local specialist and their DME company:

> "They [specialist and DME] pretty much take care of all that stuff. As long as they do all that, then I'm pretty comfortable with that. But if they don't, which I've never seen them not, we titrate the machines and do all that. And then they will follow them only if they have an underlying COPD or something like that, I think pulmonary gets involved. But other than that, once they're diagnosed and their machines are titrated and all that good stuff, they [patients] just stay with us."

Patient Characteristics: Providers felt that patients are generally receptive to discussion of OSA and open to referral for evaluation. Patients have the most trust in their local provider and when their provider takes time to discuss OSA testing and CPAP treatment they are more likely to follow-up with the referral. Providers also stated that there is more awareness in the community with regard to OSA which facilitates diagnosis and successful management. As one provider explained the receptivity of patients to treatment for OSA:

> "I've never had any patient that closed the door on that discussion with me in my practice. They're usually very open. They feel so bad, and they want to figure out why, whether they believe that or not is the question, but they're open to the possibilities [of getting assessed for OSA]."

Theme 3: Community-based Care Needs to Improve OSA Management in the Targeted Rural Areas.

Community Programming: Providers felt that a special community program for OSA would need to focus on patient education. Patients are not aware of the adverse impact of OSA and poor sleep on health. Patients tend to just accept bad sleep as something that is not changeable. In general patients are hesitant to share what's wrong or that there is a problem, especially if they are male as Appalachian culture prizes toughness as a feature of masculinity. As one provider explained the receptivity of patients to treatment for OSA:

> "A lot of them [patients] are these big burly gentlemen that are very manly, and they don't want to say that, 'Yeah. Well, maybe something's not right. I'm not tired'. But yet they can't lift five pounds, because they are so tired. So, you have this, no disrespect, but this 'man mentality' to some of these guys."

Provider Preferences: Providers felt they could develop comfort with home sleep testing but would need specific education about CPAP devices. In general, providers would not mind oversight of home tests, although some felt that the specialist should order the appropriate diagnostic tests. Providers noted that patients will often call them with CPAP issues and felt comfortable addressing easy equipment issues, but many times felt that they needed more training to respond.

> "I mean, it's my responsibility, but since you're conducting this study, I would be interested in more education on it [OSA and CPAP]".

Educational Needs: Providers wanted more education regarding OSA screening, diagnosis and management. The main concern was the limited time for patient visits and whether OSA management could be practically accomplished in a rural primary care clinic. As one provider explained:

"I probably would consider learning how to manage it [OSA] more myself and prescribe CPAP. Um, I'm sort of hesitant to say that 'cause I, you know, you, you worry about getting overwhelmed with things. My worry with that would be the clinical time to do it".

3.3. EMR Analysis

The EMR analysis identified 21,701 unique patients who sought care from July 1 2019 to October 19 2021. Among those patients, 507 (2.3%) had an ICD-10 code (G47.31, G47.33, G47.39) for sleep apnea. Almost all (99.6%) were diagnosed with "obstructive sleep apnea (adult) (pediatric)" as represented by ICD-10 code G47.33. We compared this result to expected prevalence rates based on national datasets and previous work assessing OSA prevalence in the WV Medicaid population (Table 5). The expected prevalence for OSA in the targeted population is 25% [15]. Our analysis demonstrated a prevalence rate of 2.3% based on diagnostic coding.

Table 5. National Estimate and Statewide OSA Prevalence Data Compared to Rural WV FQHC OSA Prevalence Data.

Data Source	OSA Prevalence
Expected WV Adult Medicaid OSA Prevalence from National Data Sources [15]	25%
Observed WV Adult Medicaid OSA Prevalence from State Database Analysis [15]	8.8%
FQHC Specific OSA Prevalence from Local EMR Database Analysis	2.3%

4. Discussion

Our results showed that primary care providers from Appalachia feel OSA is an important disease to consider and have reasonable knowledge but lack the confidence to assume primary management (Figure 1). The OSAKA questionnaire also identified some specific knowledge gaps that could be easily addressed through targeted training. Utilizing a low-cost education and training intervention identified by the focus group sessions may have a significant impact on increasing the OSA workforce. While providers reported not being comfortable reviewing sleep study results or managing positive airway pressure therapy, studies have demonstrated that primary care providers can be effectively trained in the management of OSA including the use of these technologies with non-inferior outcomes compared to specialists' care [19–21]. A challenge in the clinics we evaluated is the high prevalence of cardiopulmonary disease in the population. These patients were excluded from these previous studies assessing primary care management of OSA. The current American Academy of Sleep Medicine guidelines recommend management of OSA in patients with significant cardiorespiratory disease be through a specialized sleep center [22]. However, the COVID pandemic has led to paradigm shift in this thinking and these complex patients may be managed by primary care providers in collaboration with specialists through telemedicine [23].

Our findings suggest that the current OSA care model in rural WV has significant barriers that prevent successful navigation through the diagnostic testing and treatment pathways. The majority of providers stated they refer to specialty sleep centers or specialists for diagnostic testing and treatment, but given healthcare access issues in these communities related to patient financial constraints, transportation issues and geographic isolation, this approach alone cannot address the OSA disparities in rural WV and in other rural settings. Similar challenges have been identified in rural communities both inside and outside the United States [14,24–26]. Implementation of a three-pronged strategy may provide a possible solution to this issue of limited access decreasing this inequity in the targeted region and other rural areas. This strategy includes: (1) training of local providers in OSA care (2) distribution of portable sleep testing through rural health clinics, and (3) management of auto-titrating continuous positive airway pressure (APAP) treatment program through rural health clinics in partnership with local DMEs. Implementation of this three-pronged approach would likely require some support from specialists. Fortunately sleep medicine has been at the forefront of telemedicine for years including remote diagnostics, teleconsultation and telemonitoring of therapy [27–29]. These well-developed technologies could not only address rural care disparity for sleep apnea, but could also serve as a model for addressing respiratory health inequity in other disease states and communities [30].

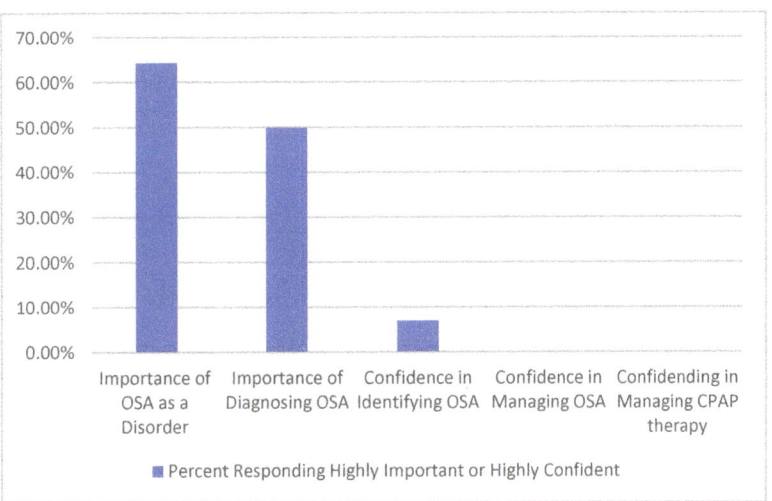

Figure 1. Percentage of Participants ($n = 14$) Responding OSA is Highly Important or Have High Confidence in OSA Management.

The providers in the current study felt targeted education on OSA management including training on portable sleep testing and APAP management could empower them to take primary ownership of OSA care and they would be enthusiastic for this training. The main concern with OSA management was with regard to feasibility; specifically lack of healthcare provider time and clinic resources. This important theme warrants further consideration. Based on recent data OSA is becoming as prevalent as other common conditions such as DM and HTN managed through primary care [11]. A mindset change for primary care and paradigm shift in OSA management pathways may be required. As with DM and HTN, PCPs will need to manage "straightforward" OSA cases to address this growing epidemic. Specialists support would only be required in more complex OSA presentations analogous to current care for refractory hypertension or brittle diabetes. As discussed above this care pathway could be well supported through specialist collaboration via telemedicine [30–32].

Analysis of EMR data demonstrated only a 2.3% prevalence of OSA based on ICD-10 codes. Our previous work estimated a 25% OSA prevalence in the WV adult population while analysis of the WV Medicaid database (>400,000 patients) demonstrated that only 8.8% of the population had an OSA diagnosis based on claims data [15]. A 2.3% prevalence in the current study suggests a significantly larger OSA care gap in challenged rural WV communities primarily served by FQHCs than previously described. This finding further demonstrates the urgent need for a redesign of the current OSA care model. These communities likely have nuanced deficiencies that will require out of the box thinking to address. Unfortunately, evidence-based practice guidelines are not developed specifically for rural communities and few guidelines have been adapted to meet the needs of rural dwelling patients. As discussed by Afifi et al., robust community engaged approaches and implementation science will be required for health equity in these regions [33].

Despite the high disease burden of OSA worldwide and growing evidence of its negative health impacts, many healthcare systems have failed to adopt effective diagnostic and management strategies to address this growing problem. This care gap is amplified in rural WV communities (and likely other rural communities) and of critical importance given the high prevalence of comorbid cardiopulmonary conditions. The specialty workforce is very limited and cannot alone feasibly address the growing OSA problem. Engaging primary care providers in OSA diagnosis and management will be essential to addressing health disparities in WV and other highly vulnerable regions with limited healthcare resources. The current work provides insight into barriers and facilitators to OSA care from rural providers' perspectives. Community engagement studies such as the current study will be essential to the creation of feasible, practical, relevant and culturally competent care pathways for providers serving rural communities with OSA and other respiratory disease to achieve health equity.

While our study provides important insight into the thoughts, beliefs, and barriers to OSA care in rural WV communities, our findings are subject to certain limitations. First, it was conducted at 4 small clinics within two FQHCs serving the southern coalfields of WV. The unique care challenges in this region—poverty, high comorbid disease burden, limited transportation access, few specialists—could limit the generalizability of our findings. However, the limited number of specialists and challenges in terms of the social determinants of health are shared by rural communities throughout the U.S. [4]. Second, although the majority of providers at each clinic participate in the focus groups, it is possible that the participants' responses may differ from those who did not participate. Third, while there is precedent for utilizing ICD-10 billing codes in our EMR analysis to assess disease prevalence, this approach relies on accurate coding by providers [14,15,34,35]. There is always some degree of error in coding, but given the large number of patient visits (>21,000) this is unlikely to dramatically alter our results. Lastly, another limitation is that the EMR analysis only captures people who actually present for care.

Finally, the identification of OSA is only the first step in improving outcomes. We did not evaluate whether the small number of individuals diagnosed with OSA were effectively treated. Previous studies suggest poor outcomes of OSA treatment in rural communities; however, further analysis is required to assess treatment outcomes in our population Appalachian population [13,14,36].

5. Conclusions

Although prior evidence suggests that primary care providers can effectively take ownership of OSA management, there are many potential challenges to implementation, particularly in rural WV communities with significant health disparities. This study suggests a lack of provider confidence in the ability to diagnose and treat OSA effectively; specific knowledge gaps related to OSA epidemiology, symptoms and treatment; overreliance and lack of access to specialty care for OSA management; and failure of new technologies to permeate rural communities (portable sleep testing, APAP). Education directed toward the identified knowledge gaps and training on new technologies would likely give rural primary care providers the confidence to take a more active role in OSA diagnosis and management, and the providers in our study were open to this intervention. An integrated model of care that incorporates primary care providers, specialists and effective use of modern technologies will be essential to address the identified OSA care disparities in rural WV and similar communities across the U.S. Community engagement studies such as the current study will be essential to the creation of feasible, practical, relevant and culturally competent care pathways for providers serving rural communities with OSA and other respiratory disease to achieve health equity.

Author Contributions: Conceptualization, R.S. (Robert Stansbury), T.R., P.J.S., S.S. and J.F.; methodology, R.S. (Robert Stansbury), T.R., R.S. (Rachel Salyer), B.K., C.D.F., A.B. and S.A.; software, R.S. (Robert Stansbury), T.R., R.S. (Rachel Salyer), B.K., C.D.F., A.B. and S.A.; validation, R.S. (Robert Stansbury), T.R., R.S. (Rachel Salyer), B.K., C.D.F., A.B. and S.A.; formal analysis, R.S. (Robert Stansbury),

T.R., R.S. (Rachel Salyer), B.K., C.D.F., A.B. and S.A.; investigation, R.S. (Robert Stansbury), T.R., P.J.S., S.S. and J.F.; resources, R.S. (Robert Stansbury)., T.R. P.J.S., S.S. and J.F.; data curation, R.S. (Robert Stansbury), T.R., R.S. (Rachel Salyer), B.K., C.D.F., A.B. and S.A.; writing—original draft preparation, R.S. (Robert Stansbury), T.R., R.S. (Rachel Salyer), B.K., C.D.F., A.B., S.A., P.J.S., S.S. and J.F.; writing—review and editing, R.S. (Robert Stansbury), T.R., R.S. (Rachel Salyer), B.K., C.D.F., A.B., S.A., P.J.S., S.S. and J.F; visualization, R.S. (Robert Stansbury), T.R., R.S. (Rachel Salyer), B.K., C.D.F., A.B., S.A., P.J.S., S.S. and J.F.; supervision, R.S. (Robert Stansbury), T.R., P.J.S., S.S. and J.F.; project administration, R.S. (Robert Stansbury), T.R., P.J.S., S.S. and J.F. funding acquisition, R.S. (Robert Stansbury), T.R., P.J.S., S.S. and J.F. All authors have read and agreed to the published version of the manuscript.

Funding: This research was funded by the West Virginia Clinical and Translational Sciences Institute. Grant Number# NIH/NIGMS 5U54GM104942-05.

Institutional Review Board Statement: The study was conducted according to the guidelines of the Declaration of Helsinki, and reviewed by the Institutional Review Board of West Virginia University (Exempt Protocol 2009107631 and approved 16 November 2020).

Informed Consent Statement: The West Virginia University Internal Review Board determined this was a minimal risk study of healthcare professionals. Based on this recommendation a minimal risk cover letter was provided to participants outlining the study and potential minimal risk involved with participation in the focus groups.

Data Availability Statement: The data quantitative data presented in this study are available on request from the corresponding author. The data are not publicly available due to data agreement between the Federally Qualified Health Center and the West Virginia University School of Public Health.

Acknowledgments: We wish to thank the West Virginia Practice Based Research Network and Dan Doyle for their support of this project.

Conflicts of Interest: Stansbury receives a consulting fee for service on the ResMed Inc. Clinician Advisory Board. Dr. Sharma serves on the American Academy of Sleep Medicine Hospital Sleep Medicine Task Force. The remainder of authors declare no conflict of interest.

References

1. Centers for Disease Control and Prevention. Adult Obesity Prevalence Maps for All 50 States, the District of Columbia, and US Territories. Available online: https://www.cdc.gov/obesity/data/prevalence-maps.html (accessed on 10 January 2022).
2. Centers for Disease Control and Prevention. Heart Disease Mortality by State. Available online: https://www.cdc.gov/nchs/pressroom/sosmap/heart_disease_mortality/heartdisease.htm (accessed on 10 January 2022).
3. Centers for Disease Control and Prevention. COPD Prevalence by State in the United States. Available online: https://www.cdc.gov/copd/data.html (accessed on 10 January 2022).
4. Rural Health Information Hub. Provides Wide Range of Data on Health Disparities, Health Workforce, Demographics, and More. Explore How Metropolitan and Nonmetro Counties Compare, Nationwide and by State. Available online: https://www.ruralhealthinfo.org/data-explorer (accessed on 11 January 2022).
5. Naranjo, M.; Willes, L.; Prillaman, B.A.; Quan, S.F.; Sharma, S. Undiagnosed OSA May Significantly Affect Outcomes in Adults Admitted for COPD in an Inner-City Hospital. *Chest* **2020**, *158*, 1198–1207. [CrossRef] [PubMed]
6. Sharma, S.; Mather, P.J.; Efird, J.T.; Kahn, D.; Shiue, K.Y.; Cheema, M.; Malloy, R.; Quan, S.F. Obstructive Sleep Apnea in Obese Hospitalized Patients: A Single Center Experience. *J. Clin. Sleep Med.* **2015**, *11*, 717–723. [CrossRef] [PubMed]
7. Shahar, E.; Whitney, C.W.; Redline, S.; Lee, E.T.; Newman, A.B.; Nieto, F.J.; O'Connor, G.T.; Boland, L.L.; Schwartz, J.E.; Samet, J.M. Sleep-Disordered Breathing and Cardiovascular Disease: Cross-Sectional Results of the Sleep Heart Health Study. *Am. J. Respir. Crit. Care Med.* **2001**, *163*, 19–25. [CrossRef] [PubMed]
8. Sharma, S.; Mather, P.; Gupta, A.; Reeves, G.; Rubin, S.; Bonita, R.; Chowdhury, A.; Malloy, R.; Willes, L.; Whellan, D. Effect of Early Intervention with Positive Airway Pressure Therapy for Sleep Disordered Breathing on Six-Month Readmission Rates in Hospitalized Patients with Heart Failure. *Am. J. Cardiol.* **2016**, *117*, 940–945. [CrossRef] [PubMed]
9. Channick, J.E.; Jackson, N.J.; Zeidler, M.R.; Buhr, R.G. Effects of Obstructive Sleep Apnea and Obesity on Thirty-Day Readmissions in Patients with Chronic Obstructive Pulmonary Disease: A Cross-Sectional Mediation Analysis. *Ann. Am. Thorac. Soc.* **2021**, *19*, 462–468. [CrossRef] [PubMed]
10. Peppard, P.E.; Young, T.; Barnet, J.H.; Palta, M.; Hagen, E.W.; Hla, K.M. Increased Prevalence of Sleep-Disordered Breathing in Adults. *Am. J. Epidemiol.* **2013**, *177*, 1006–1014. [CrossRef] [PubMed]

11. Benjafield, A.V.; Ayas, N.T.; Eastwood, P.R.; Heinzer, R.; Ip, M.S.M.; Morrell, M.J.; Nunez, C.M.; Patel, S.R.; Penzel, T.; Pépin, J.L.; et al. Estimation of the Global Prevalence and Burden of Obstructive Sleep Apnoea: A Literature-Based Analysis. *Lancet Respir Med.* **2019**, *7*, 687–698. [CrossRef]
12. Epstein, L.J.; Kristo, D.; Strollo, P.J., Jr.; Friedman, N.; Malhotra, A.; Patil, S.P. Clinical Guideline for The Evaluation, Management and Long-Term Care of Obstructive Sleep Apnea in Adults. *J. Clin. Sleep Med.* **2009**, *5*, 263–276. [CrossRef]
13. Stansbury, R.; Abdelfattah, M.; Chan, J.; Mittal, A.; Alqahtani, F.; Sharma, S. Hospital Screening for Obstructive Sleep Apnea in Patients Admitted to A Rural, Tertiary Care Academic Hospital with Heart Failure. *Hosp Pract.* **2020**, *48*, 266–271. [CrossRef]
14. Dunietz, G.L.; Yu, Y.; Levine, R.S.; Conceicao, A.S.; Burke, J.F.; Chervin, R.D.; Braley, T.J. Obstructive Sleep Apnea in Older Adults: Geographic Disparities in PAP Treatment and Adherence. *J. Clin. Sleep Med.* **2021**, *17*, 421–427. [CrossRef]
15. Stansbury, R.; Strollo, P.; Pauly, N.; Sharma, I.; Schaaf, M.; Aaron, A.; Feinberg, J. Under-Recognition of Sleep-Disordered Breathing and Other Common Health Conditions in The West Virginia Medicaid Population: A Driver of Poor Health Outcomes. *J. Clin. Sleep Med.* **2021**, *18*, 817–824. [CrossRef]
16. Health Resources and Services Administration Eligibility Requirements for Federally Qualified Health Centers. Available online: https://www.hrsa.gov/opa/eligibility-and-registration/health-centers/fqhc/index.html (accessed on 28 January 2022).
17. United States Census Bureau West Virginia Data Page. Available online: https://www.census.gov/quickfacts/WV (accessed on 15 June 2022).
18. Schotland, H.M.; Jeffe, D.B. Development of the Obstructive Sleep Apnea Knowledge and Attitudes (OSAKA) Questionnaire. *Sleep Med.* **2003**, *4*, 443–450. [CrossRef]
19. Chai-Coetzer, C.L.; Antic, N.A.; Rowland, L.S.; Reed, R.L.; Esterman, A.; Catcheside, P.G.; Eckermann, S.; Vowles, N.; Williams, H.; Dunn, S.; et al. Primary Care Vs Specialist Sleep Center Management of Obstructive Sleep Apnea and Daytime Sleepiness and Quality of Life: A Randomized Trial. *JAMA* **2013**, *309*, 997–1004. [CrossRef] [PubMed]
20. Pendharkar, S.R.; Dechant, A.; Bischak, D.P.; Tsai, W.H.; Stevenson, A.M.; Hanly, P.J. An Observational Study of the Effectiveness of Alternative Care Providers in the Management of Obstructive Sleep Apnea. *J. Sleep Res.* **2016**, *25*, 234–240. [CrossRef] [PubMed]
21. Tarraubella, N.; Sánchez-de-la-Torre, M.; Nadal, N.; De Batlle, J.; Benítez, I.; Cortijo, A.; Urgelés, M.C.; Sanchez, V.; Lorente, I.; Lavega, M.M.; et al. Management of Obstructive Sleep Apnoea in A Primary Care Vs Sleep Unit Setting: A Randomised Controlled Trial. *Thorax* **2018**, *73*, 1152–1160. [CrossRef] [PubMed]
22. Kapur, V.K.; Auckley, D.H.; Chowdhuri, S.; Kuhlmann, D.C.; Mehra, R.; Ramar, K.; Harrod, C.G. Clinical Practice Guideline for Diagnostic Testing for Adult Obstructive Sleep Apnea: An American Academy of Sleep Medicine Clinical Practice Guideline. *J. Clin. Sleep Med.* **2017**, *13*, 479–504. [CrossRef]
23. Grote, L.; McNicholas, W.T.; Hedner, J. ESADA Collaborators. Sleep Apnoea Management in Europe During The COVID-19 Pandemic: Data from The European Sleep Apnoea Database (ESADA). *Eur. Respir. J.* **2020**, *55*, 2001323. [CrossRef]
24. Spagnuolo, C.M.; McIsaac, M.; Dosman, J.; Karunanayake, C.; Pahwa, P.; Pickett, W. Distance to Specialist Medical Care and Diagnosis of Obstructive Sleep Apnea in Rural Saskatchewan. *Can. Respir. J.* **2019**, *2019*, 1683124. [CrossRef] [PubMed]
25. Allen, A.J.; Amram, O.; Tavakoli, H.; Almeida, F.R.; Hamoda, M.; Ayas, N.T. Relationship Between Travel Time from Home to A Regional Sleep Apnea Clinic in British Columbia, Canada, And the Severity of Obstructive Sleep. *Ann. Am. Thorac. Soc.* **2016**, *13*, 719–723. [CrossRef]
26. Billings, M.E. Regional Differences in PAP Care: More Questions Than Answers. *J. Clin. Sleep Med.* **2021**, *17*, 363–364. [CrossRef]
27. Bruyneel, M. Telemedicine in the Diagnosis and Treatment of Sleep Apnoea. *Eur. Respir. Rev.* **2019**, *28*, 151. [CrossRef]
28. Singh, J.; Badr, M.S.; Diebert, W.; Epstein, L.; Hwang, D.; Karres, V.; Khosla, S.; Mims, K.N.; Shamim-Uzzaman, A.; Kirsch, D.; et al. American Academy of Sleep Medicine (AASM) Position Paper for the Use of Telemedicine for the Diagnosis and Treatment of Sleep Disorders. *J. Clin. Sleep Med.* **2015**, *11*, 1187–1198. [CrossRef] [PubMed]
29. Haleem, A.; Javaid, M.; Singh, R.P.; Suman, R. Telemedicine for Healthcare: Capabilities, Features, Barriers, and Applications. *Sens. Int.* **2021**, *2*, 100117. [CrossRef] [PubMed]
30. Billings, M.E.; Cohen, R.T.; Baldwin, C.M.; Johnson, D.A.; Palen, B.N.; Parthasarathy, S.; Patel, S.R.; Russell, M.; Tapia, I.E.; Williamson, A.A.; et al. Disparities in Sleep Health and Potential Intervention Models: A Focused Review. *Chest* **2021**, *159*, 1232–1240. [CrossRef] [PubMed]
31. Phillips, B. Improving Access to Diagnosis and Treatment of Sleep-Disordered Breathing. *Chest* **2007**, *132*, 1418–1420. [CrossRef]
32. Shamim-Uzzaman, Q.A.; Bae, C.J.; Ehsan, Z.; Setty, A.R.; Devine, M.; Dhankikar, S.; Donskoy, I.; Fields, B.; Hearn, H.; Hwang, D.; et al. The Use of Telemedicine for the Diagnosis and Treatment of Sleep Disorders: An American Academy of Sleep Medicine Update. *J. Clin. Sleep Med.* **2021**, *17*, 1103–1107. [CrossRef]
33. Afifi, R.A.; Parker, E.A.; Dino, G.; Hall, D.M.; Ulin, B. Reimagining Rural: Shifting Paradigms About Health and Well-Being in the Rural United States. *Annu. Rev. Public Health* **2022**, *43*, 135–154. [CrossRef] [PubMed]
34. Chhatre, S.; Chang, Y.H.A.; Gooneratne, N.S.; Kuna, S.; Strollo, P.; Jayadevappa, R. Association Between Adherence to Continuous Positive Airway Pressure Treatment and Cost Among Medicare Enrollees. *Sleep* **2020**, *43*, zsz188. [CrossRef]
35. Benjafield, A.V.; Oldstone, L.M.; Willes, L.A.; Kelly, C.; Nunez, C.M.; Malhotra, A.; On Behalf of the medXcloud Group. Positive Airway Pressure Therapy Adherence with Mask Resupply: A Propensity-Matched Analysis. *J. Clin. Med.* **2021**, *10*, 72. [CrossRef]
36. Weaver, T.E.; Grunstein, R.R. Adherence to Continuous Positive Airway Pressure Therapy: The Challenge to Effective treatment. *Proc. Am. Thorac. Soc.* **2008**, *5*, 173–178. [CrossRef] [PubMed]

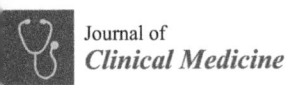

Systematic Review

Association between Obstructive Sleep Apnea and Heart Failure in Adults—A Systematic Review

Agnieszka Polecka [1,*], Natalia Olszewska [2], Łukasz Danielski [2] and Ewa Olszewska [3]

[1] Doctoral School of the Medical University of Bialystok, 15-089 Bialystok, Poland
[2] Student Research Group, Department of Otolaryngology, Medical University of Bialystok, 15-089 Bialystok, Poland
[3] Sleep Apnea Surgery Center, Department of Otolaryngology, Medical University of Bialystok, 15-089 Bialystok, Poland
* Correspondence: agnieszka.polecka@sd.umb.edu.pl

Abstract: Background: Heart failure (HF) patients commonly experience obstructive sleep apnea (OSA), which may worsen their condition. We reviewed a diverse range of studies to investigate the prevalence of OSA in HF patients, the effects of positive airway pressure (PAP) treatment, and the potential impact of sodium-glucose cotransporter-2 inhibitors (SGLT2i) and sacubitril/valsartan on OSA outcomes. Methods: We analyzed case-control, observational studies, and randomized controlled trials. Prevalence rates, PAP treatment, and HF pharmacotherapy were assessed. Results: Numerous studies revealed a high prevalence of OSA in HF patients, particularly with preserved ejection fraction. PAP treatment consistently improved an apnea-hypopnea index, left ventricular ejection fraction, oxygen saturation, and overall quality of life. Emerging evidence suggests that SGLT2i and sacubitril/valsartan might influence OSA outcomes through weight loss, improved metabolic profiles, and potential direct effects on upper airway muscles. Conclusions: The complex interplay between OSA and HF necessitates a multifaceted approach. PAP treatment has shown promising results in improving OSA symptoms and HF parameters. Additionally, recent investigations into the effects of HF pharmacotherapy on OSA suggest their potential as adjunctive therapy. This review provides insights for clinicians and researchers, highlighting the importance of addressing OSA and HF in patient management strategies.

Keywords: sleep; sleep apnea; obstructive sleep apnea; OSA; sleep-disordered breathing; heart failure

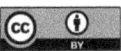

1. Introduction

Obstructive Sleep Apnea Syndrome (OSAS) is a chronic inflammatory disease characterized by episodes of total or partial obstruction of upper respiratory airways during sleep with preserved respiratory muscle effort [1]. In accordance with the American Academy of Sleep Medicine Task Force definition, obstructive sleep apnea (OSA) is characterized by the occurrence of five or more respiratory events per hour of sleep, which is measured by the apnea-hypopnea index (AHI) [2]. Clinically, OSA may manifest with the following symptoms: daytime sleepiness, loud snoring, arousals caused by gasping or choking, concentration and memory impairment, morning headaches, mood disorders, or insomnia. Moreover, the sleep partner of the patient may observe their apneas, gasping, or choking [2]. The severity of obstructive sleep apnea is classified as mild (AHI = 5–14), moderate (AHI = 15–29), or severe (AHI $\geq$ 30) [3]. The prevalence of OSA is estimated at 44% in the general European adult population, with approximately 23% of patients with moderate to severe OSA (AHI $\geq$ 15) [4]. Unfortunately, a significant number of individuals with OSA remain undiagnosed or untreated. Such patients are predisposed to an elevated risk of hypertension, cardiovascular disease (CVD), heart failure, stroke, metabolic derangements (obesity, diabetes mellitus), depression, excessive daytime sleepiness that may lead to traffic, and work-related accidents as well as absence at work [5–8]. The pathogenesis of OSA is multifactorial and remains only partially explained. It encompasses various mechanisms, including selective activation of inflammatory pathways, endothelial dysfunction, metabolic dysregulation, and oxidative stress [9–11]. Endothelial dysfunction is considered one of the earliest identifiable and potentially reversible abnormalities during the progression of atherosclerosis [12]. American Academy of Sleep Medicine (AASM) offers evidence-based recommendations for the diagnosis, management, and long-term care of patients with OSA [2].

Heart failure (HF) is characterized by structural and/or functional impairments in cardiac ejection, leading to a complex clinical syndrome with distinctive symptoms and manifestations. HF has been identified as a global pandemic, with an estimated 64.3 million individuals worldwide in 2017 [13]. The prevalence of HF is expected to increase due to enhanced survival rates following an HF diagnosis. That is attributed to the availability of HF evidence-based treatment methods and the overall extended life expectancy of the general population. According to the classification based on left ventricular ejection fraction (LVEF), heart failure was categorized into three groups: HF with reduced ejection fraction (HFrEF), HF with mildly reduced ejection fraction (HFmrEF), and HF with preserved ejection fraction (HFpEF). These categories were defined based on LVEF ranges of $\leq 40\%$, 41–49%, and $\geq 50\%$, respectively. Evidence-based recommendations for the diagnosis and management of heart failure are found in the 2022 guidelines of the American College of Cardiology/American Heart Association/Heart Failure Society of America (ACC/AHA/HFSA) and the 2021 guidelines of the European Society of Cardiology (ESC) [14,15].

OSA is highly associated with adverse outcomes in heart failure patients. It possesses a potential negative feedback loop and worsens comorbid conditions that deteriorate OSA. HF and OSA complications create a vicious circle of reciprocal correlations [16]. Among patients with symptomatic or decompensated HF, the prevalence of sleep apnea ranges up to 80%. More than half of these individuals suffer from OSA [16,17]. Sleep apnea, whether in the presence or absence of HF, is associated with a higher risk of negative cardiovascular outcomes, including aggravation of HF-related symptoms, increased hospitalizations, and higher mortality rates.

Moreover, individuals diagnosed with OSA (without a previous diagnosis of HF) meet a notably elevated risk of developing HF [18]. This association between OSA and HF is influenced by various pathophysiological mechanisms, including the activation of neurohormonal pathways, increased levels of oxidative stress and inflammation, acute changes in preload and afterload due to significant swings in intrathoracic pressure, and the exacerbation of systemic hypertension. An incident of airflow obstruction, hypoxia, and an attempted inspiratory effort result in arousal and an exaggerated drop in intrathoracic pressure. The drop in intrathoracic pressure leads to the pressure increase within the left ventricle (LV), known as transmural pressure, which subsequently raises the afterload. Additionally, intrathoracic pressure drop increases the venous return, leading to distention of the right ventricle (RV) and a leftward shift of the interventricular septum.

Consequently, a decrease in LV filling is observed. The combination of reduced LV filling and increased afterload results in a reduction in stroke volume (SV). The enlargement of the jugular vein observed in individuals with decompensated HF may significantly deteriorate OSA symptoms by exerting additional pressure on the hypopharynx, particularly in a supine position. The pathophysiological cycle showing the association between heart failure and obstructive sleep apnea is presented in Figure 1.

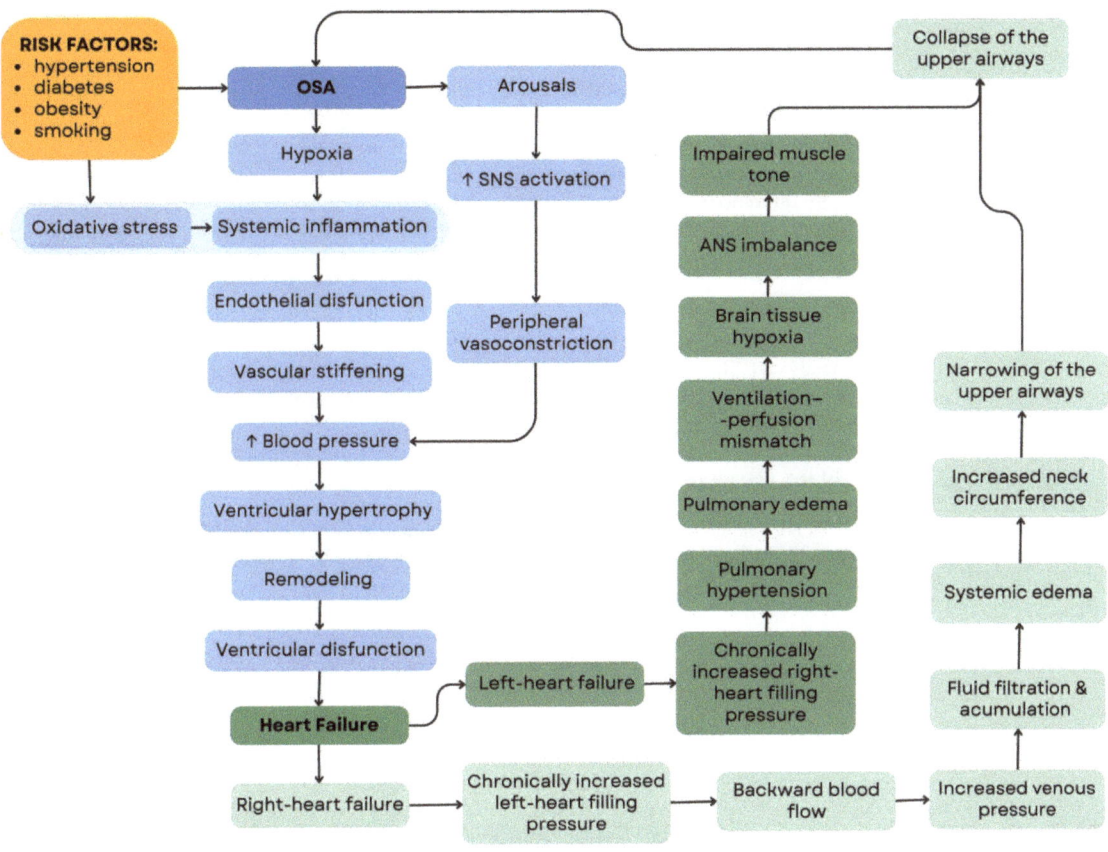

Figure 1. Pathophysiological association of heart failure and obstructive sleep apnea.

The primary objective of this systematic review is to comprehensively analyze the existing literature concerning the intricate interplay between OSA and HF (OSA + HF). By conducting this review, the authors aim to shed light on the mutual impacts of these two conditions, explaining how OSA influences the progression and outcomes of HF and vice versa. This endeavor is important as it enhances our understanding of the complex relationship between OSA and HF, ultimately contributing to improved patient management and healthcare strategies. One of the novel aspects this review brings is the exploration of the effect of emerging HF pharmacotherapies, specifically sodium-glucose cotransporter-2 inhibitors (SGLT2i) and sacubitril/valsartan (S/V), on sleep parameters in OSA + HF patients. The exploration of the impact of these HF pharmacotherapies in the treatment of HF + OSA significantly contributes to the existing body of knowledge in the following ways. Firstly, studying the effects of emerging HF medications on sleep parameters in the context of OSA addresses a complex dual health challenge many patients face. Secondly, the study aligns with the growing emphasis on holistic patient care. It acknowledges that HF + OSA patients require comprehensive treatment addressing cardiovascular health and sleep quality.

Additionally, the use of emerging HF pharmacotherapies reduces the number of hospitalizations, improves cardiac outcomes, and enhances the life quality of HF patients. Investigating how evolving HF medications impact sleep parameters may uncover synergistic benefits, enhancing the overall well-being of the patients. This correlation may help clinicians make more conscious decisions about treatment combinations, considering the cardiovascular and sleep-related aspects of care.

Moreover, it may indirectly contribute to better adherence to the prescribed treatment regimen, improving clinical outcomes. Studying these effects can contribute to the development of personalized treatment plans and adjusting medication to the individual needs of the patient. With these innovative medications revolutionizing HF management by targeting underlying pathophysiological pathways, it is imperative to elucidate whether they influence sleep characteristics in affected individuals. HF medications may indirectly impact sleep patterns. Therefore, understanding any potential changes in sleep parameters holds great clinical significance.

2. Materials and Methods

The criteria of the Preferred Reporting Items for Systematic Reviews and Meta-Analysis (PRISMA) checklist were followed in conducting and reporting this systematic review [19]. The study protocol was not registered. The PICO (population, indicator, control, outcome) questions are shown in Table 1.

Table 1. The PICO's question.

What Is the Prevalence of OSA in HF Patients?/How Do Sleep and Cardiac Parameters Change after PAP Therapy in These Patients?/Does New Cardiological Pharmacotherapy (SGLT2i and Sacubitril/Valsartan) Play a Role in the Treatment of OSA?	
The population	Patients with OSA and HF (OSA + HF)/patients with OSA and SGLT2i or sacubitril/valsartan in treatment
The indicator	AHI, LVEF, NT-proBNP concentration.
The control	Groups of patients without OSA or patients with other SDB/ patients without PAP treatment/patients without SGLT2i or sacubitril/valsartan in the treatment
The outcome	The difference in AHI/LVEF/NT-proBNP/BNP concentration
The study design	Peer-reviewed English articles. Adult (>18 years) human subjects. Case–control studies, randomized control trials, and observational studies.

Abbreviations: OSA, obstructive sleep apnea; SDB, sleep-disordered breathing; HF, heart failure; PAP, positive airway pressure; SGLT2i, sodium/glucose cotransporter-2 inhibitors; AHI, apnea-hypopnea index; LVEF, left ventricle ejection fraction; NT-proBNP, N-Terminal pro-Brain Natriuretic Peptide.

We searched PubMed, Scopus Library and Cochrane for case-control studies, randomized control trials (RCTs) and observational studies concerning the prevalence of obstructive sleep apnea syndrome in heart failure patients, changes in sleep and cardiological parameters after PAP therapy, and the role of new cardiac pharmacotherapy in OSA + HF patients. The search was performed using the words "sleep apnea", "disordered breathing", "heart failure", "preserved ejection fraction", "mildly reduced ejection fraction" and "reduced ejection fraction" in different combinations.

We searched the PubMed database using the following string: ((sleep apnea) OR (OSA) OR (disordered breathing)) AND (heart failure)) and ((sleep apnea) OR (OSA) OR (disordered breathing) AND (sglt2i) OR (dapagliflozin) OR (empagliflozin) OR (ertugliflozin) OR (canagliflozin) and (sleep apnea) AND (sacubitril/valsartan)). Filters: Randomized Control Trials.

To obtain literature from the Scopus library, we used the following string: TITLE-ABS-KEY ((sleep AND apnea OR obstructive AND sleep AND apnea OR sleep AND disordered AND breathing AND heart AND failure AND (LIMIT-TO (OA, "all") OR LIMIT-TO (OA, "Randomized Control Trials")) AND (LIMIT-TO (PUBSTAGE, "final")) AND (LIMIT-TO (SUBJAREA, "MEDI")) AND (LIMIT-TO (DOCTYPE, "ar")) AND (LIMIT-TO (LANGUAGE, "English")) AND (LIMIT-TO (EXACTKEYWORD, "Human")) and ((sleep apnea OR obstructive sleep apnea OR sleep disordered breathing AND empagliflozin OR dapagliflozin OR canagliflozin OR ertugliflozin OR sotagliflozin OR sacubitril valsartan AND (LIMIT-TO (OA,"all") OR LIMIT-TO (OA, "Randomized Control Trials"))

AND (LIMIT-TO (PUBSTAGE, "final")) AND (LIMIT-TO (SUBJAREA, "MEDI")) AND (LIMIT-TO (DOCTYPE,"ar")) AND (LIMIT-TO (LANGUAGE,"English")) AND (LIMIT-TO (EXACTKEYWORD,"Human")).

We searched Cochrane using the following string: "OSA" and "heart failure", "heart failure" and "SDB", "heart failure" and "sleep apnea", "OSA" and "dapagliflozin", "OSA" and "empagliflozin", "OSA" and "canagliflozin", "OSA and ertugliflozin", and "OSA and sotagliflozin".

The search results were exported to the Mendeley reference manager for the records' initial title and abstract screening. Duplicate articles were removed by the "remove duplicates" function of Mendeley. The literature search was performed between 2 June 2023 and 20 June 2023 and again on 2 July 2023. To obtain articles that were not received from databases, bibliographies of published articles were manually reviewed to identify additional studies. Two authors (A.P. and N.O.) independently performed the literature search and evaluated articles for inclusion. Discrepancies, if any, were resolved through discussion.

During the initial screening of titles and abstracts, the retrieved studies had to meet the following criteria for inclusion in full-text eligibility assessment: (1) randomized control trials, case-control studies or observational studies; (2) papers concerning adult human subjects with HF; (3) papers concerning adult human subjects diagnosed with OSA (AHI $\geq$ 5), (4) studies evaluating a combination of sleep and/or cardiological parameters, (5) clearly defined experimental and control groups. Exclusion criteria were: (1) studies in other than English language, (2) studies on pediatric population (i.e., age < 18 years), (3) the studies were classified as article review, letter, poster, conference summary or editorial, (4) the studies were not a randomized control trial/case-control/observational study. After the initial screening, two investigators (A.P. and N.O.) retrieved and independently assessed full-text manuscripts.

The process for selecting the studies is provided in the flow chart in Figure 2.

The Quality Assessment Tool EPHPP (Effective Public Healthcare Panacea Project) was used to evaluate the quality of the studies included in our systematic review. Two authors (A.P. and N.O.) performed an independent search and evaluation of the studies following the Quality Assessment Tool for Quantitative Studies Dictionary. Any discrepancies or concerns that arose during this process were thoroughly discussed by the authors to ensure consistency and accuracy in the evaluation process. This tool enabled us to thoroughly assess the quality of various study types (e.g., randomized controlled trial, controlled clinical trial, cohort, case-control) by offering customizable criteria based on study design. It facilitated a comprehensive evaluation of study quality by examining selection bias, study design, data collection methods, blindings, and potential confounding variables. Quality assessment of included studies is presented in Supplementary Material, Table S1. Comprehensive information on the assessment process and the specific questions used for evaluation are presented in Supplementary Material, Table S2.

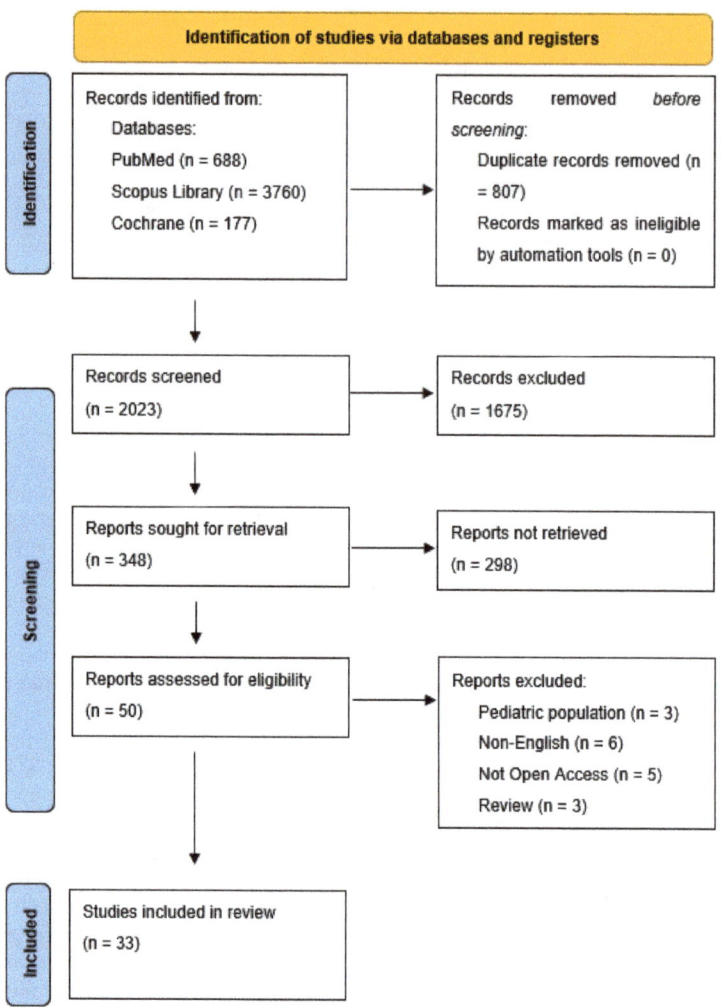

Figure 2. PRISMA flow diagram of the literature selection process.

3. Results

3.1. The Prevalence of Obstructive Sleep Apnea in the Heart Failure Population

The prevalence of OSA in HF patients was estimated by Wang et al. and depended on the LVEF [20]. Among 252 HF patients enrolled in the study, 48% presented OSA as well. When comparing the HFrEF, HFmrEF, and HFpEF groups, there were 42%, 47%, and 49% of OSA participants, respectively ($p = 0.708$). Additionally, the prevalence and the severity of sleep-disordered breathing (SDB) were significantly higher in HFrEF and HFmrEF. The above-mentioned types of heart failure were associated with central sleep apnea (CSA). OSA was found to be more common in individuals with HFpEF.

Wang et al. conducted another study with 248 patients diagnosed with heart failure to explore the prevalence of sleep-disordered breathing in patients with HF of different etiologies. The overall prevalence of SDB in the HF population was 70.6%, with OSA accounting for 47.6%. The patients were categorized into five groups based on the underlying cause of HF: ischemic, hypertensive, myocardial, valvular, and arrhythmic. The prevalence of SDB across these five groups was 75.3%, 81.4%, 77.8%, 51.9%, and 58.5%, respectively ($p = 0.014$).

Regarding OSA, the prevalence among the five groups was 42.7%, 72.1%, 36.1%, 37.0%, and 49.1%, respectively ($p = 0.009$) [21]. An analysis of sleep data across the five groups revealed that AHI, the longest duration of hypopnea, and the proportion of Cheyne-Stokes respiration (CSR) were higher in the ischemic, hypertensive, and myocardial groups compared to the valvular and arrhythmic groups (18.3 (5.0–31.4); 12.8 (6.1–28.0); 20.3 (9.3–34.5), respectively; $p < 0.05$). The myocardial group had the lowest LVEF values, followed by the ischemic group, whereas the other three groups demonstrated higher LVEF values (0.43 (0.31–0.52); 0.58 (0.43–0.68), respectively; $p < 0.001$).

Gupta et al. screened two groups of patients for SDB: 25 individuals previously diagnosed with HFpEF and 25 age and sex-matched controls of healthy subjects. SDB was observed in 64% of the case patients and 12% of the control group ($p < 0.001$). Among HFpEF patients with SDB (16/25), 13 were diagnosed with OSA and 3 with CSA. There was a significant difference between the patients and controls in AHI ($p < 0.001$), NT-ProBNP ($p < 0.001$), and polysomnography parameters (PSG WASO, PSG N1, N2, N3). A positive correlation between the AHI score and the degree of diastolic dysfunction was observed ($r = 0.67$; $p < 0.001$) [22].

The German multicenter SchlaHF (Sleep-Disordered Breathing in Heart Failure) registry by Arzt et al. enrolled 1557 HFrEF patients and estimated OSA as 29% of all included individuals [23].

Oldenburg et al. screened 700 patients with HF for SDB and presented 76% of SDB in the studied population, including 36% of OSA [16]. Patients with no SDB (including OSA) experienced less severe symptoms (New York Heart Association (NYHA) class 2.57 ± 0.5; $p < 0.05$) compared to the individuals with CSA (NYHA class 2.9 ± 0.5). Additionally, OSA patients had significantly higher LVEF values ($p < 0.05$) than CSA patients.

Bitter et al. investigated the prevalence and type of SDB in patients with HFpEF. The authors enrolled 244 patients with HFpEF and documented SDB in 169 patients (69.3%), of which 97 (39.8%) had OSA. The severity of OSA was mild in 40%, moderate in 36%, and severe in 24% of the cases [24].

A study conducted by Chan et al. screened 20 patients with HFpEF for SDB. 55% of participants were diagnosed with significant sleep-disordered breathing. In this group, 63.64% of patients had predominantly OSA with a mean AHI of 10.9 ± 5.1 [25].

Yumino et al. enrolled 218 patients with HF (with LVEF $\leq 45\%$) and screened them for SDB. Using AHI cutoff ≥ 10, ≥ 15, and ≥ 20, the prevalence of sleep apnea was estimated as 60%, 47%, and 39%, respectively. The prevalence of OSA was 37%, 26%, and 21%, respectively. The results of the OSA population were BMI (31.0 ± 5.0), LVEF (25.7 ± 9.1), and NYHA Class (class III + IV: OSA 31) [26].

Herrscher et al. assessed the prevalence of SDB in HF patients independent of systolic left ventricular function. In a cohort of 115 patients (62% with reduced EF and 38% with preserved EF), individuals were classified as New York Heart Association Class II–IV. The prevalence of SDB was 81%, including 54% of OSA. Among the HFpEF patients, SDB was present in 80% of the cases, with OSA occurring in 62%. Furthermore, the group of HFpEF patients also revealed a significantly higher incidence of hypertension. When comparing patients with preserved EF to the ones with reduced EF, both groups had nearly the same high prevalence of sleep apnea (80% vs. 82%). Additionally, within the HFpEF group, there were more patients with OSA than CSA (62% vs. 18%) [27].

Kalaydzhiev et al. screened 100 individuals and found 61 sleep-disordered breathing patients. In this study population, 50 individuals were diagnosed with OSA (82%), and 52% were male. The following parameters were estimated: left ventricular ejection fraction at $49.6 \pm 8.5\%$, AHI at 41.8 ± 23.2, BMI at 38.5 ± 7.1, NTproBNP at 1359.12 ± 740.64 pg/mL, mean oxygen saturation (MOS) at $83.9 \pm 6.8\%$, and the lowest oxygen saturation (LOS) at $65.3 \pm 12.7\%$ [28].

The summarized data of chosen studies is presented in Table 2. Figure 3 presents OSA prevalence over the years.

Table 2. The characteristics and results of chosen studies populations.

Author, Year	N	Sex, M/F	Age, Years	BMI, kg/m²	EF, %	AHI	OSA Prevalence, %	Overall OSA Prevalence, %	SDB Prevalence, %
Kalaydzhiev et al., 2023 [28]	100 screened; 61 SDB; 50 OSA, 11 CSA	32/29	66.2 ± 9.1 OSA; 66.1 ± 11.9 CSA	38.5 ± 7.1 OSA; 31.9 ± 4.5 CSA	49.6 ± 8.5 OSA; 41.8 ± 11.4 CSA	41.8 ± 23.2 OSA; 37.7 ± 12.6 CSA	81.97 (50/61)	50 (50/100)	61 (61/100)
Wang et al., 2022 [20]	252; 36 r; 43 mr; 173 p	134/118	70.1, 68.3 ± 12.6 r; 65.0 ± 14.7 mr; 71.8 ± 11.8 p	24.8 24.0 (21.1, 27.3)r; 24.8 (23.1, 27.0)mr; 24.5(22.0, 26.9)p	<40 r; 40–50 mr; ≥50 p	26.4 ± 16.2 r; 26.1 ± 15.2 mr; 14.4 ± 15.6 p *◊	42 (15/36)r; 47 (20/43)mr; 49 (85/173)p	48 (120/252)	86 (31/252) r; 86 (37/252) mr; 62 (108/252) p *◊
Wang et al., 2022 [21]	248, 89 I; 43 H; 36 M; 27 V; 53 A	132/116	70.4 ± 12.4, I:73.0 (66.0–81.5); H: 75.0 (68.0–82.0); M: 67.0 (56.0–75.0); V: 73.0 (62.0–82.0); A: 70.0 (61.5–79.0)	24.5, I:24.0 (21.9–26.7); H: 25.5 (22.9–28.7); M: 24.3 (21.2–27.2); V: 23.9 (20.1–25.8); A: 24.8 (22.2–27.8)	ND	I: 18.3 (5.0–31.4); H: 12.8 (6.1–28.0); M: 20.3 (9.3–34.5); V: 6.6 (1.7–22.5) ◊; A: 6.9 (3.6–20.5)	ND	47.6, 38 (42.7%)I; 31 (72.1%)H; 13 (36.1%)M; 10 (37.0%)V; 26 (49.1%)A	70.6 (175/248)
Gupta et al., 2020 [22]	50 (25P/25C)	40/10	58.4 ± 9.8 OSA; 60 + 10 CSA	27.9 + 1.6 OSA; 29.4 + 0.6 CSA	55.84 + 2.01 ◊ SDB; 52.08 + 3.24 ◊ noSDB	9.9 + 4.2 ◊ SDB; 3.7 + 1.1 ◊ noSDB	52 (13/25)	26 (13/50)	32 (16/50)
Arzt et al., 2017 [23]	9221screened, 1557SDB; 452 OSA, 624 OSA + CSA; 481 CSA	1353/204	66 ± 11 OSA; 69 ± 10 OSA + CSA; 69 ± 10 CSA	31 ± 6 OSA; 29 ± 5 OSA + CSA; 28 ± 4 CSA	35 ± 8 OSA; 34 ± 8 OSA + CSA; 32 ± 8 CSA	37 ± 19 OSA; 36 ± 16 OSA + CSA; 38 ± 15 CSA	29 (452/1557)	4.90 (452/9221)	16.89 (1557/9221)
Herrscher et al., 2011 [27]	115, 62 OSA, 31 CSA, 22 noSDB	91/24	62.0 ± 9.7; 62.46 ± 9.2 OSA; 62.26 ± 10.6 CSA; 60.26 ± 10.0 noSDB	30.2 ± 6.0 OSA; 28.4 ± 4.2 CSA; 27.1 ± 4.8 noSDB	40.4 ± 13.2 OSA; 34.0 ± 12.5 CSA; 37.3 ± 12.0 noSDB	25.06 ± 21.7 OSA #◊; 26.86 ± 13.1 CSA #◊; 2.36 ± 1.5 noSDB	66.67 (62/93)	53.91 (62/115)	80.87 (93/115)

Table 2. Cont.

Author, Year	N	Sex, M/F	Age, Years	BMI, kg/m²	EF, %	AHI	OSA Prevalence, %	Overall OSA Prevalence, %	SDB Prevalence, %
Bitter et al., 2009 [24]	244, 72 CSA; 97 OSA; 75 noSDB	157/87	65.3 ± 1.4; 66.9 ± 2.4 CSA ‡; 66.8 ± 1.9 OSA †; 61.6 ± 3.3 noSDB	29.3 ± 0.9 CSA ‡; 29.3 ± 1.1 OSA †; 26.42 ± 1 noSDB	>55	impaired relaxation: 15.0 ± 3.6; pseudonormal: 20.0 ± 3.3 †; restrictive: 23.4 ± 6.2 ‡	57.4 (97/169)	39.75 (97/244)	69.3 (169/244)
Yumino et al., 2009 [26]	218, 56 OSA; 45 CSA; 117 M-NSA	168/50	55.66 ± 12.7 56.36 ± 12.1 OSA; 60.46 ± 8.9 CSA; 53.46 ± 13.6 M-NSA	29.26 ± 5.3 31.0 ± 5.0 ˆ OSA; 27.8 ± 5.4 CSA **; 28.9 ± 5.3 M-NSA	25.76 ± 9.1 OSA; 21.36 ± 9.5 CSA; 25.56 ± 10.3 M-NSA	33.6 ± 14.5 ˆ OSA; 34.8 ± 15.6 ´ CSA; 6.8 ± 3.9 M-NSA	55.45 (56/101)	25.69 (56/218)	46.33 (101/218)
Oldenburg et al., 2007 [16]	700, 253 OSA; 278 CSA; 169 noSDB	139/561	65.02 ± 9.5 OSA ᵃ; 65.86 ± 10.5 CSA ᵃ; 61.45 ± 11.0 noSDB	27.84 ± 4.7 OSA ᵃ; 26.30 ± 4.1 CSA ᵇ; 25.77 ± 3.7 noSDB	29.3 ± 2.6 OSA; 27.4 ± 6.6 CSA ᵃ; 28.2 ± 7.3 noSDB	18.45 ± 13.3 ᵃ OSA; 30.15 ± 15.2 ᵃ,ᵇ CSA; 2.28 ± 1.6 noSDB	48.21 (256/531)	36 (256/700)	76 (531/700)
Chan et al., 1997 [25]	20, 11 SDB, 9 noSDB	7/13	65 ± 6.0 7.3 ± 1.3 SDB; 7.2 ± 0.8 noSDB	ND	28 ± 3.2 29.1 ± 4.2 SDB; 27.6 ± 1.3 noSDB	19.5 ± 10.8 SDB ◊; 3.9 ± 3.5 noSDB ◊	63.64 (7/11)	35 (7/20)	55 (11/20)

Abbreviations: r, reduced ejection fraction; mr, mildly-reduced ejection fraction; p, preserved ejection fraction; ND, no data; ◊, significant difference, $p < 0.05$; *, $p < 0.05$, p/mr group vs. r group and $p < 0.05$, p group vs. mr group; M/F, n Male/Female; H, hypertensive group; M, myocardial group; V, valvular group; A, arrhythmic group; EF, ejection fraction; M-NSA, mild or no sleep apnea; OSA, obstructive sleep apnea; CSA, central sleep apnea; P, patients with sleep disordered breathing; C, controls; SDB, sleep disordered breathing; noSDB, no sleep-disordered breathing; #◊, $p < 0.05$, OSA/CSA vs. noSDB; †, $p < 0.05$ OSA vs. noSDB; ‡, $p < 0.05$ CSA vs. noSDB; ´, $p < 0.05$ M-NSA vs. OSA; ˆ, $p < 0.05$ M-NSA vs. CSA; **, $p < 0.05$ OSA vs. CSA; ᵃ, $p < 0.05$ vs. no SDB; ᵇ, $p < 0.05$ vs. OSA; overall OSA prevalence, number (n) of OSA/n all study participants; OSA prevalence, n OSA/n SDB participants. Data is presented as the percentage of cohort or mean ± standard deviation or median.

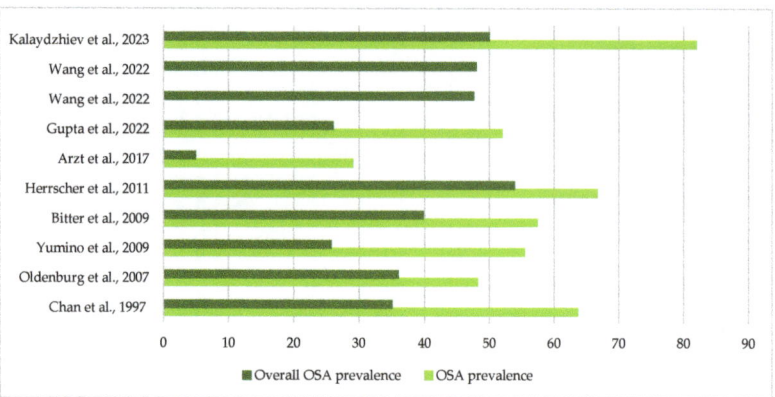

Figure 3. OSA prevalence in chosen studies. Abbreviations: Overall OSA prevalence, number (n) of OSA/n all study participants; OSA prevalence, n OSA/n SDB participants [16,20–28].

3.2. Does Positive Airway Pressure Play a Role in HF Patients?

3.2.1. Obstructive Sleep Apnea and Heart Failure with Preserved Ejection Fraction

Arikawa et al. collected data from 58 patients with new-onset HFpEF. In these patients, LVEF and plasma BNP concentration at the baseline were 61 ± 5% and 391 (218–752) pg/mL, respectively. Obstructive sleep apnea, with a mean AHI score of 43 ± 16, was found in 39 subjects (67%). Furthermore, none of these patients showed evidence of CSA. All of them were treated for OSA with CPAP and were advised lifestyle modifications over a 36-month observational period. The baseline plasma brain natriuretic peptide concentration in the studied groups was 444 (233–752) pg/mL in OSA and 316 (218–703) pg/mL in the non-OSA group. After 36 months of the follow-up period, the BNP concentration decreased in both groups. However, the reduction was less significant in patients with sleep apnea. While the BNP concentration was similar at the one-month cutoff in both groups, they were notably higher in the sleep apnea group after six months ($p < 0.05$), 12 months ($p < 0.05$), and 36 months ($p < 0.05$) [29]. This research demonstrated that in patients with HFpEF, obstructive sleep apnea leads to elevated BNP levels during extended follow-up periods compared to non-OSA subjects. These findings indicate that even with appropriate CPAP treatment, OSA might negatively impact long-term cardiac function and prognosis. Table 3 presents data from the study.

Table 3. The characteristics and results of a chosen study population with OSA and HFpEF.

Author, Year	N	Sex, M/F	Age, Years	EF, % Pre	EF, % Post	OSA Prevalence, %	CPAP Adherence	AHI Pre	AHI Post	BNP Pre, pg/mL	BNP Post, pg/mL
Arikawa et al., 2016 [29]	58	31/19	66 ± 15 (OSA) 65 ± 11 (nOSA)	61 ± 5 (OSA) 63 ± 9 (nOSA)	ND	67% (39/58)	ND	ND	ND	444 (233–752) (OSA) 316 (218–703) (nOSA)	1 m: 302 (202–350) (OSA) 212 (180–405) (nOSA) 6 m: 222 (137–324) ◊ (OSA) 76 (38–96) ◊ (nOSA) 12 m: 123 (98–197) ◊ (OSA) 52 (38–76) ◊ (nOSA) 36 m: 115 (64–174) ◊ (OSA) 56 (25–74) ◊ (nOSA)

Abbreviations: ND, no data; ◊, significant difference; M/F, Male/Female; EF, ejection fraction; OSA, obstructive sleep apnea; nOSA, no obstructive sleep apnea. Data is presented as a percentage of cohort or mean ± standard deviation or median.

3.2.2. Obstructive Sleep Apnea and Heart Failure with Reduced Ejection Fraction

The prospective, single-arm, open-label study conducted by Naito et al. analyzed 55 Japanese patients with HFrEF and moderate-to-severe OSA [30]. After one month of

CPAP treatment, the AHI decreased from 45.3 ± 16.1 to 5.4 ± 4.1 and the arousal index from 43.9 ± 19.6 to 15.7 ± 10.3. The LVEF improved from $37.2\% \pm 9.8$ to $43.2\% \pm 11.7$. Additionally, a significant decrease in heart rate (76.3 ± 11.2 vs. 70.7 ± 9.0, $p < 0.001$), systolic (131.3 ± 13.3 vs. 126.2 ± 12.2, $p < 0.001$), and diastolic (78.4 ± 10.5 vs. 74.3 ± 10.3, $p < 0.001$) blood pressure after the treatment was noted. However, there were no significant changes in the BMI. Univariate regression analysis showed that age ($p < 0.001$), BMI ($p < 0.001$), atrial fibrillation ($p = 0.0443$), LOS ($p = 0.0266$), and pressure levels of CPAP ($p = 0.0013$) were positively associated with improvements in LVEF at the baseline. After adjusting for confounding variables, age ($p = 0.008$) and BMI ($p < 0.001$) became the most significant factors for LVEF improvement. There was no correlation between pharmacotherapy (ACE inhibitors, AR blockers, Beta-blockers, diuretics, spironolactone, nitrates, digoxin) and LVEF improvement in HFrEF patients. The multivariate regression analyses indicated that young patients with obesity are inclined to LVEF enhancement. The degree of improvement was estimated at 6% in this population. The results are consistent with other studies.

Kaneko et al. conducted a study on 24 patients previously diagnosed with OSA and HFrEF [31]. The subjects were randomly assigned to control (N = 12) and CPAP group (N = 12). After one month, a significant reduction in the following sleep parameters was observed in the CPAP group: AHI (from 31.7 ± 6.4 to 8.3 ± 2.8, $p < 0.001$), arousal index (from 31.4 ± 6.1 to 12.8 ± 1.7, $p = 0.003$) and desaturation index (from 12.7 ± 3.2 to 0.8 ± 0.5, $p < 0.001$). Moreover, the LOS improved from 82.3 ± 1.2 to 89.6 ± 1.1 ($p = 0.004$). Additionally, there was a decrease in cardiological parameters, such as: daytime systolic blood pressure (from 126 ± 6 to 116 ± 5 mmHg, $p = 0.02$) and heart rate (from 68 ± 3 to 64 ± 3 beats per minute, $p = 0.007$). Furthermore, the LVEF value increased from $25.0 \pm 2.8\%$ to $33.8 \pm 2.4\%$. There were no significant improvements in the control group in the above-mentioned parameters. In conclusion, patients who received HF treatment and managed concurrent OSA through CPAP presented systolic blood pressure and HR reduction, as well as left ventricular systolic function improvement.

Mansfield et al. enrolled 55 individuals formerly diagnosed with both OSA and HFrEF. The study was randomized: 28 subjects were assigned to the CPAP group and 27—to the control group. The results indicated that three months of CPAP treatment was associated with significant improvements in LVEF ($\Delta 1.5 \pm 1.4\%$ vs. $5.0 \pm 1.0\%$, respectively, $p = 0.04$), AHI ($\Delta -8.4 \pm 3.6$ vs. -21.1 ± 3.8, $p < 0.001$), LOS ($\Delta 0.0 \pm 1.6$ vs. 11.5 ± 2.7, $p = 0.001$), reductions in overnight urinary norepinephrine excretion ($\Delta 1.6 \pm 3.7$ vs. -9.9 ± 3.6 nmol/mmol creatinine, $p = 0.036$), and improvements in quality of life (in the domains of physical role ($p = 0.03$), vitality ($p = 0.02$), social functioning ($p = 0.03$), and mental health ($p = 0.01$). Overall, the treatment of OSA among HF patients leads to improvement in cardiac function, sympathetic activity, and quality of life [32].

Fox et al. randomized 58 patients with HFrEF and OSA to automatic positive airway pressure (Auto-PAP) (N = 25) or nasal strips (controls) (N = 33) [33]. The study indicated significant LVEF improvement in the Auto-PAP group (from $38 \pm 9\%$ at baseline to $40 \pm 9\%$ at six months) compared with controls ($40 \pm 9\%$ to $40 \pm 8\%$; $p < 0.01$). AHI decreased significantly from baseline to 6 months in the Auto-PAP group (from $34 \pm 17/h$ to $9 \pm 8/h$; $p < 0.001$) but remained unchanged in the control group (from $35 \pm 13/h$ to $33 \pm 20/h$). Additionally, patients with Auto-PAP treatment experienced a greater improvement in the MOS (controls: from 92.03 ± 2.23 to 92.00 ± 2.97, $p = 0.857$; Auto-PAP group: from 92.47 ± 2.62 to 93.82 ± 1.92, $p = 0.001$) when compared to both initial levels and the control group. In summary, Auto-PAP intervention demonstrated a significant improvement compared to the control group, especially in terms of percent-predicted cardiopulmonary exercise capacity (peak VO2), a well-established marker for cardiovascular prognosis in HFrEF. Additionally, Auto-PAP showed beneficial effects on hypoxemia, cardiac function, and overall quality of life.

A randomized sham-controlled trial conducted by Kim et al. on 52 patients with severe OSA and reduced ejection fraction analyzed left ventricle (LV) and right ventricle (RV) function by conventional and speckle-tracking echocardiography before and after three months of CPAP (N = 26) or sham treatment (N = 26) [34]. CPAP treatment significantly improved LV global longitudinal strain (GLS) compared to the sham treatment (−20.0% ± 2.1% vs. −18.0% ± 2.5%; p = 0.004). There were no differences in LV dimension or ejection fraction. CPAP treatment reduced RV size and improved the fractional area change (51.3% ± 7.9% vs. 46.9% ± 6.7%; p = 0.038) compared with the sham treatment but did not improve the RV GLS compared with the sham treatment. Overall, in individuals diagnosed with severe OSA, three months of CPAP therapy resulted in enhancement of LV and RV function when compared to the sham treatment. CPAP treatment significantly improved, especially in LV mechanical function and RV fractional area change evaluated through speckle-tracking and two-dimensional echocardiography.

Gilman et al. performed a substudy of a larger randomized controlled trial on 19 OSA and HFrEF individuals and randomized them to CPAP treatment (N = 12) or control (N = 7) group for one month [35]. In the control group, there were no significant changes in the AHI (from 41 ± 13 to 37 ± 18) and other sleep parameters (LOS) from 82.4 ± 6.9 to 78.5 ± 12.4; arousals from 34.1 ± 13.5 to 35.1 ± 15.8) between the baseline and the follow-up. However, in contrast, CPAP intervention, with an average pressure of 8.8 ± 2.4 cm H_2O and a nightly usage duration of 6.3 ± 1.5 h, resulted in significant reductions in AHI (from 30 ± 15 to 7 ± 6), arousal index (from 26.7 ± 10.3 to 11.6 ± 3.6) (all p < 0.001). Furthermore, CPAP therapy led to improvements in MOS (from 94.8 ± 1.0 to 96.1 ± 1.6, p = 0.022) and LOS (from 82.5 ± 5.1 to 90.5 ± 3.6, p < 0.001). In the control group, there was no significant change in LVEF between baseline and follow-up. In contrast, the CPAP group presented an increase in LVEF, significantly greater than the control group (p = 0.028).

Servantes et al. conducted a study to examine the effects of exercise training and CPAP in patients with HFrEF (LVEF < 40%) and OSA. A total of sixty-five participants enrolled in four groups: control group (N = 18), exercise group (N = 17), CPAP group (N = 15), and exercise + CPAP group (N = 15), completed the study protocol. CPAP adherence and average daily use were similar between the groups. When comparing the baseline measurements with the three-month follow-up, there was no significant change in the mean AHI in the control group. However, the exercise group demonstrated a moderate decrease in AHI from 28 ± 17 to 18 ± 12 (p < 0.03). In contrast, both the CPAP group and the exercise + CPAP group exhibited a significant reduction in AHI, from 32 ± 25 to 8 ± 11 (p < 0.007) and from 25 ± 15 to 10 ± 16 (p < 0.007), respectively. No significant changes were observed in NYHA functional class distribution, excessive daytime sleepiness, quality of life, or sexual function in the control group. However, in the other intervention groups, there was an improvement in the NYHA functional class (classes II and III moved into class I, p < 0.05) and a reduction in daytime sleepiness (p < 0.05). Significant improvements in quality of life were observed in the exercise and exercise + CPAP groups compared to the control group (p < 0.05). Sexual function improved in the exercise + CPAP group compared to baseline, with no significant differences among the groups [36].

Egea et al. selected 60 patients with HF with LVEF < 45% and sleep apnea (83% OSA, 17% CSA) with AHI > 10/h and evaluated them at baseline and after three months of treatment with optimal CPAP or sham-CPAP. An improvement in AHI and LVEF was observed in the CPAP group but not in the sham group. In patients with HF and OSA, there was an improvement in the LVEF in the patients treated with CPAP but no changes in the sham-CPAP group after three months of treatment (p = 0.03) [37].

Ryan et al. enrolled 18 patients with OSA and HF with LVEF < 45% and randomized them to the control group (N = 8) and the CPAP group (N = 10). Over one month, there were no changes in participants' BMI, diastolic blood pressure, or heart rate. After one month, a significant reduction in AHI was observed in the CPAP group (p < 0.001), with no improvement in controls (p = 0.77). The improvement in LVEF was observed in the CPAP group (p = 0.03), and no improvement in controls (p = 0.18). Additionally, in the CPAP group, there was a reduction in arousal index (p = 0.004), ventricular premature beats (VPBs) (p = 0.037), and an increase in minimum SaO2 (p = 0.05) [38].

Table 4 summarizes data from the above-mentioned studies.

Table 4. The characteristics and results of chosen OSA and HFrEF studies.

Author, Year	N	Sex, M/F	Age, Years	Ef, % Pre	EF, % Post	CPAP Duration	AHI pre	AHI Post	NT-proBNP Pre	NT-proBNP Post
Naito et al., 2022 [30]	55 OSA	52/3	60.7 ± 12.2	37.2 ± 9.8 ◇	43.2 ± 11.7 ◇	1 m	45.3 ± 16.1	5.4 ± 4.1	ND	ND
Kaneko et al., 2003 [31]	24 12 c/12 p	21/3	55.2 ± 3.6 c 55.9 ± 2.5 p	28.5 ± 1.8 c 25.0 ± 2.8 p	ND	1 m	45.2 ± 5.3 c 37.1 ± 6.4 p◇	44.7 ± 6.8 c 8.3 ± 2.8 p◇	ND	ND
Mansfield et al., 2004 [32]	55 27 c/28 p	52/3	57.5 ± 1.6 c 57.2 ± 1.7 p	33.6 ± 2.6 c 37.6 ± 2.5 p Δ1.5 ± 1.4 ◇	35.1 ± 3.1 c 42.6 ± 0.3 p Δ5.0 ± 1.0 ◇	3 m	26.6 ± 4.5 c 25.0 ± 4.1 p Δ−8.4 ± 3.6 ◇	18.2 ± 2.8 c 2.9 ± 0.8 p Δ−21.1 ± 3.8	ND	ND
Fox et al., 2023 [33]	58 33 c/25 pa	51/7	64.9 ± 10.1 c 67.4 ± 9.8 pa	36.31 ± 6.91 c 39.29 ± 6.51 p◇	39.23 ± 9.41 c 44.35 ± 8.96 p◇	6 m	35 ± 13 c 34 ± 17 p◇	33 ± 20 c 9 ± 8 p◇	ND	ND
Kim et al., 2019 [34]	52 26 c/26 p	48/4	48.8 ± 10.7 c 49.1 ± 11.4 p	64 ± 6 c 66 ± 5 p	64 ± 6 c 65 ± 6 p	3 m	53.4 ± 20.5 c 64.2 ± 20.5 p	ND	ND	ND
Gilman et al., 2008 [35]	19 7 c/12 p	17/2	58.1 ± 7.1 c 56.7 ± 8.0 p	30.4 ± 10.5 c 26.4 ± 10.3 p◇	29.5 ± 6.3 c 34.8 ± 8.3 p◇	1 m	41 ± 13 c 30 ± 15 p◇	37 ± 18 c 7 ± 6 p◇	ND	ND
Servantes et al., 2018 [36]	65 18 c/17 e/15 p/ 15 e,p	43/65	57 ± 8 c 51 ± 9 e 57 ± 7 p 53 ± 10 e,p	29 ± 6 c 31 ± 5 e 31 ± 6 p 33 ± 5 e,p	ND	3 m	29 ± 17 c 28 ± 17 e◇ 32 ± 25 p 25 ± 15 e,p	31 ± 14 c 18 ± 12 e◇ 8 ± 11 p◇ 10 ± 16 e,p◇	ND	ND
Egea et al., 2008 [37]	60 32 c/28 p	56/60	63 ± 1.6 c 64 ± 0.9 p	28.1 ± 1.5 c 28.0 ± 0.5 p	28.1 ± 1.7 c 30.5 ± 0.8 p◇	3 m	35.3 ± 3.1 c 43.7 ± 4.4 p	28.0 ± 4.6 c 10.8 ± 2.2 p	ND	ND
Ryan et al., 2005 [38]	18 8 c/10 p	16/2	60.3 ± 4.1 c 57.6 ± 2.2 p	34.1 ± 3.0 c 27.6 ± 3.4 p◇	29.6 ± 3.1 c 34.3 ± 2.8 p◇	1 m	57.9 ± 5.50 c 29.3 ± 4.8 p◇	56.2 ± 5.3 c 6.1 ± 1.1 p◇	ND	ND

Abbreviations: OSA, obstructive sleep apnea; ND, no data; ◇, significant difference; M/F, Male/Female; EF, ejection fraction; p, participants receiving CPAP; pa, participants receiving APAP; c, controls; m, month(s); e, exercise; e,p, exercise, and CPAP. Data is presented as a percentage of cohort or mean ± standard deviation or median.

3.3. Healthcare Resources Utilization in Heart Failure and Obstructive Sleep Apnea Patients

Cistulli et al. conducted a retrospective observational study of 4237 patients with HFpEF who received a new diagnosis of OSA. The adherence to Positive Airway Pressure (PAP) therapy was associated with improvements in healthcare resource use, including reductions in general hospitalization rate (adherent to PAP 0.33 ± 0.84 vs. nonadherent 0.53 ± 1.08, $p < 0.001$), cardiovascular hospitalizations (adherent to PAP 0.06 ± 0.28 vs. nonadherent 0.11 ± 0.41, $p < 0.004$.), and emergency room visits (adherent to PAP 0.83 ± 1.49 vs. nonadherent 1.21 ± 1.82, $p < 0.001$). The study observed the clinical and economic benefits of OSA treatment in patients with heart failure with preserved ejection fraction, particularly among individual's adherent to therapy. Adherent patients had lower total healthcare costs than moderately adherent and nonadherent patients, with \$12,676 vs. \$16,157 vs. \$16,173, respectively ($p < 0.001$ for both comparisons). Furthermore, adherent patients had significantly reduced costs associated with inpatient hospitalizations (\$3880 vs. \$6409, vs. \$7025, respectively; $p < 0.001$ for both comparisons) and emergency room visits (\$741 vs. \$1142, vs. \$1168, respectively; $p < 0.001$ for both comparisons) [39].

The correlation between OSA and the risk of hospitalization in patients with HF was analyzed by Abdullah et al. The researchers examined data from the National Inpatient Sample (NIS), Healthcare Cost and Utilization Project, and Agency for Healthcare Research and Quality database, specifically focusing on records between 2012 and 2014. A total of 12,608,637 hospital discharges of adult patients were included in the analysis. Among the data, there were 147,463 patients with a primary diagnosis of HFpEF. There were 653,762 (5.2%) patients with OSA. The prevalence of OSA in patients with HFpEF and without HFpEF was estimated at 16.8% and 5.0%, respectively. Patients with OSA were older (62.5 $\pm$ 13.7 vs. 58.6 $\pm$ 20.8, $p < 0.001$) and predominantly male, smoked (35.4% vs. 28.0%, $p < 0.001$) and had a higher incidence of comorbidities, including hypertension (78.1% vs. 53.9%, $p < 0.001$), coronary artery disease (35.3% vs. 20.7%, $p < 0.001$), prior myocardial infarction (8.9% vs. 5.2%, $p < 0.001$), atrial fibrillation (26.1% vs. 14.1%, $p < 0.001$), chronic kidney disease (28.1% vs. 15.5%, $p < 0.001$), acute kidney injury (18.7% vs. 12.3%, $p < 0.001$), diabetes mellitus (52.8% vs. 25.9%, $p < 0.001$), obesity with BMI = 30–40 (18.7% vs. 6.0%, $p < 0.001$), and morbid obesity with BMI > 40 (31.8% vs. 3.7%, $p < 0.001$). The primary endpoint, a discharge with HFpEF diagnosis, occurred in 3.8% of patients in the OSA group and 1.0% in the non-OSA group ($p < 0.001$). Multivariable logistic regression analysis confirmed that OSA was independently associated with higher odds of admission with HFpEF. This association remained significant in both women and men, with adjusted odds ratios of 2.3 (95% CI 2.27 to 2.36) and 2.0 (95% CI 1.98 to 2.08), respectively [40].

Malhotra et al. enrolled 3182 patients with OSA and HFrEF and assessed the impact of adherence to PAP therapy on healthcare resource utilization. During the first year of therapy, 39% of patients (N = 1252) were considered adherent to PAP therapy, 29% (N = 935) had intermediate adherence, and 31% (N = 995) were nonadherent. After one year of initiating positive airway pressure treatment, patients adherent to the treatment had a lower number of combined healthcare visits compared to nonadherent patients (0.92 $\pm$ 1.59 and 1.15 $\pm$ 1.83, respectively, $p = 0.006$). This reduction was primarily attributed to a 24% decrease in emergency room visits. Additionally, the cost of combined healthcare visits was found to be statistically lower in adherent patients (\$3500) compared to nonadherent patients (\$5879, $p = 0.031$) [41]. Significant predictors of adhering to PAP included older age (>55 years), presence of atrial fibrillation, and adherence to β-blocker medication. Table 5 presents data on costs and hospitalization and ER risk of OSA + HF patients.

Table 5. Effect of PAP adherence on costs, hospitalizations, and ER visits in OSA and HFpEF/HFrEF.

Author, Year	N	Sex, M/F	Age, Years	PAP Adherence	PAP Usage	Effect of PAP Adherence on Hospitalizations and ER Visits
Cistulli et al., 2023 [39]	4237	1950/2287	64.1	64.1% Adherent (n = 1701) Intermediate (n = 1250) Nonadherent (n = 1286)	Hours per day: A: 6.8 ± 1.5 ◊ I: 2.9 ± 1.4 ◊ N: 0.4 ± 0.6 ◊ Days per week: A: 6.6 ± 0.5 ◊ I: 3.8 ± 1.7 ◊ N: 0.9 ± 1.2 ◊ Hours per use day: A: 7.2 ± 1.4 ◊ I: 5.4 ± 1.3 ◊ N: 2.9 ± 1.7 ◊	Composite: A: 1.22 ± 2.06; I: 1.88 ± 3.12; N: 1.99 ± 3.21 A-N ◊ A-I ◊ I-N ER: A: 0.89 ± 1.66; I: 1.37 ± 2.54, N: 1.41 ± 2.68 A-N ◊ A-I ◊ I-N All-cause hospitalization: A: 0.33 ± 0.84; I: 0.51 ± 1.23, N: 0.59 ± 1.17 A-N ◊ A-I ◊ I-N Cardiovascular hospitalization: A: 0.06 ± 0.27, I: 0.13 ± 0.61, N: 0.13 ± 0.47 A-N ◊ A-I ◊ I-N
Malhotra et al., 2023 [41]	3182	2223/959	59.7 ± 11.2	Adherent 39%, (n = 1252); Intermediate 29%, (n = 935); Nonadherent 31%, (n = 995)	Hours per day: A: 6.6 ± 1.5 ◊ I: 2.8 ± 1.4 ◊ N: 0.4 ± 0.6 ◊ Days per week: A: 6.6 ± 0.5 ◊ I: 3.8 ± 1.7 ◊ N: 0.9 ± 1.1 ◊ Hours per use day: A: 7.1 ± 1.4 ◊ I: 5.4 ± 1.3 ◊ N: 2.9 ± 1.6 ◊	Composite: A: 1.00 ± 1.73; I: 1.30 ± 2.09; N: 1.37 ± 2.56 A-N ◊ A-I ◊ I-N ER: A: 0.71 ± 1.38; I: 0.91 ± 1.65; N: 1.00 ± 2.06 A-N ◊ A-I ◊ I-N All-cause hospitalization: A: 0.29 ± 0.77; I: 0.38 ± 0.93; N: 0.37 ± 0.99 A-N A-I I-N Cardiovascular hospitalization: A: 0.10 ± 0.43; I: 0.12 ± 0.47; N: 0.12 ± 0.47 A-N A-I I-N
Abdullah et al., 2018 [40]	12,608,637, OSA 653,762; nOSA 11,954,875	5,442,091/7,166,546	OSA 62.5 ± 13.7 nOSA 58.6 ± 20.8	ND	ND	ND

Abbreviations: OSA, obstructive sleep apnea patients; nOSA, no obstructive sleep apnea patients; ◊, statistically significant; M/F, Male/Female; ER, emergency room; A, adherent; I, intermediate; N, non-adherent; A-N, adherent-to-nonadherent; A-I, adherent-to-intermediate; I-N, intermediate-to-nonadherent; ND, no data. Data is presented as a percentage of cohort or mean ± standard deviation.

3.4. Do New Medicaments in Heart Failure Pharmacotherapy Play a Role in Sleep-Disordered Breathing Patients?

3.4.1. Sodium/Glucose Cotransporter-2 Inhibitors (SGLT2i)

Wojeck et al., in VERTIS CV exploratory study, evaluated the impact of ertugliflozin (5 mg, 15 mg, and control group) on the prevalence of OSA. Out of 8246 enrolled patients, 93.3% (N = 7697) had no baseline OSA (placebo N = 2561; ertugliflozin N = 5136; mean age 64.4 years; BMI 31.7 kg/m^2; HbA1c 8.2%; 69.2% male; 88.3% White). The results were: OSA incidence rate: 1.44 per 1000 person-years for ertugliflozin vs. 2.61 per 1000 person-years for placebo, resulting in a 48% relative risk reduction (HR 0.52; 95% CI 0.28–0.96; p = 0.04). In summary, in the VERTIS CV study, the use of the SGLT2 inhibitor ertugliflozin resulted in a decreased occurrence of OSA in individuals with type 2 diabetes [42].

In a recent post-hoc analysis of the EMPA-REG OUTCOME trial to explore the effects of empagliflozin (EMPA) on the incidence of OSA, it was found that approximately 6% of the enrolled population had OSA at baseline. Patients with OSA were more likely to have moderate to severe obesity (55.2% vs. 18.2%) and a higher prevalence of coronary artery disease (CAD). Additionally, patients with OSA had an increased risk of cardiovascular and kidney events and higher overall all-cause mortality compared to those without OSA. The analysis also indicated a trend towards greater weight loss (adjusted for baseline body weight) in patients with OSA treated with empagliflozin compared to those without OSA. Interestingly, patients treated with EMPA had a 52% lower likelihood of developing new-onset OSA than those treated with a placebo. No AHI measurements were made. The diagnosis of OSA in this study was based on patient and investigator reports rather than objective assessment using systematic polysomnography [43].

Two small prospective studies assessed dapagliflozin (DAPA) in individuals with SDB. In the first study, DAPA (5 mg/day) was administered to 30 obese diabetes type 2 (T2D) patients for 24 weeks. SDB was categorized based on the 3% oxygen desaturation index (ODI). After treatment, weight loss was 1.7 kg and 2.56 kg in mild and moderate/severe SDB groups, respectively. DAPA significantly improved 3% ODI only in the moderate/severe SDB group (baseline: 25.0 ± 3.8; end: 18.5 ± 6.1, p = 0.017). Notably, weight loss and neck circumference reduction did not correlate with a 3% ODI improvement. Polysomnography, AHI data, and a control group were lacking in this study [44].

In the second study, 36 OSA and T2D patients were divided into two groups: the dapagliflozin (DAPA) arm (N = 18) received 5 mg/day DAPA (increased to 10 mg after one week), and the control arm (N = 18) received 2 mg/day glimepiride (titrated up to 4 mg if needed). Both groups received metformin 850 mg twice daily for 24 weeks. DAPA resulted in significant reductions in BMI, Homeostatic Model Assessment for IR (HOMA-IR), and AHI, improved minimum SpO$_2$, and decreased ESS scores compared to glimepiride (p < 0.05). Limitations include small sample size, short duration, and absence of neck circumference and other obesity-related data. Sulfonylurea use in the control group may have affected BMI differences [45].

A retrospective study (with no control group) conducted by Sawada et al. examined the effects of SGLT2 inhibitors on 18 T2D patients with OSA (12/18 with severe OSA) regarding weight reduction and changes in AHI. SGLT2 inhibitors were administered for a median of 21 weeks. Body weight, BMI, and AHI (from 31.9 ± 18.0 to 18.8 ± 11.5, p = 0.003) significantly improved after treatment. The number of participants with severe OSA decreased from 12 to 4. However, greater body weight reduction was associated with less AHI improvement in severe OSA patients. Compensatory hyperphagia and concurrent diuretic therapy were suggested as possible explanations [46].

DAHOS, a 3-month, multicentric, prospective, randomized controlled clinical study by Xie et al., is conducted to assess the changes in OSA-related indicators and the treatment of heart failure and to verify the effectiveness of dapagliflozin (10 mg) in the treatment of HFrEF with coexisted OSA. Inclusion criteria are adults with LVEF $\leq$ 40% AHI $\geq$ 15. Patients will be randomized to optimized HF therapy plus a standard dose of dapagliflozin, while the controls will receive only optimized HF therapy. Participants will be evaluated at baseline and 3-month follow-up after dapagliflozin administration. The primary endpoint of the main study is the decreasing value of AHI. The secondary outcomes of the study include assessing the proportion of patients experiencing a 20% and 50% decrease in the AHI before and after dapagliflozin treatment, evaluating changes in Epworth Sleepiness Scale (ESS) scores, examining echocardiographic measures of structure and function (ejection fractions, left ventricular diameters, atrial surface, diastolic function, and filling pressures) pre- and post-dapagliflozin, analyzing serum BNP and pro-BNP concentrations before and after dapagliflozin, measuring laboratory parameters such as creatinine, potassium, sodium, hemoglobin, alanine, and aspartate transaminase levels, assessing the quality of life using the Minnesota Living with Heart Failure Questionnaire and EQ-5D-3L Questionnaire, and evaluating levels of inflammatory and oxidative stress factors (IL-6, CRP) before and after dapagliflozin [47].

The summarized data of the chosen studies is presented in Table 6.

Table 6. Characteristics from SGLT2i studies.

Author, Year	N	Sex, M/F	Age, Years	Rate/1000 Patient-Years	3P-MACE	CV Death	HHF	All-Case Mortality	Incident or Worsening Nephropaty	Changes in Sleep Parameters
Wojeck et al., 2023 [42]	5126 E, 2557 P	69.2(%)	64.3	1.4 E 2.6 P ◊	ND	ND	ND	ND	ND	ND
Neeland et al., 2020 [43]	7020 w/OSA: 4421 Em, 2208 P; 391 OSA: 266 Em, 125 P	5016/2004	63.1 ± 8.6 w/OSA, Em; 63.2 ± 8.9 w/OSA, P; 63.7 ± 7.7 OSA, Em; 63.7 ± 7.3 OSA, P	2.2 E; 4.6 P ◊	490/4687 Em; 282/2333 P ◊	172/4687 Em; 137/2333 P ◊	126/4687 Em; 95/2333P ◊	269/4687 Em; 194/2333 P ◊	525/4687 Em; 388/2333 P ◊; 459/4687 Em; 330/2333 P ◊	ND
Furukawa et al., 2018 [44]	30, 24 mSDB; 6 m-sSDB	20/10	59.0 ± 10.7 mSDB; 58.3 ± 11.7 m-sSDB	ND	ND	ND	ND	ND	ND	3% ODI, baseline: 25.0 ± 3.8; follow-up: 18.5 ± 6.1 ◊
Tang et al., 2019 [45]	36, 18 dapa; 18 w/dapa	22/14	56.10 ± 7.2 dapa; 57.8 ± 10.07 w/dapa	ND	ND	ND	ND	ND	ND	AHI dapa: baseline 37.45 ± 6.04 vs. follow-up 26.72 ± 4.69 ◊; w/dapa: baseline 38.11 ± 6.27 vs. follow-up 36.1 ± 4.50; LSpO2: dapa: baseline 84.06 ± 14.58 vs. follow-up 87.16 ± 13.56 ◊; w/dapa: baseline 83.72 ± 13.77 follow-up 84.12 ± 13.83
Sawada et al., 2018 [46]	18	14/4	64 ± 13	ND	ND	ND	ND	ND	ND	AHI baseline: 31.9 ± 18.0, follow-up 18.8 ± 11.5 ◊

Abbreviations: E, patients with ertugliflozin; Em, empagliflozin; dapa, patients with dapagliflozin; w/dapa, patients without dapagliflozin; P, placebo; OSA, obstructive sleep apnea patients; w/OSA, patients without obstructive sleep apnea; ◊, significant difference; M/F, Male/Female; 3P-MACE, 3-point major adverse CV events; HHF, hospitalization for heart failure; mSDB, mild sleep disordered breathing; m-sSDB, moderate-to-severe sleep disordered breathing; ODI, oxygen desaturation index; LSpO2, lowest oxygen saturation, AHI, apnea/hypopnea index; ND, no data. Data is presented as a percentage of cohort or mean ± standard deviation.

3.4.2. Sacubitril/Valsartan

Owens et al. conducted AWAKE-HF randomized, double-blind study conducted in 23 centers in the United States. Participants with HFrEF (N = 140) were randomly allocated to receive either sacubitril/valsartan (N = 70) or enalapril (N = 70) treatment. Subjects presented with undiagnosed, untreated, moderate-to-severe sleep-disordered breathing (≥15 events/h), and nearly all had OSA (N = 1 CSA). Baseline and 8-week follow-up assessments were conducted to evaluate all endpoints. After eight weeks of treatment, the mean 4% AHI changed minimally from 16.3/h to 15.2/h in the sacubitril/valsartan group and from 16.8/h to 17.6/h in the enalapril group. Mean total sleep time decreased slightly in both treatment groups at week 8 (−14 and −11 min for sacubitril/valsartan and enalapril, respectively) [48].

The study conducted by Pelaia et al. in 2022 evaluated the effects of a 6-month therapy with sacubitril/valsartan on hemodynamic and metabolic parameters in patients with HFrEF and sleep apnea already under treatment with CPAP. Additionally, apnea/hypopnea occurrence and oxygen saturation were examined. The authors enrolled 132 consecutive patients with HFrEF and analyzed them at baseline and 6-month follow-up. Fifty-five patients (41.7%) were diagnosed with OSA, and 77 (58.3%) had CSA. Each participant received CPAP treatment. During a temporary CPAP interruption, the sleep parameters evaluation demonstrated significant improvements. There was a notable reduction in the overall AHI (from 26.5 ± 10.4 to 21.7 ± 8.3, $p < 0.0001$), ODI (from 18.0 ± 3.7 to 13.5 ± 4.9, $p < 0.0001$), and time spent with oxygen saturation below 90% (TC90) (from 14.1 ± 4.5% to 6.8 ± 3.9%, $p < 0.0001$). Additionally, there were significant increases in mean oxygen saturation, which improved from 91.3 ± 1.9% to 92.0 ± 2.0% ($p < 0.0001$). There were significant decreases in BMI ($p < 0.0001$) and NT-proBNP concentration ($p < 0.0001$) [49].

The ENTRESTO-SAS trial is a six-center, prospective, open-label, real-life cohort study by Jaffuel et al., which was conducted to evaluate the sacubitril/valsartan impact on sleep apnea in HFrEF patients [50]. The authors analyzed 118 patients at baseline and 3-month follow-up. The nocturnal ventilatory polygraphy was performed. Based on the initial results, three groups were established: G1: AHIcentral ≥ 5/h and AHIobstructive <15/h; G2: AHIobstructive ≥ 15/h regardless of the AHIcentral; and G3: AHIcentral <5/h and AHIobstructive <15/h. A significant decrease in AHI was observed in G1 + G2 patients, with a median reduction of −7.10/h (range: −16.10 to 0.40), $p < 0.001$. In G1 patients, who primarily exhibited a central pattern of irregular breathing, AHI significantly decreased from a median of 22.90 (range: 16.00–43.50)/h to 19.20 (range: 12.70–31.10)/h ($p = 0.002$). The median AHI difference was −6.60 (range: −11.70 to 0.40). For G2 patients, who predominantly had an obstructive pattern, AHI decreased from a median of 30.10 (range: 26.40–47.60) to 22.75 (range: 14.60–36.90) (statistically non-significant, $p = 0.059$). The median AHI difference was −12.40 (range: −23.60 to 0.35). Around 24.4% of patients experienced a ≥50% decrease in AHI (21.6% for G1 and 37.5% for G2). Additionally, 20% of patients had an initial AHI < 15, which increased to 37.78% at three months (24.3% for G1, $p = 0.146$; 0% for G2, $p = 0.5$). NT-proBNP concentration significantly decreased in all three groups (median change of −301.00 pg/mL for G1, $p = 0.001$; −309.00 pg/mL for OSA-G2, $p = 0.043$; and −299.50 pg/mL for G3, $p < 0.001$). Approximately 51.72% of the population showed a change of over 30% in NT-proBNP values after initiating SV, with no significant differences between groups. LVEF significantly increased in G1 and G3 (median change of 2% for G1, $p = 0.001$; median change of 2% for G3, $p = 0.016$) [50].

Wang et al. conducted a study to evaluate the effect of sacubitril-valsartan on 18 HFrEF patients. Out of the total 18 patients, 50% (9 patients) had OSA, 39% (7 patients) had CSA, and 11% (2 patients) had normal breathing. After three months of sacubitril-valsartan therapy, there was a reduction in NT-pro BNP concentration ($p < 0.001$) and an improvement in LVEF ($p < 0.001$). Portable apnea monitoring showed a significant decrease in the respiratory event index (REI) following sacubitril-valsartan treatment ($p = 0.003$). Subgroup analysis based on the type of apneas revealed that both REI and the time spent below 90% saturation decreased in patients with both OSA and CSA (all $p < 0.05$) [51].

Passino et al. enrolled 51 stable HFrEF patients and switched them from an ACE-i/ARB to sacubitril-valsartan [52]. The baseline characteristics were age 65 ± 9 years, 39 males, 45% of ischemic etiology, LVEF 28.6 ± 6%, 41%, NYHA class III. Fifteen patients had OSA (29%), and 33 had CSA (65%) at nighttime. Among patients with OSA, 4 (8%), 7 (13%), and 4 (8%) had mild (i.e., AHI $\geq$ 5, <15), moderate (i.e., AHI $\geq$ 15, < 30) and severe (i.e., AHI $\geq$ 30) apneas, respectively. Among those with CSA,12 (23%), 8 (16%) and 13 (26%) had mild, moderate, and severe apneas, respectively. After six months of S/V administration, cardiac parameters improved. There was a relevant decrease in NTproBNP ($p < 0.001$) and an increase in LVEF ($p < 0.001$). When assessing the effects on sleep parameters in the overall population, sacubitril-valsartan administration was associated with a significant decrease in the daytime AHI ($p < 0.001$), nighttime AHI ($p = 0.026$) and the 24-h AHI ($p < 0.001$). Within the subset of individuals with OSA, the impact of medication administration did not display any nocturnal effect ($p > 0.05$). In contrast, the utilization of sacubitril-valsartan showed a significant reduction in daytime occurrences ($p = 0.007$), primarily attributed to a decrease in hypopneas (80 events (33–128) to 23 events (10–41), $p = 0.011$), rather than apneas (1 event (0–9) to 0 events (0–3), $p = 0.51$). Table 7 presents summarized data from the above-mentioned studies.

Table 7. Characteristics from Sacubitril/Valsartan studies.

Author, Year	N	Sex, M/F	Age, Years	Rate/1000 Patient-Years	AHI Pre	AHI Post	N-TproBNP	MOS	ODI
Owens et al., 2021 [48]	140, 70 S/; 70 E	108/32	62.3 ± 8.8 S/V; 64.2 ± 11.6 E	ND	16.3 ± 14.2 S/V; 16.8 ± 14.3 E	15.2 ± 15.6 S/V; 17.6 ± 16.3 E	ND	ND	ND
Pelaia et al., 2022 [49]	132	107/25	67.0 ± 9.8	ND	26.5 ± 10.4	21.7 ± 8.3 ◊	baseline: 1840 (886.0–3378); follow-up: 970.0 (571.3–2870) ◊	baseline: 91.3 ± 1.9; follow-up: 92.0 ± 2.0 ◊	baseline: 18.0 ± 3.7; follow-up: 13.5 ± 4.9 ◊
Jaffuel et al., 2021 [50]	118, 49G1; 27G2; 42G3	96/22	66.00 (56.00–73.00)	ND	24.20 (16.40–43.50) G1 + G2; 22.90 (16.00–43.50) G1; 30.10 (26.40–47.60) G2	20.40 (12.70–31.10) G1 + G2 ◊; 19.20 (12.70–31.10) G1◊; 22.75 (14.60–36.90) G2	G1 baseline: 1811.00 (987.00; 3958.00), follow-up: 1104.00 (391.00; 3075.00) ◊; G2 baseline: 2043.00 (845.0; 3445.00), follow-up: 1351.00 (44.00; 2164.00) ◊; G3 baseline: 852.00 (244.0; 2102.0), follow-up: 591.50 (205.0; 1128.5) ◊	G1 + G2 baseline: 92.30 (91.35–94.55), follow up: 93.05 (91.60–94.70); G1 baseline: 93.00 (91.80–94.60), follow-up: 93.40 (92.20–94.90) G2 baseline: 91.3 (90.00–93.00), follow-up: 91.80 (91.00–92.10)	G1 + G2 baseline: −6.32 (±15.79), follow-up: −6.20 (−12.70 to 0.90) ◊; G1 baseline: 11.90 (7.10–14.65), follow-up: 7.65 (4.90–13.65); G2 baseline: 31.00 (15.30–55.90), follow-up: 24.00 (11.00–45.90)
Wang et al., 2023 [51]	18, 9 OSA, 7 CSA, 2 NB	15/3	66.7 ± 10.7	ND	overall population 20 ± 23 *◊; OSA 14 ± 6 *◊; CSA 36 ± 32 ◊*	overall population 7 ± 7 ◊*; OSA 7 ± 7 ◊*; CSA 7 ± 8 ◊*	baseline 1792.1 ± 1271.3; Three months follow-up 876.9 ± 984.2	ND	ND

Table 7. Cont.

Author, Year	N	Sex, M/F	Age, Years	Rate/1000 Patient-Years	AHI Pre	AHI Post	N-TproBNP	MOS	ODI
Passino et al., 2021 [52]	51, 15 OSA, 33 CSA	39/12	65 ± 9	ND	overall population: daytime 7 (2–20); nighttime 19 (7–37); 24 h 13 (5–26); OSA: daytime 6 (2–12); nighttime 18 (10–30); 24 h 13 (5–16); CSA: daytime 10 (2–22); nighttime 23 (9–41); 24 h 14 (6–31)	overall population: daytime 3 (0–7) ◊; nighttime 16 (7–23) ◊; 24 h 8 (3–14) ◊; OSA: daytime 1 (0–3) ◊; nighttime 15 (9–27); 24 h 7 (3–8) ◊; CSA: daytime 3 (1–10) ◊; nighttime 16 (7–23) ◊; 24 h 7 (3–16) ◊	baseline 1439 (701–3015); Six months follow-up 604 (320–1268)	ND	ND

Abbreviations: E, patients with enalapril; S/V, patients with sacubitril/valsartan; En, empagliflozin; dapa, patients with dapagliflozin; w/dapa, patients without dapagliflozin; P, placebo; OSA, obstructive sleep apnea patients; w/OSA, patients without obstructive sleep apnea; CSA, central sleep apnea; NB, normal breathing; ◊, statistically significant; M/F, Male/Female; 3P-MACE, 3-point major adverse CV events; HHF, hospitalization for heart failure; mSDB, mild sleep disordered breathing; m-sSDB, moderate-to-severe sleep disordered breathing; ODI, oxygen desaturation index; MOS, mean oxygen saturation; LSpO2, lowest oxygen saturation; AHI, apnea/hypopnea index; ND, no data; G1, group 1, AHI central ≥ 5/h and AHI obstructive < 15/h; G2: group 2, AHI obstructive ≥ 15/h regardless of the AHI central; G3: group 3, AHI central < 5/h and AHI obstructive < 15/h; *, REI, respiratory events index (events/hour); 24 h, 24-h AHI. Data is presented as a percentage of cohort or mean ± standard deviation or median.

4. Discussion

4.1. The Prevalence of Obstructive Sleep Apnea in Heart Failure Patients

Heart failure and obstructive sleep apnea are prevalent conditions that often coexist and interact, leading to increased morbidity and mortality [53,54]. A prior investigation indicated that approximately 75% of individuals suffering from HF experience SDB linked to daytime sleepiness, chronic bronchitis, peripheral edema, and dyspnea [55]. The prevalence of OSA in HF patients with systolic dysfunction varied from approximately 20% to 45% [56]. These findings highlight the importance of considering OSA as a potential comorbidity in HF patients, given its impact on disease progression and outcomes. Overall, the prevalence of obstructive sleep apnea among heart failure patients has exhibited a varied trajectory over the years. Especially OSA prevalence rates within the HF population, as demonstrated by studies conducted in 1997, 2007, and 2009 by Chan et al., Oldenburg et al. and Yumino et al., were reported as 63.64%, 48.21%, and 55.45%, with corresponding overall OSA prevalence rates of 35%, 36%, and 25.69% [16,25,26]. However, it's essential to consider that the more recent investigation by Kalaydzhiev et al. in 2023 reported a notably higher OSA prevalence of 81.97% among HF patients, while the overall OSA prevalence remained at 50% [28]. It's worth highlighting that the study by Kalaydzhiev et al. had a sample size of 100, which could potentially introduce a risk of bias due to its limited size [28]. These findings underscore a dynamic shift in OSA prevalence among the HF population across the analyzed years and emphasize the need for caution when interpreting results from studies with smaller sample sizes.

Interestingly, the prevalence of OSA in HF patients appears to vary depending on the type of HF, but these differences are not significant. However, the studies consistently show that HFrEF and HFmrEF patients tend to have higher rates of sleep-disordered breathing, particularly CSA. On the other hand, HFpEF patients exhibit a higher prevalence of OSA [22,24,27,29,40,57–60]. Additionally, it is noteworthy that the underlying etiology of HF may also influence the prevalence of sleep-disordered breathing, with ischemic and hypertensive groups having higher rates of SDB compared to valvular and arrhythmic groups [21]. Moreover, the studies suggest that OSA patients with HF have higher LVEF values than CSA patients, indicating potential differences in the pathophysiology and mechanisms of these two types of sleep-disordered breathing in HF [20]. In instances of right heart failure, fluid accumulation in the body, including the cervical region, leads to edema. This, in turn, contributes to an escalation in upper airway obstruction.

Furthermore, the inadequacy of the right ventricle impairs the circulation of blood within the pulmonary vessels, culminating in reduced perfusion of the lung tissue. Consequently, there is a decline in oxygenation levels, exacerbating desaturation during episodes of apnea. Conversely, left heart failure prompts the occurrence of pulmonary edema, impacting the optimal perfusion of the alveoli and the ensuing gas exchange process. This, in effect, leads to a reduction in oxygen (O_2) levels in the blood and an elevation in carbon dioxide (CO_2) levels. The malfunction of the left ventricle further results in compromised renal perfusion, thereby fostering the development of hypertension and heightened fluid retention within the body, consequently exacerbating generalized edema.

In summary, the findings from these studies underscore the importance of considering sleep-disordered breathing, particularly OSA, in the management and treatment of heart failure patients. The data from the cited studies collectively emphasize the strong association between HFpEF and OSA. The prevalence of OSA in HFpEF patients is significant and highlights the need for routine screening and management of OSA in this population. There is no screening program for OSA in HF patients, and it is primarily attributed to the elevated costs associated with polysomnography and the constrained accessibility of sleep centers, even within well-developed regions. Early diagnosis and appropriate interventions for OSA in HF patients may play a role in improving patient outcomes and quality of life. However, further research is warranted to understand better the mechanisms and implications of sleep-disordered breathing in different types of heart failure and its impact on patient prognosis and management strategies.

4.2. The Impact of Positive Airway Pressure Therapy in Heart Failure and Obstructive Sleep Apnea Patients

Sleep-disordered breathing presents a potent stimulant for the upregulation of adrenergic activity. Disrupted sleep patterns and episodes of intermittent hypoxia can potentially initiate excessive sympathetic activity, oxidative stress, vascular inflammation, endothelial dysfunction, arterial stiffness and hypercoagulation [59]. Following the American Academy of Sleep Medicine guidelines, positive airway pressure therapy (CPAP, Auto-PAP and, BiPAP, bilevel positive airway pressure) is recommended in adult patients with OSA [2]. Considering the multifactorial benefits and its targeting of shared pathophysiological pathways in heart failure and obstructive sleep apnea, evaluating the impact of PAP therapy on HF outcomes becomes crucial. CPAP has the strongest evidence for a beneficial cardiovascular effect [61]. Investigations involving PAP treatment have indicated that effective therapy could alleviate the heightened sympathetic activity observed in patients with OSA [62,63]. Studies have demonstrated that each occurrence of breathing cessation during sleep triggers significant elevations in muscle sympathetic nerve activity (MSNA) among individuals with OSA. Comparatively, HF patients with coexisting OSA have demonstrated an increase of 11 bursts per 100 heartbeats in MSNA compared to those without sleep apnea [64]. Notably, a subanalysis of a randomized controlled trial revealed a reduction of 12 bursts per 100 heartbeats in patient MSNA following CPAP therapy, underscoring the potential of distinct sympathoexcitatory mechanisms (HF and OSA) to synergistically heighten MSNA through additive summative effects.

A moderate confirmation level suggests that OSA is associated with increased serum and plasma inflammatory cytokines, oxidative stress indicators, adhesion molecules, adipose tissue hormones, and abnormal lipid profiles, which can be reduced with PAP treatment [65]. Additionally, PAP may help to maintain sinus rhythm after ablation or electrical cardioversion in patients with atrial fibrillation [66]. Moreover, analyzed studies reported reductions in NT-proBNP concentration after follow-up in HFpEF patients treated with PAP [22,29]. However, it is worth noting that the reduction in NT-proBNP concentration was less significant in patients with OSA compared to non-OSA patients, indicating that OSA may have a modifying effect on the response to treatment. Studies with HFrEF patient groups and PAP treatment also showed a consistent trend toward improvement in LVEF. The LVEF changes suggest that PAP therapy might positively impact cardiac function and improve outcomes in HF patients with coexisting OSA. Gupta et al. also assessed the correlation between the severity of OSA measured by the AHI and diastolic dysfunction in HFpEF patients [22]. The study found a positive correlation between AHI severity and the degree of diastolic dysfunction. This suggests that the presence and severity of OSA may be associated with worsening diastolic function in HFpEF patients.

When analyzing HFrEF patients, studies consistently show significant reductions in the AHI and arousal index after PAP treatment [30–33,35,37,38]. These improvements indicate successful management of OSA and relief of sleep-disordered breathing in HF patients. Additionally, PAP therapy leads to significant enhancements in desaturation index, LOS, and MOS levels, promoting better sleep quality and increased oxygenation during sleep. Most importantly, studies indicated that PAP treatment was associated with reduced daytime systolic blood pressure and heart rate in HF patients with OSA [30,31,38] among the observational studies and RCTs included in a well-summarized review by Peker et al. PAP treatment significantly reduces blood pressure, especially nocturnal, in OSA patients. Lowering blood pressure is crucial for patients with HF to reduce the workload afterload, prevent cardiac strain, minimize fluid retention, and improve coronary blood flow [67].

Moreover, maintaining a low heart rate reduces myocardial oxygen demand, enhances diastolic filling, optimizes cardiac output, and improves synchronization [68]. A clinical trial conducted on individuals with HFrEF, known as the Ivabradine and Outcomes in Chronic Heart Failure (SHIFT) study, demonstrated the advantageous effects of ivabradine in HF patients with heart rates exceeding 70 beats per minute (bpm) persisted even when patients were already undergoing recommended therapeutic approaches, including beta-blocker therapy [69]. The incidence of major adverse cardiovascular events, such as hospitalization for heart failure and cardiovascular-related mortality, exhibited a noteworthy decrease in the ivabradine-treated group compared to the placebo-treated group. This reduction was particularly prominent among those participants with initially higher baseline heart rates. Additionally, these findings are crucial as hypertension and increased heart rate are common complications in HF, and PAP therapy might play a role in mitigating further cardiovascular risk among OSA patients with heart failure at baseline.

Age and BMI are significant determinants of LVEF improvement in HF patients with OSA after PAP treatment [30]. Younger patients with obesity demonstrated a higher degree of improvement in LVEF. These observations highlight the importance of patient-specific factors in predicting the response to PAP therapy and suggest that younger, obese patients may benefit more from the intervention. Additionally, several studies indicated that PAP treatment is associated with improved quality of life, NYHA functional class, and daytime sleepiness in HF + OSA patients [31,32,36]. These improvements suggest that PAP may have broader benefits beyond cardiovascular parameters, enhancing these patients' overall well-being and functional status.

Moreover, in contemporary medical practice, assessing the treatment-related costs and the potential risk of hospitalization in OSA + HF patients has become essential, particularly considering that the HF population tends to have a higher frequency of hospital visits than the general population. Furthermore, it is crucial to investigate whether PAP treatment could contribute to reducing the aforementioned utilization of medical resources in individuals with OSA and HF. Cistulli et al. found that good adherence to PAP therapy resulted in significant improvements in healthcare utilization [39]. Adherent patients experienced reduced hospitalization rates, emergency room visits, and cardiovascular hospitalizations compared to non-adherent patients. Additionally, adherent patients had lower total healthcare costs. Moreover, adherence to PAP therapy in HFrEF patients was associated with reduced healthcare resource utilization, including decreased emergency room visits and healthcare costs [41]. These findings highlight the potential economic benefits of PAP treatment, which may lead to cost-effective management of this patient population.

4.3. The Heart Failure Medications on Sleep Parameters: Correlation and Potential Mechanisms

Worsening of HF symptoms can elevate the tendency to obstructive and central apneas. HF can potentially worsen or unmask latent OSA through heightened upper airway instability, particularly during supine sleep due to cervical venous congestion [70]. Research has demonstrated a link between volume redistribution during sleep and AHI in HF patients with OSA [71]. Increased volume load could lead to cervical venous congestion, thus aggravating OSA. Consequently, optimizing HF therapy emerges as the pivotal approach, as it diminishes preload and interstitial lung pressure, thus mitigating the hyperventilation that drives OSA. Preload reduction concurrently alleviates cervical venous congestion and upper airway instability. Given the fluid retention and rostral fluid shift in HF patients, interventions aimed at reducing intravascular volume and venous congestion hold promise in alleviating the severity of both OSA and CSA.

Pharmacological intervention is a cornerstone in HF management, guided by established protocols. Beta-blockers and ACE inhibitors enhance cardiac output and confer symptomatic relief in OSA [72]. Diuretics effectively curtail OSA severity by impeding fluid retention and curtailing fluid translocation to the oral cavity [73]. For instance, a three-day regimen of spironolactone and furosemide heightened upper airway caliber and decreased AHI ($p < 0.001$) in individuals with diastolic HF and severe OSA [74]. Addressing HF complications warrants particular attention. Pharmacotherapy for HF offers a beneficial impact on OSA by mitigating volume shifts and lung and cervical region volume overload. Cardiac resynchronization therapy has been observed to ameliorate CSA in congestive heart failure patients by reducing AHI. However, significant reductions are yet to be found in subjects with OSA [75]. These initial investigations have occurred against notable transformations in heart failure treatment, leading to improved prognoses in HF.

American Heart Association and European Society of Cardiology new guidelines have added a class of diabetes drugs called SGLT-2 inhibitors (empagliflozin, dapagliflozin) to the list of treatments for heart failure [14,15]. Canagliflozin, ertugliflozin and sotagliflozin are other SGLT2 inhibitors. Conducting studies on the effects of new pharmacotherapy, SGLT2 inhibitors and sacubitril/valsartan in patients with OSA and HF is paramount due to several compelling reasons. These medications represent novel therapeutic approaches in HF treatment, and their potential benefits extend beyond cardiovascular parameters. The SGLT2 inhibitors have gained prominence in the treatment of both HF and type 2 diabetes. Their multifaceted effects encompass cardiovascular benefits, renal protection, and metabolic improvements. Since sleep disturbances are intricately linked to metabolic dysregulation and cardiovascular dysfunction, studying the impact of SGLT2 inhibitors on sleep quality and OSA parameters in HF patients becomes pivotal. The proven positive effects of SGLT2 inhibitors on sleep in diabetes patients underscore the need to explore their potential benefits in the HF population, shedding light on yet unexplored avenues for enhancing patient well-being. When analyzing the effects of SGLT2-i on OSA incidence, Wojeck et al. reported a 48% relative risk reduction in the development of OSA in HF patients treated with ertugliflozin compared to placebo [42]. This finding suggests a potential protective effect of this SGLT2 inhibitor against the development of OSA in HF patients. Additionally, an analysis of the EMPA-REG OUTCOME trial revealed that patients with OSA were at increased risk of cardiovascular and kidney events and higher all-cause mortality [43]. Interestingly, treatment with empagliflozin was associated with a lower likelihood of developing new-onset OSA. These findings suggest a potential benefit of empagliflozin in reducing the risk of OSA and improving outcomes in HF patients with coexisting OSA. Given the constrained availability of data regarding SGLT2 inhibitors in individuals with heart failure and obstructive sleep apnea, our inclusion criteria encompassed studies involving these medications among patients with OSA and other conditions, e.g., diabetes, where more comprehensive data were obtained. Small prospective studies on dapagliflozin indicated potential improvements in sleep parameters in obese type 2 diabetes (T2D) patients with OSA [44,45]. The first study showed a significant improvement in the oxygen desaturation index in the moderate/severe SDB group after dapagliflozin treatment. However, the second study's small sample size limits the conclusions that can be drawn. Sawada et al.'s retrospective study demonstrated that SGLT2 inhibitors, including dapagliflozin, were associated with weight reduction and improvements in AHI in T2D patients with OSA [46]. However, severe OSA may attenuate the AHI improvement with increasing body weight reduction, suggesting the importance of personalized approaches in this population. Additional evidence of the favorable impact on the pathophysiology of OSA arises from the established influence of SGLT2 inhibitors on visceral and subcutaneous adipose tissue, as demonstrated in previous studies [76–78]. This phenomenon is exemplified in animal models of type 2 diabetes mellitus and metabolic syndrome, where the alteration in energy substrates from carbohydrates to lipids results in heightened lipolysis and beta-oxidation of fatty acids [79–81]—changes that contribute to the aforementioned positive effects. SGLT2i have also exhibited efficacy in countering liver steatosis in individuals and animals with T2DM [82–87]. Notably, the SGLT2 inhibitor, canagliflozin, has been proven to decrease the accumulation of epicardial fat [88], a factor closely linked to coronary heart disease [89,90]. There have been suggestions that SGLT2 inhibitors might yield beneficial outcomes for individuals with obstructive sleep apnea due to a fascinating, albeit debated, mechanism [91]. This mechanism involves the inhibition of leptin activation [92], a hormone found at elevated levels in individuals with OSA [93,94]. Indeed, reinforcing this notion, a recent meta-analysis involving ten randomized controlled trials highlighted that the use of SGLT2i in individuals with type 2 diabetes mellitus was linked to reductions in circulating leptin levels and increases in adiponectin levels [95]. There is a potential link between leptin and obstructive sleep apnea, although the relationship is complex and not fully understood. Leptin concentration tends to be higher in individuals with more adipose tissue, and obesity is associated with leptin resistance. The resistance may contribute to disruptions in appetite regulation and potentially impact the regulation of breathing during sleep. Moreover, hypoxia can influence the production and release of various hormones, including leptin. Increased sympathetic activity in OSA individuals can impact hormonal regulation, including leptin production and signaling. Disrupted sympathetic activity due to OSA might influence leptin's actions and further complicate metabolic pathways [96]. The results of the ongoing DAHOS trial will provide further insights into the potential role of dapagliflozin in managing OSA and heart failure in this specific patient population.

Another new medicament in HF pharmacotherapy, sacubitril/valsartan, was assessed in several studies with OSA patients. Sacubitril/valsartan, a neprilysin inhibitor combined with an angiotensin receptor blocker, has demonstrated remarkable efficacy in HF therapy. S/V acts by inhibiting neprilysin, thereby preventing the degradation of natriuretic peptides. This, in turn, amplifies their natriuretic and vasodilatory impacts, leading to decreased pulmonary congestion [97,98]. The treatment also positively affects cardiac reverse remodeling, a phenomenon linked to improved LVEF, potentially augmenting cardiac output [99,100]. These combined effects can enhance respiratory efficiency and optimize gas exchange.

Furthermore, the treatment may influence the chemoreflex by diminishing pulmonary stretch receptor activation and enhancing peripheral chemoreceptor perfusion [101]. Another conceivable outcome of increased cardiac output is reduced circulation time, which limits the chemoreflex system's capacity to recognize and react to fluctuations in CO_2 levels [102]. Lastly, this medication has demonstrated the capacity to mitigate the upward shift of fluids towards the head that typically occurs when an individual is in a reclined position [103]. To the best of our knowledge, Fox et al. identified the first case of a 71-year-old male with heart failure and sleep-disordered breathing, in which administering sacubitril/valsartan therapy was linked to enhanced cardiac function, evidenced by a reduction in NT-proBNP levels and an improvement in LVEF and a substantial decrease in the AHI. This instance marks the inaugural presentation of amelioration in both HF and SDB subsequent to the initiation of SV treatment [104]. In another analyzed study, we found minimal changes in the AHI and total sleep time after eight weeks of S/V treatment, suggesting that these medications might not have a significant impact on OSA parameters [48]. However, the effects of a 6-month therapy with sacubitril/valsartan on hemodynamic, sleep and metabolic parameters demonstrated significant improvements in AHI, oxygen desaturation index, and time spent with oxygen saturation below 90% [49].

Additionally, there were significant decreases in BMI, NT-proBNP concentration, and improvements in LVEF. Moreover, patients primarily exhibiting a central pattern of irregular breathing and an obstructive pattern of breathing showed a decrease in AHI. These findings from the ENTRESTO-SAS trial suggest that sacubitril/valsartan might have a positive impact on sleep parameters in patients with both CSA and OSA [50]. Additionally, the medication was associated with improved cardiac biomarkers and left ventricular function, further supporting its potential benefits in managing sleep apnea and heart failure with reduced ejection fraction. However, further studies with larger sample sizes and longer follow-up periods are necessary to confirm these observations and provide more definitive evidence.

Incorporating an investigation into the effects of SGLT-2i and sacubitril/valsartan on sleep parameters aligns with contemporary patient-centered care, where a holistic approach encompasses the management of cardiac function and the overall well-being of HF patients. Recognizing any modifications in sleep patterns due to these medications can aid healthcare providers in optimizing treatment plans and improving patient outcomes.

4.4. OSA and HF—Clinical Relevance, Clinical Practice and Patient Care

The relationship between OSA, HF, and cardiovascular medications (like SGLT2i and sacubitril/valsartan) significantly impacts clinical practice and patient care. Incorporating this correlation into healthcare strategies may enhance the efficiency of screening and treating patients with the above-mentioned interconnected conditions. Regarding screening strategies, it is important to identify OSA in HF patients, particularly those with preserved ejection fraction, due to the high prevalence of OSA in this population. Routine OSA screening and using tools such as the STOP-BANG questionnaire or portable sleep study devices may facilitate early detection and successful intervention. Additionally, acknowledgement of common risk factors (obesity, hypertension, daytime sleepiness) shared between OSA and HF may guide clinicians to perform OSA evaluation for particular patients. Managing HF should include not only traditional HF medications but also treatments addressing comorbid conditions like OSA. Effective management of OSA may contribute to the improvement of HF outcomes.

Furthermore, cardiovascular medications like SGLT2i and sacubitril/valsartan have displayed promise in enhancing cardiac function among HF patients. Thus, clinicians should consider incorporating these medications into their HF + OSA management strategy. Exploring combination therapy is essential, as these medications may offer synergistic benefits for HF patients with OSA. Apart from the primary indications, the above-mentioned pharmacotherapy may also be used to reduce OSA-related cardiovascular risks. In patient-centered care, recognizing the diversity among HF patients is crucial. Personalized treatment plans should include the presence of OSA and the choice of cardiological medications based on individual patient's characteristics and comorbidities. The role of effective follow-up is worth emphasizing. Patients with HF and OSA may benefit from long-term monitoring of both conditions to assess treatment effectiveness. Regular follow-up appointments may help clinicians adjust treatment strategies as needed to optimize patients' outcomes. Lastly, education of the patients is a key to therapeutic success. Patients should know the interplay between OSA, HF, and cardiological medications. Overall outcomes of the therapy may be significantly improved by encouraging patients to report sleep-related symptoms and engage in discussions with their healthcare providers about treatment options.

In conclusion, this systematic review is a valuable effort to advance our understanding of the intricate relationship between OSA and HF. By exploring the bidirectional influences between these conditions and examining the impact of innovative pharmacotherapies of HF on sleep parameters, the authors aspire to contribute significantly to the expanding knowledge base in this field. This undertaking is pivotal in guiding evidence-based clinical decisions, fostering multidisciplinary approaches, and ultimately improving the quality of life for individuals grappling with the complexities of both OSA and HF.

Importantly, the current AASM recommendations for optimal sleep breathing disorders treatment include, among others, body mass reduction, PAP therapy, oral appliances, and surgical methods. Medicaments used in the treatment of heart failure do not reverse airway obstruction. Analyzing data from randomized controlled trials might only enable selecting an appropriate method of pharmacotherapy and sleep apnea management dedicated to patients co-suffering from HF and OSA. Optimized therapy could potentially and maximally reduce OSA and HF complications, extend life expectancy, improve the quality of life and sleep, and reduce the risk of hospitalization. Nevertheless, treating patients with multi-chronic conditions should target all the diseases' causes. Patients with comorbid OSA and HF should obtain proper HF treatment and OSA management.

Despite the promising results, the current systematic review has some limitations that should be acknowledged. Firstly, substantial heterogeneity across included studies, stemming from differences in study populations and outcome measures, may hinder the comprehensive pooling of results for meaningful analysis. Additionally, randomized controlled trials are limited in the context of novel HF pharmacotherapy on OSA outcomes. Including different study types allowed for a more comprehensive exploration of this intricate relationship between pharmacotherapy and sleep parameters in HF patients with coexisting OSA. Secondly, the review's potential language bias, resulting from the restriction of the search to the English language, raises the possibility of omitting relevant studies conducted in other languages, introducing a source of bias into the analysis. Thirdly, the inherent publication bias in the literature, wherein studies with significant findings are more likely to be published, might lead to an unintentional overrepresentation of positive results in the review. Lastly, the limited availability of long-term data in most of the included studies might impede a thorough understanding of the potential long-term effects of interventions, particularly if the majority of studies are short-term in nature. These limitations should be considered when interpreting the findings and implications of the review. Therefore, additional large-scale, well-controlled clinical trials are necessary to confirm and further investigate the effects of these medications on sleep parameters and clinical outcomes in HF patients.

Overall, the evidence presented in these studies underscores the importance of recognizing and managing OSA in patients with heart failure to optimize their overall outcomes and quality of life. Multidisciplinary approaches that incorporate cardiovascular and sleep medicine specialists may benefit the comprehensive management of these patients. Future research will likely provide more insights and pave the way for more effective therapeutic strategies for heart failure patients with coexisting obstructive sleep apnea.

5. Conclusions

The evidence presented in the above-mentioned studies strongly supports the association between heart failure and obstructive sleep apnea, highlighting the need for early detection and appropriate management of sleep-disordered breathing in heart failure patients. The data suggest that implementing effective interventions for obstructive sleep apnea, such as PAP treatment, might lead to significant improvements in sleep parameters, cardiac function, and overall patient well-being. Furthermore, using PAP in heart failure patients with coexisting OSA can optimize patient outcomes, reduce HF-related hospitalizations, and lower healthcare costs. Additionally, the integration of novel pharmacotherapeutic agents such as SGLT2 inhibitors and sacubitril/valsartan in the treatment regimen for heart failure holds promise for ameliorating sleep parameters in patients with OSA + HF. Exploring these innovative therapeutic modalities offers the potential to reveal favorable effects on sleep disruptions associated with OSA in the context of heart failure pathology. Multidisciplinary collaboration between cardiovascular and sleep medicine specialists is most likely beneficial in providing comprehensive care to heart failure patients with coexisting obstructive sleep apnea.

Supplementary Materials: The following supporting information can be downloaded at: https://www.mdpi.com/article/10.3390/jcm12196139/s1, Table S1: Quality assessment of included studies. Table S2. Effective Public Healthcare Panacea Project—Quality Assessment Tool for Quantitative Studies Dictionary.

Author Contributions: Conceptualization, A.P. and E.O.; methodology, A.P. and E.O.; software, A.P. and N.O.; validation, A.P., N.O. and E.O.; formal analysis, A.P.; investigation, A.P., N.O. and E.O.; resources, Ł.D.; data curation, Ł.D.; writing—original draft preparation, A.P. and N.O.; writing—review and editing, E.O.; visualization, A.P. and N.O.; supervision, E.O.; project administration, A.P. All authors have read and agreed to the published version of the manuscript.

Funding: This research received no external funding.

Institutional Review Board Statement: Not applicable.

Conflicts of Interest: The authors declare no conflict of interest.

References

1. Heatley, E.M.; Harris, M.; Battersby, M.; McEvoy, R.D.; Chai-Coetzer, C.L.; Antic, N.A. Obstructive sleep apnoea in adults: A common chronic condition in need of a comprehensive chronic condition management approach. *Sleep Med. Rev.* **2013**, *17*, 349–355. [CrossRef]
2. Epstein, L.J.; Kristo, D.; Strollo, P.J.; Friedman, N.; Malhotra, A.; Patil, S.P.; Ramar, K.; Rogers, R.; Schwab, R.J.; Weaver, E.M.; et al. Clinical guideline for the evaluation, management and long-term care of obstructive sleep apnea in adults. *J. Clin. Sleep Med.* **2009**, *5*, 263–276. [PubMed]

3. American Academy of Sleep Medicine Task Force. Sleep-related breathing disorders in adults: Recommendations for syndrome definition and measurement techniques in clinical research. The report of an American Academy of Sleep Medicine task force. *Sleep* **1999**, *22*, 667–689. [CrossRef]
4. Malhotra, A.; Heinzer, R.; Morrell, M.J.; Penzel, T.; Pepin, J.-L.; Valentine, K.; Nunez, C.; Benjafield, A. Late Breaking Abstract—European prevalence of OSA in adults: Estimation using currently available data. *Eur. Respir. J.* **2018**, *52*, OA4961. [CrossRef]
5. Kapur, V.K.; Auckley, D.H.; Chowdhuri, S.; Kuhlmann, D.C.; Mehra, R.; Ramar, K.; Harrod, C.G. Clinical Practice Guideline for Diagnostic Testing for Adult Obstructive Sleep Apnea. *J. Clin. Sleep Med.* **2017**, *1313*, 479–504. [CrossRef]
6. Milicic Ivanovski, D.; Milicic Stanic, B.; Kopitovic, I. Comorbidity Profile and Predictors of Obstructive Sleep Apnea Severity and Mortality in Non-Obese Obstructive Sleep Apnea Patients. *Medicina* **2023**, *59*, 873. [CrossRef]
7. McKee, Z.; Auckley, D.H. A sleeping beast: Obstructive sleep apnea and stroke. *Clevel. Clin. J. Med.* **2019**, *86*, 407–415. [CrossRef]
8. Redline, S. Screening for Obstructive Sleep Apnea Implications for the Sleep Health of the Population. *J. Am. Med. Assoc.* **2017**, *317*, 368–370. [CrossRef]
9. McNicholas, W.T.; Bonsignore, M.R. Sleep Apnoea as an Independent Risk for Cardiovascular Disease: Current Evidence, Basic Mechanisms and Research Priorities. *Eur. Respir. J.* **2007**, *29*, 156–178. [CrossRef]
10. McNicholas, W.T. Obstructive Sleep Apnea and Inflammation. *Prog. Cardiovasc. Dis.* **2009**, *51*, 392–399. [CrossRef]
11. Olszewska, E.; Rogalska, J.; Brzóska, M.M. The Association of Oxidative Stress in the Uvular Mucosa with Obstructive Sleep Apnea Syndrome: A Clinical Study. *J. Clin. Med.* **2021**, *10*, 1132. [CrossRef] [PubMed]
12. Bonetti, P.O.; Lerman, L.O.; Lerman, A. Endothelial Dysfunction: A Marker of Atherosclerotic Risk. *Arterioscler. Thromb. Vasc. Biol.* **2003**, *23*, 168–175. [CrossRef] [PubMed]
13. GBD 2017 Disease and Injury Incidence and Prevalence Collaborators. Global, regional, and national incidence, prevalence, and years lived with disability for 354 diseases and injuries for 195 countries and territories, 1990–2017: A systematic analysis for the Global Burden of Disease Study 2017. *Lancet* **2018**, *392*, 1789–1858.
14. Heidenreich, P.A.; Bozkurt, B.; Aguilar, D.; Allen, L.A.; Byun, J.J.; Colvin, M.M.; Deswal, A.; Drazner, M.H.; Dunlay, S.M.; Evers, L.R.; et al. 2022 AHA/ACC/HFSA Guideline for the Management of Heart Failure: A Report of the American College of Cardiology/American Heart Association Joint Committee on Clinical Practice Guidelines. *J. Am. Coll. Cardiol.* **2022**, *79*, e263–e421. [CrossRef]
15. McDonagh, T.A.; Metra, M.; Adamo, M.; Gardner, R.S.; Baumbach, A.; Böhm, M.; Burri, H.; Butler, J.; Čelutkienė, J.; Chionce, O.; et al. ESC Guidelines for the diagnosis and treatment of acute and chronic heart failure: Developed by the Task Force for the diagnosis and treatment of acute and chronic heart failure of the European Society of Cardiology (ESC) with the special contribution of the Heart Failure Association (HFA) of the ESC. *Eur. Heart J.* **2021**, *42*, 3599–3726. [CrossRef]
16. Oldenburg, O.; Lamp, B.; Faber, L.; Teschler, H.; Horstkotte, D.; Töpfer, V. Sleep-disordered breathing in patients with symptomatic heart failure: A contemporary study of prevalence in and characteristics of 700 patients. *Eur. J. Heart Fail.* **2007**, *9*, 251–257. [CrossRef]
17. Bekfani, T.; Schöbel, C.; Pietrock, C.; Valentova, M.; Ebner, N.; Döhner, W.; Schulze, P.C.; Anker, S.D.; von Haehling, S. Heart failure and sleep-disordered breathing: Susceptibility to reduced muscle strength and preclinical congestion (SICA-HF cohort). *ESC Heart Fail.* **2020**, *7*, 2063–2070. [CrossRef]
18. Holt, A.; Bjerre, J.; Zareini, B.; Koch, H.; Tønnesen, P.; Gislason, G.H.; Nielsen, O.W.; Schou, M.; Lamberts, M. Sleep apnea, the risk of developing heart failure, and potential benefits of continuous positive airway pressure (CPAP) therapy. *J. Am. Heart Assoc.* **2018**, *7*, e008684. [CrossRef]
19. Page, M.J.; McKenzie, J.E.; Bossuyt, P.M.; Boutron, I.; Hoffmann, T.C.; Mulrow, C.D.; Shamseer, L.; Tetzlaff, J.M.; Akl, E.A.; Brennan, S.E.; et al. The PRISMA 2020 statement: An updated guideline for reporting systematic reviews. *BMJ* **2021**, *372*, n71. [CrossRef]
20. Wang, T.; Yu, F.C.; Wei, Q.; Chen, L.; Xu, X.; Ding, N.; Tong, J.Y. Prevalence and clinical characteristics of sleep-disordered breathing in patients with heart failure of different left ventricular ejection fractions. *Sleep Breath.* **2022**, *27*, 245–253. [CrossRef]
21. Wang, T.; Yu, F.C.; Wei, Q.; Xu, X.; Xie, L.; Ding, N.; Tong, J.Y. Sleep-disordered breathing in heart failure patients with different etiologies. *Clin. Cardiol.* **2022**, *45*, 778–785. [CrossRef] [PubMed]
22. Gupta, N.; Agrawal, S.; Goel, A.D.; Ish, P.; Chakrabarti, S.; Suri, J.C. Profile of sleep disordered breathing in heart failure with preserved ejection fraction. *Monaldi Arch. Chest Dis.* **2020**, *90*, 660–665. [CrossRef]
23. Arzt, M.; Oldenburg, O.; Graml, A.; Erdmann, E.; Teschler, H.; Wegscheider, K.; Suling, A.; Woehrle, H. SchlaHF Investigators. Phenotyping of Sleep-Disordered Breathing in Patients With Chronic Heart Failure With Reduced Ejection Fraction-the SchlaHF Registry. *J. Am. Heart Assoc.* **2017**, *6*, e005899. [CrossRef] [PubMed]
24. Bitter, T.; Faber, L.; Hering, D.; Langer, C.; Horstkotte, D.; Oldenburg, O. Sleep-disordered breathing in heart failure with normal left ventricular ejection fraction. *Eur. J. Heart Fail.* **2009**, *11*, 602–608. [CrossRef] [PubMed]
25. Chan, J.; Sanderson, J.; Chan, W.; Lai, C.; Choy, D.; Ho, A.; Leung, R. Prevalence of sleep-disordered breathing in diastolic heart failure. *Chest* **1997**, *111*, 1488–1493. [CrossRef] [PubMed]
26. Yumino, D.; Wang, H.; Floras, J.S.; Newton, G.E.; Mak, S.; Ruttanaumpawan, P.; Parker, J.D.; Bradley, T.D. Prevalence and physiological predictors of sleep apnea in patients with heart failure and systolic dysfunction. *J. Card. Fail.* **2009**, *15*, 279–285. [CrossRef]

27. Herrscher, T.E.; Akre, H.; Øverland, B.; Sandvik, L.; Westheim, A.S. High prevalence of sleep apnea in heart failure outpatients: Even in patients with preserved systolic function. *J. Card. Fail.* **2011**, *17*, 420–425. [CrossRef] [PubMed]
28. Kalaydzhiev, P.; Poroyliev, N.; Somleva, D.; Ilieva, R.; Markov, D.; Kinova, E.; Goudev, A. Sleep apnea in patients with exacerbated heart failure and overweight. *Sleep Med. X* **2023**, *5*, 100065. [CrossRef]
29. Arikawa, T.; Toyoda, S.; Haruyama, A.; Amano, H.; Inami, S.; Otani, N.; Sakuma, M.; Taguchi, I.; Abe, S.; Node, K.; et al. Impact of Obstructive Sleep Apnoea on Heart Failure with Preserved Ejection Fraction. *Heart Lung Circ.* **2016**, *25*, 435–441. [CrossRef] [PubMed]
30. Naito, R.; Kasai, T.; Dohi, T.; Takaya, H.; Narui, K.; Momomura, S.I. Factors Associated With the Improvement of Left Ventricular Systolic Function by Continuous Positive Airway Pressure Therapy in Patients With Heart Failure With Reduced Ejection Fraction and Obstructive Sleep Apnea. *Front. Neurol.* **2022**, *13*, 781054. [CrossRef]
31. Kaneko, Y.; Floras, J.S.; Usui, K.; Plante, J.; Tkacova, R.; Kubo, T.; Ando, S.; Bradley, T.D. Cardiovascular effects of continuous positive airway pressure in patients with heart failure and obstructive sleep apnea. *N. Engl. J. Med.* **2003**, *348*, 1233–1241. [CrossRef] [PubMed]
32. Mansfield, D.R.; Gollogly, N.C.; Kaye, D.M.; Richardson, M.; Bergin, P.; Naughton, M.T. Controlled trial of continuous positive airway pressure in obstructive sleep apnea and heart failure. *Am. J. Respir. Crit. Care Med.* **2004**, *169*, 361–366. [CrossRef] [PubMed]
33. Fox, H.; Bitter, T.; Sauzet, O.; Rudolph, V.; Oldenburg, O. Automatic positive airway pressure for obstructive sleep apnea in heart failure with reduced ejection fraction. *Clin. Res. Cardiol.* **2021**, *110*, 983–992. [CrossRef] [PubMed]
34. Kim, D.; Shim, C.Y.; Cho, Y.J.; Park, S.; Lee, C.J.; Park, J.H.; Cho, H.J.; Ha, J.W.; Hong, G.R. Continuous Positive Airway Pressure Therapy Restores Cardiac Mechanical Function in Patients With Severe Obstructive Sleep Apnea: A Randomized, Sham-Controlled Study. *J. Am. Soc. Echocardiogr.* **2019**, *32*, 826–835. [CrossRef]
35. Matthew, P.; Gilman JS Floras, K.U.; Yasuyuki, K.; Richard, S.T.L.; Douglas, T.B. Continuous positive airway pressure increases heart rate variability in heart failure patients with obstructive sleep apnoea. *Clin. Sci.* **2008**, *114*, 243–249. [CrossRef]
36. Servantes, D.M.; Javaheri, S.; Kravchychyn, A.C.P.; Storti, L.J.; Almeida, D.R.; de Mello, M.T.; Cintra, F.D.; Tufik, S.; Bittencourt, L. Effects of Exercise Training and CPAP in Patients With Heart Failure and OSA: A Preliminary Study. *Chest* **2018**, *154*, 808–817. [CrossRef]
37. Egea, C.J.; Aizpuru, F.; Pinto, J.A.; Ayuela, J.M.; Ballester, E.; Zamarrón, C.; Sojo, A.; Montserrat, J.M.; Barbe, F.; Alonso-Gomez, A.M.; et al. Cardiac function after CPAP therapy in patients with chronic heart failure and sleep apnea: A multicenter study. *Sleep Med.* **2008**, *9*, 660–666. [CrossRef]
38. Ryan, C.M.; Usui, K.; Floras, J.S.; Bradley, T.D. Effect of continuous positive airway pressure on ventricular ectopy in heart failure patients with obstructive sleep apnoea. *Thorax* **2005**, *60*, 781–785. [CrossRef]
39. Cistulli, P.A.; Malhotra, A.; Cole, K.V.; Malik, A.S.; Pépin, J.L.; Sert Kuniyoshi, F.H.; Benjafield, A.V.; Somers, V.K.; medXcloud group. Positive Airway Pressure Therapy Adherence and Health Care Resource Use in Patients With Obstructive Sleep Apnea and Heart Failure With Preserved Ejection Fraction. *J. Am. Heart Assoc.* **2023**, *8*, e028733. [CrossRef]
40. Abdullah, A.; Eigbire, G.; Salama, A.; Wahab, A.; Nadkarni, N.; Alweis, R. Relation of Obstructive Sleep Apnea to Risk of Hospitalization in Patients With Heart Failure and Preserved Ejection Fraction from the National Inpatient Sample. *Am. J. Cardiol.* **2018**, *122*, 612–615. [CrossRef]
41. Malhotra, A.; Cole, K.V.; Malik, A.S.; Pépin, J.L.; Sert Kuniyoshi, F.H.; Cistulli, P.A.; Benjafield, A.V.; Somers, V.K.; medXcloud group. Positive Airway Pressure Adherence and Health Care Resource Utilization in Patients With Obstructive Sleep Apnea and Heart Failure with Reduced Ejection Fraction. *J. Am. Heart Assoc.* **2023**, *12*, e028732. [CrossRef] [PubMed]
42. Wojeck, B.S.; Inzucchi, S.E.; Neeland, I.J.; Mancuso, J.P.; Frederich, R.; Masiukiewicz, U.; Cater, N.B.; McGuire, D.K.; Cannon, C.P.; Yaggi, H.K. Ertugliflozin and incident obstructive sleep apnea: An analysis from the VERTIS CV trial. *Sleep Breath.* **2023**, *27*, 669–672. [CrossRef] [PubMed]
43. Neeland, I.J.; Eliasson, B.; Kasai, T.; Marx, N.; Zinman, B.; Inzucchi, S.E.; Wanner, C.; Zwiener, I.; Wojeck, B.S.; Yaggi, H.K.; et al. EMPA-REG OUTCOME Investigators. The Impact of Empagliflozin on Obstructive Sleep Apnea and Cardiovascular and Renal Outcomes: An Exploratory Analysis of the EMPA-REG OUTCOME Trial. *Diabetes Care* **2020**, *43*, 3007–3015. [CrossRef] [PubMed]
44. Furukawa, S.; Miyake, T.; Senba, H.; Sakai, T.; Furukawa, E.; Yamamoto, S.; Niiya, T.; Matsuura, B.; Hiasa, Y. The effectiveness of dapagliflozin for sleep-disordered breathing among Japanese patients with obesity and type 2 diabetes mellitus. *Endocr. J.* **2018**, *65*, 953–961. [CrossRef]
45. Tang, Y.; Sun, Q.; Bai, X.Y.; Zhou, Y.F.; Zhou, Q.L.; Zhang, M. Effect of dapagliflozin on obstructive sleep apnea in patients with type 2 diabetes: A preliminary study. *Nutr. Diabetes* **2019**, *9*, 32. [CrossRef]
46. Sawada, K.; Karashima, S.; Kometani, M.; Oka, R.; Takeda, Y.; Sawamura, T.; Fujimoto, A.; Demura, M.; Wakayama, A.; Usukura, M.; et al. Effect of sodium glucose cotransporter 2 inhibitors on obstructive sleep apnea in patients with type 2 diabetes. *Endocr. J.* **2018**, *65*, 461–467. [CrossRef]
47. Xie, L.; Song, S.; Li, S.; Wei, Q.; Liu, H.; Zhao, C.; Yu, F.; Tong, J. Efficacy of dapagliflozin in the treatment of HFrEF with obstructive sleep apnea syndrome (DAHOS study): Study protocol for a multicentric, prospective, randomized controlled clinical trial. *Trials* **2023**, *24*, 318. [CrossRef]

48. Owens, R.L.; Birkeland, K.; Heywood, J.T.; Steinhubl, S.R.; Dorn, J.; Grant, D.; Fombu, E.; Khandwalla, R. Sleep Outcomes from AWAKE-HF: A Randomized Clinical Trial of Sacubitril/Valsartan vs Enalapril in Patients With Heart Failure and Reduced Ejection Fraction. *J. Card. Fail.* **2021**, *27*, 1466–1471. [CrossRef]
49. Pelaia, C.; Armentaro, G.; Volpentesta, M.; Mancuso, L.; Miceli, S.; Caroleo, B.; Perticone, M.; Maio, R.; Arturi, F.; Imbalzano, E.; et al. Effects of Sacubitril-Valsartan on Clinical, Echocardiographic, and Polygraphic Parameters in Patients Affected by Heart Failure with Reduced Ejection Fraction and Sleep Apnea. *Front. Cardiovasc. Med.* **2022**, *9*, 861663. [CrossRef]
50. Jaffuel, D.; Nogue, E.; Berdague, P.; Galinier, M.; Fournier, P.; Dupuis, M.; Georger, F.; Cadars, M.P.; Ricci, J.E.; Plouvier, N.; et al. Sacubitril-valsartan initiation in chronic heart failure patients impacts sleep apnea: The ENTRESTO-SAS study. *ESC Heart Fail.* **2021**, *8*, 2513–2526. [CrossRef]
51. Wang, Y.; Branco, R.F.; Salanitro, M.; Penzel, T.; Schöbel, C. Effects of sacubitril-valsartan on central and obstructive apneas in heart failure patients with reduced ejection fraction. *Sleep Breath.* **2023**, *27*, 283–289. [CrossRef] [PubMed]
52. Passino, C.; Sciarrone, P.; Vergaro, G.; Borrelli, C.; Spiesshoefer, J.; Gentile, F.; Emdin, M.; Giannoni, A. Sacubitril-valsartan treatment is associated with decrease in central apneas in patients with heart failure with reduced ejection fraction. *Int. J. Cardiol.* **2021**, *330*, 112–119. [CrossRef] [PubMed]
53. Khayat, R.N.; Jarjoura, D.; Porter, K.; Sow, A.; Wannemacher, J.; Dohar, R.; Pleister, A.; Abraham, W.T. Sleep disordered breathing and post-discharge mortality in patients with acute heart failure. *Eur. Heart J.* **2015**, *36*, 1463–1469. [CrossRef] [PubMed]
54. Khayat, R.N.; Javaheri, S.; Porter, K.; Sow, A.; Holt, R.; Randerath, W.; Abraham, W.T.; Jarjoura, D. In-Hospital Management of Sleep Apnea During Heart Failure Hospitalization: A Randomized Controlled Trial. *J. Card. Fail.* **2020**, *26*, 705–712. [CrossRef]
55. Ambrosy, A.P.; Gheorghiade, M.; Chioncel, O.; Mentz, R.J.; Butler, J. Global perspectives in hospitalized heart failure: Regional and ethnic variation in patient characteristics, management, and outcomes. *Curr. Heart Fail. Rep.* **2014**, *11*, 416–427. [CrossRef]
56. Suen, C.; Wong, J.; Ryan, C.M.; Goh, S.; Got, T.; Chaudhry, R.; Lee, D.S.; Chung, F. Prevalence of Undiagnosed Obstructive Sleep Apnea Among Patients Hospitalized for Cardiovascular Disease and Associated In-Hospital Outcomes: A Scoping Review. *J. Clin. Med.* **2020**, *9*, 989. [CrossRef]
57. Javaheri, S.; Brown, L.K.; Abraham, W.T.; Khayat, R. Apneas of Heart Failure and Phenotype-Guided Treatments: Part One: OSA. *Chest* **2020**, *157*, 394–402. [CrossRef]
58. Kishan, S.; Rao, M.S.; Ramachandran, P.; Devasia, T.; Samanth, J. Prevalence and Patterns of Sleep-Disordered Breathing in Indian Heart Failure Population. *Pulm. Med.* **2021**, *2021*, 9978906. [CrossRef]
59. Javaheri, S.; Barbe, F.; Campos-Rodriguez, F.; Dempsey, J.A.; Khayat, R.; Javaheri, S.; Malhotra, A.; Martinez-Garcia, M.A.; Mehra, R.; Pack, A.I.; et al. Sleep Apnea: Types, Mechanisms, and Clinical Cardiovascular Consequences. *J. Am. Coll. Cardiol.* **2017**, *69*, 841–858. [CrossRef]
60. Javaheri, S.; Javaheri, S. Obstructive Sleep Apnea in Heart Failure: Current Knowledge and Future Directions. *J. Clin. Med.* **2022**, *11*, 3458. [CrossRef]
61. Donovan, L.M.; Boeder, S.; Malhotra, A.; Patel, S.R. New developments in the use of positive airway pressure for obstructive sleep apnea. *J. Thorac. Dis.* **2015**, *7*, 1323–1342. [CrossRef] [PubMed]
62. Henderson, L.A.; Fatouleh, R.H.; Lundblad, L.C.; McKenzie, D.K.; Macefield, V.G. Effects of 12 Months Continuous Positive Airway Pressure on Sympathetic Activity Related Brainstem Function and Structure in Obstructive Sleep Apnea. *Front. Neurosci.* **2016**, *10*, 90. [CrossRef] [PubMed]
63. Jullian-Desayes, I.; Joyeux-Faure, M.; Tamisier, R.; Launois, S.; Borel, A.L.; Levy, P.; Pepin, J.L. Impact of obstructive sleep apnea treatment by continuous positive airway pressure on cardiometabolic biomarkers: A systematic review from sham CPAP randomized controlled trials. *Sleep Med. Rev.* **2015**, *21*, 23–38. [CrossRef] [PubMed]
64. Spaak, J.; Egri, Z.J.; Kubo, T.; Yu, E.; Ando, S.; Kaneko, Y.; Usui, K.; Bradley, T.D.; Floras, J.S. Muscle sympathetic nerve activity during wakefulness in heart failure patients with and without sleep apnea. *Hypertension* **2005**, *46*, 1327–1332. [CrossRef]
65. Fiedorczuk, P.; Polecka, A.; Walasek, M.; Olszewska, E. Potential Diagnostic and Monitoring Biomarkers of Obstructive Sleep Apnea-Umbrella Review of Meta-Analyses. *J. Clin. Med.* **2022**, *12*, 60. [CrossRef]
66. Peker, Y.; Balcan, B. Cardiovascular outcomes of continuous positive airway pressure therapy for obstructive sleep apnea. *J. Thorac. Dis.* **2018**, *10* (Suppl. S34), S4262–S4279. [CrossRef]
67. Franco, O.H.; Peeters, A.; Bonneux, L.; de Laet, C. Blood pressure in adulthood and life expectancy with cardiovascular disease in men and women: Life course analysis. *Hypertension* **2005**, *46*, 280–286. [CrossRef]
68. Reil, J.C.; Custodis, F.; Swedberg, K.; Komajda, M.; Borer, J.S.; Ford, I.; Tavazzi, L.; Laufs, U.; Bohm, M. Heart rate reduction in cardiovascular disease and therapy. *Clin. Res. Cardiol.* **2011**, *100*, 11–19. [CrossRef]
69. Bohm, M.; Swedberg, K.; Komajda, M.; Borer, J.S.; Ford, I.; Dubost-Brama, A.; Lerebours, G.; Tavazzi, L.; Investigators, S. Heart rate as a risk factor in chronic heart failure (shift): The association between heart rate and outcomes in a randomised placebo-controlled trial. *Lancet* **2010**, *376*, 886–894. [CrossRef]
70. Shepard, J.W., Jr.; Pevernagie, D.A.; Stanson, A.W.; Daniels, B.K.; Sheedy, P.F. Effects of changes in central venous pressure on upper airway size in patients with obstructive sleep apnea. *Am. J. Respir. Crit. Care Med.* **1996**, *153*, 250–254. [CrossRef]
71. Yumino, D.; Redolfi, S.; Ruttanaumpawan, P.; Su, M.C.; Smith, S.; Newton, G.E.; Mak, S.; Bradley, T.D. Nocturnal rostral fluid shift: A unifying concept for the pathogenesis of obstructive and central sleep apnea in men with heart failure. *Circulation* **2010**, *121*, 1598–1605. [CrossRef] [PubMed]

72. Carmo, J.; Araújo, I.; Marques, F.; Fonseca, C. Sleep-disordered breathing in heart failure: The state of the art after the SERVE-HF trial. *Rev. Port. Cardiol.* **2017**, *36*, 859–867. [CrossRef] [PubMed]
73. Revol, B.; Jullian-Desayes, I.; Bailly, S.; Tamisier, R.; Grillet, Y.; Sapène, M.; Joyeux-Faure, M.; Pépin, J.L. Who May benefit from diuretics in OSA?: A propensity score-match observational study. *Chest* **2020**, *158*, 359–364. [CrossRef] [PubMed]
74. Bucca, C.B.; Brussino, L.; Battisti, A.; Mutani, R.; Rolla, G.; Mangiardi, L.; Cicolin, A. Diuretics in obstructive sleep apnea with diastolic heart failure. *Chest* **2007**, *132*, 440–446. [CrossRef]
75. Lamba, J.; Simpson, C.S.; Redfearn, D.P.; Michael, K.A.; Fitzpatrick, M.; Baranchuk, A. Cardiac resynchronization therapy for the treatment of sleep apnoea: A meta-analysis. *EP Eur.* **2011**, *13*, 1174–1179. [CrossRef]
76. Bolinder, J.; Ljunggren, Ö.; Kullberg, J.; Johansson, L.; Wilding, J.; Langkilde, A.M.; Sugg, J.; Parikh, S. Effects of dapagliflozin on body weight, total fat mass, and regional adipose tissue distribution in patients with type 2 diabetes mellitus with inadequate glycemic control on metformin. *J. Clin. Endocrinol. Metab.* **2012**, *97*, 1020–1031. [CrossRef]
77. Bolinder, J.; Ljunggren, Ö.; Johansson, L.; Wilding, J.; Langkilde, A.M.; Sjöström, C.D.; Sugg, J.; Parikh, S. Dapagliflozin maintains glycaemic control while reducing weight and body fat mass over 2 years in patients with type 2 diabetes mellitus inadequately controlled on metformin. *Diabetes Obes. Metab.* **2014**, *16*, 159–169. [CrossRef]
78. ČertíkováChábová, V.; Zakiyanov, O. Sodium glucose cotransporter-2 inhibitors: Spotlight on favorable effects on clinical outcomes beyond diabetes. *Int. J. Mol. Sci.* **2022**, *23*, 2812. [CrossRef]
79. Yokono, M.; Takasu, T.; Hayashizaki, Y.; Mitsuoka, K.; Kihara, R.; Muramatsu, Y.; Miyoshi, S.; Tahara, A.; Kurosaki, E.; Li, Q.; et al. SGLT2 selective inhibitor ipragliflozin reduces body fat mass by increasing fatty acid oxidation in high-fat diet-induced obese rats. *Eur. J. Pharmacol.* **2014**, *15*, 66–74. [CrossRef]
80. Liang, Y.; Arakawa, K.; Ueta, K.; Matsushita, Y.; Kuriyama, C.; Martin, T.; Du, F.; Liu, Y.; Xu, J.; Conway, B.; et al. Effect of canagliflozin on renal threshold for glucose, glycemia, and body weight in normal and diabetic animal models. *PLoS ONE* **2012**, *7*, e30555. [CrossRef]
81. Suzuki, M.; Takeda, M.; Kito, A.; Fukazawa, M.; Yata, T.; Yamamoto, M.; Nagata, T.; Fukuzawa, T.; Yamane, M.; Honda, K.; et al. Tofogliflozin, a sodium/glucose cotransporter 2 inhibitor, attenuates body weight gain and fat accumulation in diabetic and obese animal models. *Nutr. Diabetes* **2014**, *4*, e125. [CrossRef] [PubMed]
82. Ferrannini, E.; Muscelli, E.; Frascerra, S.; Baldi, S.; Mari, A.; Heise, T.; Broedl, U.C.; Woerle, H.J. Metabolic response to sodium–glucose cotransporter 2 inhibition in type 2 diabetic patients. *J. Clin. Investig.* **2014**, *124*, 499–508. [CrossRef] [PubMed]
83. Itani, T.; Ishihara, T. Efficacy of canagliflozin against nonalcoholic fatty liver disease: A prospective cohort study. *Obes. Sci. Pract.* **2018**, *4*, 477–482. [CrossRef] [PubMed]
84. Raj, H.; Durgia, H.; Palui, R.; Kamalanathan, S.; Selvarajan, S.; Kar, S.S.; Sahoo, J. SGLT-2 inhibitors in non-alcoholic fatty liver disease patients with type 2 diabetes mellitus: A systematic review. *World J. Diabetes* **2019**, *10*, 114–132. [CrossRef]
85. Choi, D.H.; Jung, C.H.; Mok, J.O.; Kim, C.H.; Kang, S.K.; Kim, B.Y. Effect of dapagliflozin on alanine aminotransferase improvement in type 2 diabetes mellitus with non-alcoholic fatty liver disease. *Endocrinol. Metab.* **2018**, *33*, 387–394. [CrossRef]
86. Shimizu, M.; Suzuki, K.; Kato, K.; Jojima, T.; Iijima, T.; Murohisa, T.; Iijima, M.; Takekawa, H.; Usui, I.; Hiraishi, H.; et al. Evaluation of the effects of dapagliflozin, a sodium–glucose co-transporter-2 inhibitor, on hepatic steatosis and fibrosis using transient elastography in patients with type 2 diabetes and non-alcoholic fatty liver disease. *Diabetes Obes. Metab.* **2019**, *21*, 285–292. [CrossRef]
87. Omori, K.; Nakamura, A.; Miyoshi, H.; Takahashi, K.; Kitao, N.; Nomoto, H.; Kameda, H.; Cho, K.Y.; Takagi, R.; Hatanaka, K.C.; et al. Effects of dapagliflozin and/or insulin glargine on beta cell mass and hepatic steatosis in db/db mice. *Metabolism* **2019**, *98*, 27–36. [CrossRef]
88. Yagi, S.; Hirata, Y.; Ise, T.; Kusunose, K.; Yamada, H.; Fukuda, D.; Salim, H.M.; Maimaituxun, G.; Nishio, S.; Takagawa, Y.; et al. Canagliflozin reduces epicardial fat in patients with type 2 diabetes mellitus. *Diabetol. Metab. Syndr.* **2017**, *4*, 78. [CrossRef]
89. Shimabukuro, M.; Hirata, Y.; Tabata, M.; Dagvasumberel, M.; Sato, H.; Kurobe, H.; Fukuda, D.; Soeki, T.; Kitagawa, T.; Takanashi, S.; et al. Epicardial adipose tissue volume and adipocytokine imbalance are strongly linked to human coronary atherosclerosis. *Arter. Thromb. Vasc. Biol.* **2013**, *33*, 1077–1084. [CrossRef]
90. Mahabadi, A.A.; Lehmann, N.; Kälsch, H.; Robens, T.; Bauer, M.; Dykun, I.; Budde, T.; Moebus, S.; Jöckel, K.H.; Erbel, R.; et al. Association of epicardial adipose tissue with progression of coronary artery calcification is more pronounced in the early phase of atherosclerosis: Results from the Heinz Nixdorf recall study. *JACC Cardiovasc. Imaging* **2014**, *7*, 909–916. [CrossRef]
91. Avogaro, A.; Fadini, G.P. Counterpoint to the hypothesis that SGLT2 inhibitors protect the heart by antagonizing leptin. *Diabetes Obes. Metab.* **2018**, *20*, 1367–1368. [CrossRef]
92. Packer, M. Do sodium–glucose co-transporter-2 inhibitors prevent heart failure with a preserved ejection fraction by counterbalancing the effects of leptin? A novel hypothesis. *Diabetes Obes. Metab.* **2018**, *20*, 1361–1366. [CrossRef]
93. Pan, W.; Kastin, A.J. Leptin: A biomarker for sleep disorders? *Sleep Med. Rev.* **2014**, *18*, 283–290. [CrossRef]
94. Berger, S.; Polotsky, V.Y. Leptin and leptin resistance in the pathogenesis of obstructive sleep apnea: A possible link to oxidative stress and cardiovascular complications. *Oxidative Med. Cell. Longev.* **2018**, *2018*, 5137947. [CrossRef] [PubMed]
95. Wu, P.; Wen, W.; Li, J.; Xu, J.; Zhao, M.; Chen, H.; Sun, J. Systematic review and meta-analysis of randomized controlled trials on the effect of SGLT2 inhibitor on blood leptin and adiponectin level in patients with type 2 diabetes. *Horm. Metab. Res.* **2019**, *51*, 487–494. [CrossRef] [PubMed]
96. Imayama, I.; Prasad, B. Role of Leptin in Obstructive Sleep Apnea. *Ann. Am. Thorac. Soc.* **2017**, *14*, 1607–1621. [CrossRef]

97. Selvaraj, S.; Claggett, B.; Pozzi, A.; McMurray, J.J.; Jhund, P.S.; Packer, M.; Desai, A.S.; Lewis, E.F.; Vaduganathan, M.; Lefkowitz, M.P.; et al. Prognostic implications of congestion on physical examination among contemporary patients with heart failure and reduced ejection fraction: PARADIGM-HF. *Circulation* **2019**, *140*, 1369–1379. [CrossRef] [PubMed]
98. Giannoni, A.; Raglianti, V.; Taddei, C.; Borrelli, C.; Chubuchny, V.; Vergaro, G.; Mirizzi, G.; Valleggi, A.; Cameli, M.; Pasanisi, E.; et al. Cheyne-Stokes respiration related oscillations in cardiopulmonary hemodynamics in patients with heart failure. *Int. J. Cardiol.* **2019**, *289*, 76–82. [CrossRef]
99. Bayard, G.; Da Costa, A.; Pierrard, R.; Roméyer-Bouchard, C.; Guichard, J.B.; Isaaz, K. Impact of sacubitril/valsartan on echo parameters in heart failure patients with reduced ejection fraction a prospective evaluation. *IJC Heart Vasc.* **2019**, *25*, 100418. [CrossRef]
100. Romano, G.; Vitale, G.; Ajello, L.; Agnese, V.; Bellavia, D.; Caccamo, G.; Corrado, E.; Di Gesaro, G.; Falletta, C.; La Franca, E.; et al. The effects of sacubitril/valsartan on clinical, biochemical and echocardiographic parameters in patients with heart failure with reduced ejection fraction: The "hemodynamic recovery". *J. Clin. Med.* **2019**, *8*, 2165. [CrossRef]
101. Giannoni, A.; Raglianti, V.; Mirizzi, G.; Taddei, C.; Del Franco, A.; Iudice, G.; Bramanti, F.; Aimo, A.; Pasanisi, E.; Emdin, M.; et al. Influence of central apneas and chemoreflex activation on pulmonary artery pressure in chronic heart failure. *Int. J. Cardiol.* **2016**, *202*, 200–206. [CrossRef] [PubMed]
102. Spiesshoefer, J.; Aries, J.; Giannoni, A.; Emdin, M.; Fox, H.; Boentert, M.; Bitter, T.; Oldenburg, O. APAP therapy does not improve impaired sleep quality and sympatho-vagal balance: A randomized trial in patients with obstructive sleep apnea and systolic heart failure. *Sleep Breath.* **2020**, *24*, 211–219. [CrossRef] [PubMed]
103. White, L.H.; Bradley, T.D. Role of nocturnal rostral fluid shift in the pathogenesis of obstructive and central sleep apnoea. *J. Physiol.* **2013**, *591*, 1179–1193. [CrossRef] [PubMed]
104. Fox, H.; Bitter, T.; Horstkotte, D.; Oldenburg, O. Resolution of Cheyne-Stokes respiration after treatment of heart failure with sacubitril/valsartan: A first case report. *Cardiology* **2017**, *137*, 96–99. [CrossRef] [PubMed]

Disclaimer/Publisher's Note: The statements, opinions and data contained in all publications are solely those of the individual author(s) and contributor(s) and not of MDPI and/or the editor(s). MDPI and/or the editor(s) disclaim responsibility for any injury to people or property resulting from any ideas, methods, instructions or products referred to in the content.

Review

A Narrative Review of the Association of Obstructive Sleep Apnea with Hypertension: How to Treat Both When They Coexist?

Servet Altay [1,†], Selma Fırat [2,†], Yüksel Peker [3,4,5,6,7,*] and The TURCOSACT Collaborators [‡]

1. Department of Cardiology, Trakya University School of Medicine, Edirne 22030, Turkey; svtaltay@gmail.com
2. Department of Pulmonary Medicine, University of Health Sciences, Atatürk Sanatorium Education and Research Hospital, Ankara 06280, Turkey; selmafirat1@gmail.com
3. Department of Pulmonary Medicine, Koç University School of Medicine, Istanbul 34450, Turkey
4. Division of Sleep and Circadian Disorders, Brigham and Women's Hospital, Boston, MA 02115, USA
5. Division of Pulmonary, Allergy, and Critical Care Medicine, University of Pittsburgh School of Medicine, Pittsburgh, PA 15213, USA
6. Department of Clinical Sciences, Respiratory Medicine and Allergology, Faculty of Medicine, Lund University, 22002 Lund, Sweden
7. Department of Molecular and Clinical Medicine, Institute of Medicine, Sahlgrenska Academy, University of Gothenburg, 40530 Gothenburg, Sweden
* Correspondence: yuksel.peker@lungall.gu.se
† These authors contributed equally to this work.
‡ The Turkish Collaboration of Sleep Apnea Cardiovascular Trialists (TURCOSACT) Collaborators are provided in the Acknowledgments.

Abstract: Hypertension (HT) is a worldwide public health issue and an essential risk factor for cardiovascular and cerebrovascular diseases. Obstructive sleep apnea (OSA) is a condition characterized by recurrent episodes of apnea and hypopnea as a consequence of partial or complete obstruction of the upper airways due to anatomic and/or functional disturbances. There is mounting evidence of a relationship between OSA and HT. In patients with OSA, HT is predominantly nocturnal and characterized by high diastolic blood pressure and usually by a nondipping pattern. Optimizing the blood pressure control is recommended in the current guidelines as the first treatment option in hypertensive patients with OSA. Continuous positive airway pressure (CPAP) therapy may reduce blood pressure, albeit only slightly as a stand-alone treatment. CPAP, as an add-on treatment to antihypertensive medication, appears to be an efficient treatment modality when both conditions coexist. This narrative review aims to summarize the current perspectives on the association of OSA with HT and the treatment options available for adults with OSA-related HT.

Keywords: obstructive sleep apnea; hypertension; narrative review

1. Introduction

In general, patients with an office systolic blood pressure (SBP) ≥ 140 mm Hg and a diastolic blood pressure (DBP) ≥ 90 mmHg are deemed to have hypertension (HT). The overall prevalence of HT in adults is reportedly around 30–45% [1]. Obstructive sleep apnea (OSA) is a condition with recurrent apnea and hypopnea, frequent arousal, and hypoxemia, which can lead to serious cardiovascular consequences such as HT, heart failure, arrhythmia, and atherosclerosis [2]. As an important cause of morbidity and mortality, HT accounted for the deaths of approximately 10 million people in 2015 and over 200 million disability-adjusted life years [3]. Blood pressure normally drops during sleep. A nocturnal decrease of more than 10% in the mean blood pressure level throughout the day is defined as the "dipping pattern". The absence of this decrease indicates a nondipping pattern. One of the important causes for the nondipping pattern is OSA [4,5]. Here, the sympathetic nervous system is activated due to the obstructed airway in patients with OSA, resulting in the disruption of the natural dipping pattern and causing an increase in blood pressure [5].

Traditionally recognized risk factors for cardiovascular diseases (CVDs), such as obesity, insulin resistance, diabetes mellitus, and hyperlipidemia, are common in OSA patients, and the most common CVD in patients with OSA is HT. The coexistence of OSA and chronic obstructive pulmonary disease (COPD) is called overlap syndrome [6], and individuals with overlap syndrome have a significantly increased risk of HT compared with those with COPD alone [7].

On behalf of the Turkish Collaboration of Sleep Apnea Cardiovascular Trialists (TUR-COSACT), we recently published a position paper on OSA and cardiovascular diseases [8]. To provide in-depth analyses of the topic, the present narrative review aimed to summarize the existing perspectives on the association of OSA with HT and the treatment options available for individuals with OSA and concomitant HT.

2. Epidemiology of OSA and Hypertension

HT and OSA often coexist. Pensukan et al. found a significant relationship between OSA and elevated blood pressure (odds ratio (OR): 2.38; 95% confidence interval (CI): 1.68–3.39), and HT (OR: 2.55; 95% CI: 1.57–4.15) after adjusting for demographic characteristics [9]. OSA has been reported among 30–50% of hypertensive patients. This rate can increase to 80% among cases with drug-resistant HT [10–12]. It has also been reported that masked HT is 2.7 times more common in OSA patients [13,14].

There is a bidirectional and causal relationship between HT and OSA. Several studies have revealed a clear dose–response relationship with OSA severity and HT. The meta-analyses on the relationship between OSA and HT are summarized in Table 1 [15–18].

Table 1. Recent meta-analyses regarding the association of OSA with the risk of HT.

Author (Reference)	Year	Number of Studies	Total Sample Size	OSA (OR (95% CI)) for HT
Meng [15]	2016	6	20,367	1.41 (1.29–1.89)
Hou [16]	2018	26	51,623	1.80 (1.54–2.06)
Han [17]	2020	10	13,274	1.80 (1.36–2.38)
Yuan [18]	2021	8	3484	6.44 (5.38–7.71)

Abbreviations: CI, confidence interval; HT, hypertension; OR, odds ratio; OSA, obstructive sleep apnea.

The Sleep Heart Health Study (SHHS), a large-scale, community-based, multicenter, cross-sectional study conducted with 6152 participants, reported an increased OR of 1.37 (95% CI: 1.03–1.83) of HT in those with severe OSA after adjusting for confounding factors [12]. Different results have been reported on the relationship between OSA and HT in prospective studies. One of these studies was the Wisconsin Sleep Cohort Study, which was conducted with 709 participants. The results indicated a dose–response relationship independent of known confounding factors between sleep-disordered breathing and new-onset HT 4 years later [19]. Similarly, in the Zaragoza Sleep Cohort Study, a prospective, observational study conducted with 1889 participants for a mean follow-up duration of 12.2 years, an increased risk of new-onset HT was detected in untreated OSA patients after adjusting for confounding factors, including apnea hypopnea index (AHI), age, sex, baseline SBP, DBP, and body mass index (BMI) [20].

In contrast, in the Victoria sleep cohort study conducted with 1557 participants for a follow-up duration of 7.5 years, no relationship was found between OSA and the incidence of HT [21]. Along these lines, the 5-year follow-up study of the SHHS, conducted with 2470 participants without HT at admission, found that after adjusting for BMI, AHI was no longer a significant predictor of HT. The findings that do not support the relationship between OSA and HT were attributed to the lower rate of participants with moderate-to-severe OSA. Indeed, the vast majority (around 87%) of the participants included in the 5-year follow-up of the SHHS had mild OSA, defined as an AHI between 5 and 15 events/h [22].

A meta-analysis of seven studies by Xia W et al., published in 2018, including 6 prospective cohort studies and 1 case-control study, conducted with a total of 6098 participants, reported that high AHI values were related to a significantly increased risk of essential HT compared with low AHI values (OR 1.77, 95% CI 1.30–2.41, p = 0.001). The results of the linear dose–response meta-analysis indicated that the risk of essential HT increased by 17% for every 10 events/hour increase in the AHI (OR 1.17, 95% CI 1.07–1.27, p = 0.001). Moreover, the nonlinear dose–response found in the meta-analysis results revealed that the risk of essential HT increased with AHI [23]. Similarly, a recent meta-analysis by Yuan F. et al. published in 2021, including 8 studies conducted with a total of 3484 OSA patients, revealed a significant association between OSA and HT (OR 6.44, 95% CI 5.38–7.71, p < 0.001) and between OSA severity and HT [17].

3. Pathogenesis of Hypertension in OSA

The mechanisms promoting HT in OSA are multifactorial. Sympathetic activity due to intermittent hypoxia is one of the mechanisms triggering the elevation in blood pressure in OSA. Sympathetic activity due to the hypoxemic state causes both vasoconstriction and the stimulation of chemoreceptors. Consequently, the renin–angiotensin–aldosterone system (RAAS) is activated, the endothelin-1 level is increased, and the nitric oxide level is decreased, all of which contribute to the increase in vascular resistance and the development of HT [24,25]. In addition, RAAS activation increases the amount of angiotensin-2, a strong vasoconstrictor, in the blood and, thus, blood pressure [26]. Increased aldosterone levels also contribute to the development of HT by causing fluid and sodium retention [27]. Sympathetic hyperactivity leads to a proinflammatory state, resulting in endothelial injury and oxidative stress [28,29]. The other factors that play a role in the pathogenesis of HT in OSA are obesity, gut dysbiosis, rostral fluid shifts, pharyngeal collapse, nocturnal energy expenditure, and metabolic derangements [24] (Figure 1).

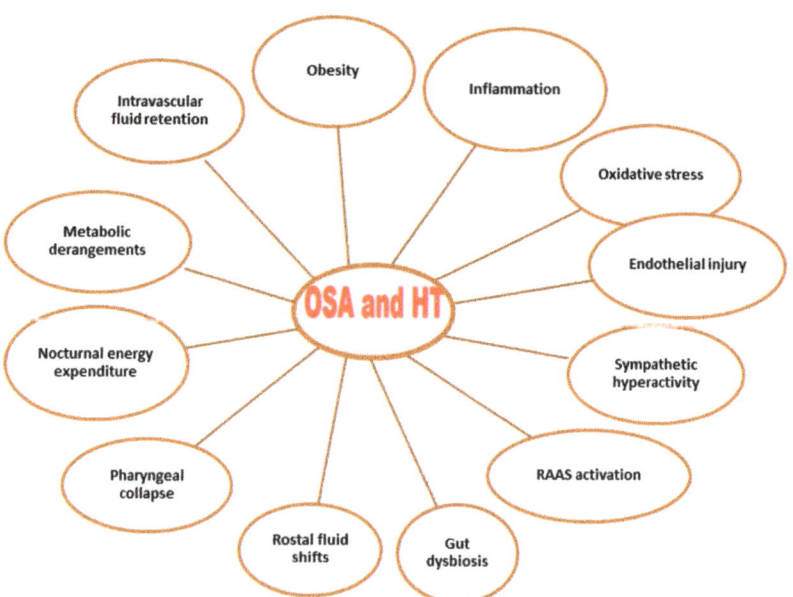

Figure 1. Conditions associated with OSA and hypertension. Abbreviations: OSA, obstructive sleep apnea; RAAS, renin–angiotensin–aldosterone system.

4. Clinical Characteristics of Hypertension in OSA

In patients with OSA, HT is predominantly nocturnal and characterized by a high DBP, masked HT, and a nondipping pattern [4]. Blood pressure is normally the highest during the mid-morning, gradually decreasing as the day progresses, down to 10% of the wakefulness value during sleep, and reaches its lowest value at 3 a.m. This dipping pattern is correlated with the duration of deep sleep. It has been reported that the expected decrease in blood pressure may not occur in the case of several diseases such as OSA. Important cardiovascular consequences may occur in patients who have such diseases who are referred to as "nondippers" [30,31].

Nocturnal blood pressure elevation is correlated with the severity of OSA [32]. The nondipping blood pressure pattern was reported at a rate of 84% in OSA patients who did not receive treatment [33]. Nocturnal and nondipping HT is closely associated with target organ damage and the development of cardiovascular diseases [34]. Additionally, it has been reported that night-time blood pressure variability, which is related to increased target organ damage, was higher in a OSA group than in a non-OSA group [35,36]. The pathogenesis of the nondipping pattern and blood pressure variability is multifactorial. Intermittent hypoxia and recurring microarousals are major events leading to sleep fragmentation, reduced slow-wave sleep, and increased sympathetic activity, resulting in elevated blood pressure and increased blood pressure variability [37].

5. Treatment Modalities

Among the treatment modalities that come to the fore in the treatment of OSA in patients with HT are CPAP, diuretics, renal denervation, use of maxillomandibular advancement devices, and hypoglossal nerve stimulation surgery for restricted airways or tonsillar enlargement. Weight loss, physical exercise, reducing alcohol consumption, and smoking cessation are among the primary lifestyle changes recommended for hypertensive patients with OSA [38].

6. Pharmacological Therapies of HT in Patients with OSA

6.1. Antihypertensive Medications

Current guidelines for HT do not make specific recommendations on the pharmacological treatment modalities for patients with concomitant OSA and HT. Given the increased sympathetic activity and renin–angiotensin–aldosterone (RAAS) activity in OSA patients, medications that block these pathways are highlights. Among the antihypertensive medications that were initially preferred were angiotensin-converting enzyme (ACE) inhibitors and angiotensin receptor blockers (ARBs) [39]. It was also demonstrated that beta-blockers mitigate night-time blood pressure rise and apnea-related tachycardias [40]. An earlier study conducted by Hedner et al. compared the effects of atenolol, hydrochlorothiazide, amlodipine, enalapril, and losartan on office and ambulatory blood pressures in 40 individuals with HT and OSA [41]. Each participant received two of the aforementioned five agents (balanced incomplete block design) for 6 weeks, with a 3-week washout period in-between. Compared with the other four drugs, atenolol lowered the office diastolic BP as well as mean night-time ambulatory SBP and DBP [41]. These findings support the hypothesis that overactivity of the sympathetic nervous system is the most important mechanism involved in the development of HT in adults with OSA [41].

6.2. Diuretics

Two small studies have suggested that the use of spironolactone, an aldosterone antagonist, may efficiently decrease blood pressure in OSA patients with treatment-resistant HT [42,43]. Similarly, eplerenone, another aldosterone antagonist, was shown to significantly decrease blood pressure in hypertensive OSA patients [44]. Recent studies have shown that primary aldosteronism is common in patients with moderate-to-severe OSA, a finding that indicates aldosterone antagonists may be beneficial in this patient group [45–47]. There are also studies suggesting that aldosterone antagonists may reduce the frequency of apnea by mitigating laryngeal edema in OSA patients [42,46]. Taken together, these findings suggest that aldosterone antagonist diuretics, especially spironolactone, may be effective in the treatment of HT in OSA patients. However, large-scale cohort studies are needed to elucidate the efficacy of aldosterone antagonist diuretics in treating HT in OSA patients.

6.3. Sodium-Glucose Cotransporter 2 (SGLT2) Inhibitors

Canagliflozin, one of the SGLT2 inhibitors that has recently been the focus in the treatment of cardiac failure, was shown to provide significant nocturnal blood pressure reductions in adults with diabetes, treatment-resistant HT, and OSA [48].

7. CPAP Therapy for OSA in Patients with HT

A number of studies have shown that CPAP therapy results in a modest reduction of 2–3 mmHg in SBP and of 1.5–2 mmHg in DBP in OSA patients (Table 2) [49–56]. On the other hand, this reduction is higher in adults with treatment-resistant HT. Although a 1–2 mmHg decrease in blood pressure may not be considered much, even such a slight decrease in blood pressure was shown to be associated with significant decrease sin cardiovascular mortality and stroke risk [57].

Table 2. Recent meta-analyses regarding the effect of OSA treatment on blood pressure values.

Author (Reference)	Year	Number of Studies	Total Sample Size	OSA Therapy	Main Findings
Liu [49]	2016	5	446	CPAP	MBP reduction: 4.78 mmHg, 95% C:I 1.61–7.95 mmHg SBP reduction: 2.95 mmHg, 95% CI: 0.53–5.37 mmHg DBP reduction: 1.53 mmHg, 95% CI: 0.00–3.07 mmHg
Pengo [50]	2020	68		CPAP or MADs	MBP reduction: 2.09 mmHg, 95% CI: 2.78–1.40 mmHg SBP reduction: 1.92 mmHg, 95% CI: 2.40–1.43 mmHg DBP reduction: 1.27 mmHg, 95% CI, 2.34–0.20 mmHg
Bratton [51]	2015	51	4888	CPAP or MADs	DBP reduction: 2.5 mmHg, 95% CI: 1.5–3.5 mmHg DBP reduction: 2.0 mm Hg, 95% CI: 1.3–2.7 mmHg
Iftikhar [52]	2013	7	399	MADs	MBP reduction: 2.4 mmHg, 95% CI: 0.8–4.0 mmHg SBP reduction: 2.7 mmHg, 95% CI: 0.8–4.6 mmHg DBP reduction: 2.7 mmHg, 95% CI: 0.9–4.6 mmHg
Schein [53]	2014	16	1166	CPAP	Office SBP reduction: 3.20 mmHg, 95% CI: 1.72–4.67 mmHg Office DBP reduction: 2.87 mmHg, 95% CI: 0.55–5.18 mmHg Night-time SBP reduction: 4.92 mmHg, 95% CI: 1.14–8.70 Mean 24 h BP reduction: 3.56 mmHg, 95% CI: 0.33–6.79 mmHg Mean night-time BP reduction: 2.56 mmHg 95% CI: 0.68–4.43 mmHg

Table 2. Cont.

Author (Reference)	Year	Number of Studies	Total Sample Size	OSA Therapy	Main Findings
Fava [54]	2014	29	1820	CPAP	24-h SBP reduction: 2.6 ± 0.6 mmHg 24 h DBP reduction: 2.0 ± 0.4 mmHg
Labarca [55]	2021	10	606	CPAP	24 h SBP reduction: 5.06 mmHg, 95% CI: 2.13–7.98 mmHg 24 h DBP reduction: 4.21 mmHg, 95% CI: 1.93–6.50 mmHg Daytime SBP reduction: 2.34 mmHg, 95% CI: 2.27–6.94 mmHg Daytime DBP reduction: 2.14 mmHg, 95% CI: 0.67–4.96 mmHg Night-time SBP reduction: 4.15 mmHg, 95% CI: 1.29–7.01 mmHg Nighttime DBP reduction: 1.95 mmHg, 95% CI: 0.57–3.32 mmHg
Shang [56]	2022	19	1904	CPAP	SBP reduction: 5.01 mmHg 95% CI: 3.08–6.94 mmHg

Abbreviations: CI, confidence interval; CPAP, continuous positive airway pressure; DBP, diastolic blood pressure; HT, hypertension; MAD, mandibular advancement device; MBP, mean blood pressure; OR, odds ratio; OSA, obstructive sleep apnea; SBP, systolic blood pressure.

The efficacy of CPAP therapy in the treatment of HT in patients with OSA has been extensively investigated in the literature. Earlier meta-analyses demonstrated a good effect of CPAP therapy in lowering blood pressure in OSA patients. Studies have shown significant reductions in day- and night-time blood pressure values, especially in OSA patients with treatment-resistant HT [58–61].

Kartali N. et al. reported that SBP decreased from 141.5 ± 12.1 mmHg to 133.5 ± 9.7 mmHg ($p = 0.007$) and that DBP decreased from 87.8 ± 6.8 to 83 ± 5.4 mmHg ($p = 0.004$) after three months of CPAP treatment [62]. Interestingly, the decrease in SBP was observed only during the night ($p = 0.031$), whereas the decrease in DBP was both during the day and night ($p = 0.024$ and $p = 0.007$, respectively). Of note, all the hypertensive participants included in the study were initially nondippers, and the dipping status was significantly improved after CPAP therapy (from 7.9 to 10.4% for SBP, $p = 0.014$; and from 8.4 to 10.5% for DBP, $p = 0.029$) [62].

In a randomized controlled trial (RCT) by Hoyos C. et al., a significant decrease was detected in blood pressure after CPAP therapy. The magnitude of the decrease was 4.1 mmHg regarding the mean central SBP ($p = 0.003$), 3.9 mmHg in mean central DBP ($p = 0.0009$), 4.1 mmHg in mean peripheral SBP ($p = 0.004$), and 3.8 mmHg in mean peripheral DBP ($p = 0.001$) [63].

In a four-year retrospective study by Yang M.C. et al., the mean blood pressure decreased from 100.8 ± 13.6 mmHg to 96.6 ± 10.8 mmHg ($p = 0.004$) in OSA patients who were adherent with CPAP [64].

A 24-week follow-up study by Campos-Rodriguez F. et al. demonstrated that dose-related beneficial effects were achieved in the long term, even in hypertensive OSA patients who were initially undertreated [65].

In an RCT comparing three months of CPAP therapy with sham-CPAP in adults with moderate-to-severe OSA and nocturnal HT, a slight decrease in 24 h SBP/DBP by 2.8/2.5 mmHg was observed, but this was not statistically significant [66]. The blood-pressure-lowering effect of CPAP was shown to depend on the baseline daytime pulse rate; and, accordingly, the reduction was significantly greater (10.1 mmHg or more) in patients with a greater daytime pulse rate [66].

A multicenter RCT comparing CPAP with sham-CPAP in 272 patients with new-onset systemic HT and moderate-to-severe OSA revealed a significant effect of CPAP on the dipping pattern [65]. CPAP therapy was associated with reductions in 24 h ambulatory blood pressure variables and night-time ambulatory blood pressure measurements only in the nondipper group, whereas no significant difference was detected in the dipper group [67].

In a recent 8-week-long parallel-group RCT conducted with 92 patients with treatment-resistant HT and OSA, the participants were randomized to CPAP and no-CPAP groups [68]. Significant decreases were observed in 24 h SBP by 4.4 mmHg, in 24 h DBP by 2.9 mmHg, in daytime SBP by 5.4 mmHg, and in daytime DBP by 3.4 mmHg, yet only in nondippers, not in dippers [68].

Other studies have evaluated the effect of antihypertensive medications vs. CPAP on blood pressure in patients with OSA, suggesting that antihypertensive drugs reduce the blood pressure better than CPAP therapy alone and that the combined use of CPAP therapy and antihypertensive medications provide better results than the stand-alone use of either treatment method [69,70].

The application of CPAP therapy for one more hour per night reportedly reduced SBP and DBP 1.5 mmHg and 0.9 mmHg more, respectively [71]. CPAP therapy reduced blood pressure more in adults with severe OSA and in those with more complaints of insomnia during the day [72].

It has been proposed that the blood-pressure-lowering effect of CPAP therapy is more prominent in patients under 60 years of age, in those with higher pretreatment blood pressure, in untreated HT, treatment-resistant HT, nocturnal or nondipping HT, severe OSA, and in those who are adherent to CPAP therapy [13,50,52,71,73]. Nonetheless, given that CPAP therapy does not correct all factors that increase blood pressure (e.g., volume overload, high salt production, etc.), CPAP alone cannot produce a significant improvement in blood pressure. According to the 2017 American Heart Association (AHA)/American College of Cardiology (ACC) blood pressure guidelines, CPAP therapy is yet not a well-established antihypertensive treatment in adults with HT and OSA (class IIb) [74].

8. Non-CPAP Treatments of OSA in Patients with HT

A number of studies, though small-scale and observational, have demonstrated that non-CPAP treatments, e.g., soft-palate lifters, tongue-retaining devices, mandibular advancement appliances, expansion sphincter pharyngoplasty, etc., provided blood pressure reduction comparable to CPAP therapy in patients with HT in patients with OSA [52].

In one of these RCTs, including 65 hypertensive patients with OSA, uvulopalatopharyngoplasty (UPPP) provided a blood pressure reduction of 4–9 mmHg compared with the control group [75]. Previous studies reported that CPAP therapy was not superior to UPPP in preventing the development of hypertension in OSA patients [76]. In contrast, a recent study conducted with 413 OSA patients demonstrated that both CPAP therapy and UPPP had a preventative effect on the development of HT in OSA patients and that CPAP treatment prevented the development of HT more than UPPP [77]. Another recent study revealed that expansion sphincter pharyngoplasty resulted in significant blood pressure reduction in OSA patients [78].

9. Renal Denervation for Treatment-Resistant HT in OSA

It has been suggested that renal sympathetic denervation, which has recently emerged as a new approach in the treatment of treatment-resistant HT, might also be used in the treatment of HT in patients with OSA. Daniels et al. conducted a prospective study in patients with OSA and treatment-resistant HT and demonstrated that renal denervation (RDN) provided a significant decrease in office and ambulatory blood pressure values after a six month follow-up period [79]. Similarly, an RCT conducted with moderate-to-severe OSA patients with treatment-resistant HT demonstrated that RDN safely provided significant blood pressure reduction compared with the control group [80]. Further large-scale studies on the efficacy of RDN in OSA patients are needed.

10. Summary, Generalization, and Inferences

Based on the current evidence about the association between OSA and HT, it appears appropriate that patients with drug-resistant or poorly controlled or nondipping hypertension should be screened for OSA [8]. Weight loss, regular physical exercise, a healthy diet, and salt restriction are important for blood pressure regulation in patients with OSA and HT. Regarding the medications, calcium channel blockers, ACEIs or ARBs, and thiazide-type diuretics are recommended as first-line therapy in patients with OSA and HT, and spironolactone should be added to the first line treatment in the presence of resistant hypertension in OSA patients. Moreover, beta-blocker therapy should be preferred in hypertensive OSA patients in the presence of CAD, arrhythmia, or heart failure, whereas SGLT-2 inhibitors and renal denervation therapy may be considered as an option in patients refractory to standard therapy. Last but not least, CPAP therapy should be considered at all stages in OSA patients with HT, and it should definitely be used, especially in cases with drug-resistant HT [8].

11. Conclusions

OSA and HT often coexist, which means OSA is one of the important factors to be considered in managing treatment-resistant HT. The current guidelines for the treatment of HT in patients with OSA adopt the general principles of HT treatment. Hence, even though it provides a modest blood pressure reduction, CPAP therapy is considered in the treatment modalities recommended for the treatment of HT, especially as an add-on treatment. In this context, high CPAP compliance is crucial for the effective treatment of HT in OSA. The number of studies on the efficacy of pharmacological treatments and surgical treatments is limited. Further large-scale studies featuring conventional and novel treatment approaches are needed to serve as a guide for future studies related to OSA and HT.

Author Contributions: Conception and design: S.A., S.F. and Y.P.; analysis and interpretation: S.A., S.F., Y.P. and the TURCOSACT Collaborators; drafting the manuscript for important intellectual content: S.A., S.F. and Y.P. All authors have read and agreed to the published version of the manuscript.

Funding: This research received no external funding.

Institutional Review Board Statement: Not applicable.

Informed Consent Statement: Not applicable.

Data Availability Statement: Not applicable.

Acknowledgments: The Turkish Collaboration of Sleep Apnea Cardiovascular Trialists (TURCOSACT) collaborators: Bahri Akdeniz; Baran Balcan; Özcan Başaran; Erkan Baysal; Ahmet Çelik; Dursun Dursunoğlu; Neşe Dursunoğlu; Canan Gündüz Gürkan; Önder Öztürk; Mehmet Sezai Taşbakan; Vedat Aytekin.

Conflicts of Interest: Y.P. declares institutional grants from ResMed Foundation, outside the submitted work. S.A., S.F., B.A., B.B., Ö.B., E.B., A.C., D.D., N.D., C.G.G., Ö.Ö., M.S.T. and V.A. have no conflicts to report.

References

1. The Task Force for the Management of Arterial Hypertension of the European Society of Cardiology (ESC); the European Society of Hypertension (ESH). 2018 ESC/ESH Guidelines for the management of arterial hypertension. *Eur. Heart J.* **2018**, *39*, 3021–3104. [CrossRef]
2. Yeghiazarians, Y.; Jneid, H.; Tietjens, J.R.; Redline, S.; Brown, D.L.; El-Sherif, N.; Mehra, R.; Bozkurt, B.; Ndumele, C.E.; Somers, V.K. Obstructive Sleep Apnea and Cardiovascular Disease: A Scientific Statement From the American Heart Association. *Circulation* **2021**, *144*, e56–e67. [CrossRef]

3. Forouzanfar, M.H.; Liu, P.; Roth, G.A.; Ng, M.; Biryukov, S.; Marczak, L.; Alexander, L.; Estep, K.; Abate, K.H.; Akinyemiju, T.F.; et al. Global burden of hypertension and systolic blood pressure of at least 110 to 115 mm Hg, 1990–2015. *JAMA* **2017**, *317*, 165–182. [CrossRef]
4. Baguet, J.P.; Hammer, L.; Lévy, P.; Pierre, H.; Rossini, E.; Mouret, S.; Ormezzano, O.; Mallion, J.M.; Pépin, J.L. Night-time and diastolic hypertension are common and underestimated conditions in newly diagnosed apnoeic patients. *J. Hypertens.* **2005**, *23*, 521–527. [CrossRef]
5. Hla, K.M.; Young, T.; Finn, L.; Peppard, P.E.; Szklo-Coxe, M.; Stubbs, M. Longitudinal association of sleep-disordered breathing and nondipping of nocturnal blood pressure in the Wisconsin sleep chort study. *Sleep* **2008**, *31*, 795–800. [CrossRef]
6. Flenley, D.C. Sleep in chronic obstructive lung disease. *Clin. Chest Med.* **1985**, *6*, 651–661. [CrossRef]
7. Shah, A.J.; Quek, E.; Alqahtani, J.S.; Hurst, J.R.; Mandal, S. Cardiovascular outcomes in patients with COPD-OSA overlap syndrome: A systematic review and meta-analysis. *Sleep Med. Rev.* **2022**, *63*, 101627. [CrossRef]
8. Shah, A.J.; Quek, E.; Alqahtani, J.S.; Hurst, J.R.; Mandal, S. Obstructive Sleep Apnea and Cardiovascular Disease: Where Do We Stand? A narrative review and position paper from the Turkish Collaboration of Sleep Apnea Cardiovascular Trialists (TURCOSACT), founded by the Turkish Society of Cardiology & Turkish Thoracic Society. *Anatol. J. Cardiol.* **2023**. Ahead of Print. [CrossRef]
9. Pensuksan, W.C.; Chen, X.; Lohsoonthorn, V.; Lertmaharit, S.; Gelaye, B.; Williams, M.A. High risk for obstructive sleep apnea in relation to hypertension among southeast Asian youngadults: Role of obesity as an efect modifier. *Am. J. Hypertens.* **2014**, *27*, 229–236. [CrossRef]
10. Tietjens, J.R.; Claman, D.; Kezirian, E.J.; De Marco, T.; Mirzayan, A.; Sadroonri, B.; Goldberg, A.N.; Long, C.; Gerstenfeld, E.P.; Yeghiazarians, Y. Obstructive sleep apnea in cardiovascular disease: A review of the literature and proposed multidisciplinary clinical management strategy. *J. Am. Heart Assoc.* **2019**, *8*, e010440. [CrossRef]
11. Muxfeldt, E.S.; Margallo, V.S.; Guimarães, G.M.; Salles, G.F. Prevalence and associated factors of obstructive sleep apnea in patients with resistant hypertension. *Am. J. Hypertens.* **2014**, *27*, 1069–1078. [CrossRef]
12. Jinchai, J.; Khamsai, S.; Chattakul, P.; Limpawattana, P.; Chindaprasirt, J.; Chotmongkol, V.; Silaruks, S.; Senthong, V.; Sawanyawisuth, K. How common is obstructive sleep apnea in young hypertensive patients? *Intern. Emerg. Med.* **2020**, *15*, 1005–1010. [CrossRef]
13. Baguet, J.P.; Lévy, P.; Barone-Rochette, G.; Tamisier, R.; Pierre, H.; Peeters, M.; Mallion, J.M.; Pépin, J.L. Masked hypertension in obstructive sleep apnea syndrome. *J. Hypertens.* **2008**, *26*, 885–892. [CrossRef]
14. Nieto, F.J.; Young, T.B.; Lind, B.K.; Shahar, E.; Samet, J.M.; Redline, S.; D'Agostino, R.B.; Newman, A.B.; Lebowitz, M.D.; Pickering, T.G.; et al. Association of sleep-disordered breathing, sleep apnea, and hypertension in a large community-based study. Sleep Heart Health Study. *JAMA* **2000**, *283*, 1829–1836. [CrossRef]
15. Meng, F.; Ma, J.; Wang, W.; Lin, B. Obstructive sleep apnea syndrome is a risk factor of hypertension. *Minerva Med.* **2016**, *107*, 294–299.
16. Hou, H.; Zhao, Y.; Yu, W.; Dong, H.; Xue, X.; Ding, J.; Xing, W.; Wang, W. Association of obstructive sleep apnea with hypertension: A systematic review and meta-analysis. *J. Glob. Health* **2018**, *8*, 010405. [CrossRef]
17. Yuan, F.; Zhang, S.; Liu, X.; Liu, Y. Correlation between obstructive sleep apnea hypopnea syndrome and hypertension: A systematic review and meta-analysis. *Ann. Palliat. Med.* **2021**, *10*, 12251–12261. [CrossRef]
18. Han, B.; Chen, W.Z.; Li, Y.C.; Chen, J.; Zeng, Z.Q. Sleep and hypertension. *Sleep Breath* **2020**, *24*, 351–356. [CrossRef]
19. Peppard, P.E.; Young, T.; Palta, M.; Skatrud, J. Prospective study of the association between sleep-disordered breathing and hypertension. *N. Engl. J. Med.* **2000**, *342*, 1378–1384. [CrossRef]
20. Marin, J.M.; Agusti, A.; Villar, I.; Forner, M.; Nieto, D.; Carrizo, S.J.; Barbé, F.; Vicente, E.; Wei, Y.; Nieto, F.J.; et al. Association between treated and untreated obstructive sleep apnea and risk of hypertension. *JAMA* **2012**, *307*, 2169–2176. [CrossRef]
21. Cano-Pumarega, I.; Durán-Cantolla, J.; Aizpuru, F.; Miranda-Serrano, E.; Rubio, R.; Martínez-Null, C.; de Miguel, J.; Egea, C.; Cancelo, L.; Alvarez, A. Obstructive sleep apnea and systemic hypertension: Longitudinal study in the general population: The Vitoria Sleep Cohort. *Am. J. Respir. Crit. Care Med.* **2011**, *184*, 1299–1304. [CrossRef] [PubMed]
22. O'Connor, G.T.; Caffo, B.; Newman, A.B.; Quan, S.F.; Rapoport, D.M.; Redline, S.; Resnick, H.E.; Samet, J.; Shahar, E. Prospective study of sleep-disordered breathing and hypertension: The Sleep Heart Health Study. *Am. J. Respir. Crit. Care Med.* **2009**, *179*, 1159–1164. [CrossRef] [PubMed]
23. Xia, W.; Huang, Y.; Peng, B.; Zhang, X.; Wu, Q.; Sang, Y.; Luo, Y.; Liu, X.; Chen, Q.; Tian, K. Relationship between obstructive sleep apnoea syndrome and essential hypertension: A dose-response meta-analysis. *Sleep Med.* **2018**, *47*, 11–18. [CrossRef]
24. Brown, J.; Yazdi, F.; Jodari-Karimi, M.; Owen, J.G.; Reisin, E. Obstructive Sleep Apnea and Hypertension: Updates to a Critical Relationship. *Curr. Hypertens. Rep.* **2022**, *24*, 173–184. [CrossRef] [PubMed]
25. Diogo, L.N.; Monteiro, E.C. The efficacy of antihypertensive drugs in chronicintermittent hypoxia conditions. *Front. Physiol.* **2014**, *5*, 361. [CrossRef] [PubMed]
26. Heitmann, J.; Greulich, T.; Reinke, C.; Koehler, U.; Vogelmeier, C.; Becker, H.F.; Schmidt, A.C.; Canisius, S. Comparison of the effects of nebivolol and valsartan on BP reduction and sleep apnoea activity in patients with essential hypertension and OSA. *Curr. Med. Res. Opin.* **2010**, *26*, 1925–1932. [CrossRef]
27. Phillips, C.L.; O'Driscoll, D.M. Hypertension and obstructive sleep apnea. *Nat. Sci. Sleep* **2013**, *5*, 43–52. [CrossRef]

28. Gonzaga, C.C.; Gaddam, K.K.; Ahmed, M.I.; Pimenta, E.; Thomas, S.J.; Harding, S.M.; Oparil, S.; Cofield, S.S.; David, A. Calhoun Severity of obstructive sleep apnea is related to aldosterone status in subjects with resistant hypertension. *J. Clin. Sleep Med.* **2010**, *6*, 363–368. [CrossRef]
29. Drager, L.F.; Polotsky, V.Y.; Lorenzi-Filho, G. Obstructive sleep apnea: An emerging risk factor for atherosclerosis. *Chest* **2011**, *140*, 534–542. [CrossRef]
30. Wolf, J.; Hering, D.; Narkiewicz, K. Non-dipping pattern of hypertension and obstructive sleep apnea syndrome. *Hypertens. Res.* **2010**, *33*, 867–871. [CrossRef] [PubMed]
31. Ma, Y.; Sun, S.; Peng, C.K.; Fang, Y.; Thomas, R.J. Ambulatory Blood Pressure Monitoring in Chinese Patients with Obstructive Sleep Apnea. *J. Clin. Sleep Med.* **2017**, *13*, 433–439. [CrossRef] [PubMed]
32. Kuwabara, M.; Tomitani, N.; Shiga, T.; Kario, K. Polysomnography-derived sleep parameters as a determinant of nocturnal blood pressure profile in patients with obstructive sleep apnea. *J. Clin. Hypertens.* **2018**, *20*, 1039–1048. [CrossRef] [PubMed]
33. Loredo, J.S.; Ancoli-Israel, S.; Dimsdale, J.E. Sleep quality and blood pressure dipping in obstructive sleep apnea. *Am. J. Hypertens.* **2001**, *14 Pt 1*, 887–892. [CrossRef]
34. Kario, K.; Hoshide, S.; Mizuno, H.; Kabutoya, T.; Nishizawa, M.; Yoshida, T.; Abe, H.; Katsuya, T.; Fujita, Y.; Okazaki, O.; et al. JAMP Study Group. Nighttime blood pressure phenotype and cardiovascular prognosis: Practitionerbased nationwide JAMP Study. *Circulation* **2020**, *142*, 1810–1820. [CrossRef]
35. Ke, X.; Sun, Y.; Yang, R.; Liang, J.; Wu, S.; Hu, C.; Wang, X. Association of 24 h-systolic blood pressure variability and cardiovascular disease in patients with obstructive sleep apnea. *BMC Cardiovasc. Disord.* **2017**, *17*, 287. [CrossRef]
36. Kario, K.; Kanegae, H.; Tomitani, N.; Okawara, Y.; Fujiwara, T.; Yano, Y.; Hoshide, S. Nighttime blood pressure measured by home blood pressure monitoring as an independent predictor of cardiovascular events in general practice. *Hypertension* **2019**, *73*, 1240–1248. [CrossRef]
37. Crinion, S.J.; Ryan, S.; McNicholas, W.T. Obstructive sleep apnoea as a cause of nocturnal nondipping blood pressure: Recent evidence regarding clinical importance and underlying mechanisms. *Eur. Respir. J.* **2017**, *49*, 1601818. [CrossRef]
38. Kario, K.; Hettrick, D.A.; Prejbisz, A.; Januszewicz, A. Obstructive Sleep Apnea–Induced Neurogenic Nocturnal Hypertension: A Potential Role of Renal Denervation? *Hypertension* **2021**, *77*, 1047–1060. [CrossRef] [PubMed]
39. Ziegler, M.G.; Milic, M.; Sun, P. Antihypertensive therapy for patients with obstructive sleep apnea. *Curr. Opin. Nephrol. Hypertens.* **2011**, *20*, 50–55. [CrossRef]
40. Wolf, J.; Drozdowski, J.; Czechowicz, K.; Winklewski, P.J.; Jassem, E.; Kara, T.; Somers, V.K.; Narkiewicz, K. Effect of beta-blocker therapy on heart rate response in patients with hypertension and newly diagnosed untreated obstructive sleep apnea syndrome. *Int. J. Cardiol.* **2016**, *202*, 67–72. [CrossRef]
41. Kraiczi, H.; Hedner, J.; Peker, Y.; Grote, L. Comparison of atenolol, amlodipine, enalapril, hydrochlorothiazide, and losartan for antihypertensive treatment in patients with obstructive sleep apnea. *Am. J. Respir. Crit. Care Med.* **2000**, *161*, 1423–1428. [CrossRef] [PubMed]
42. Gaddam, K.; Pimenta, E.; Thomas, S.J.; Cofield, S.S.; Oparil, S.; Harding, S.M.; Calhoun, D.A. Spironolactone reduces severity of obstructive sleep apnoea in patients with resistant hypertension: A preliminary report. *J. Hum. Hypertens.* **2010**, *24*, 532–537. [CrossRef]
43. Yang, L.; Zhang, H.; Cai, M.; Zou, Y.; Jiang, X.; Song, L.; Liang, E.; Bian, J.; Wu, H.; Hui, R. Effect of spironolactone on patients with resistant hypertension and obstructive sleep apnea. *Clin. Exp. Hypertens.* **2016**, *38*, 464–468. [CrossRef] [PubMed]
44. Krasinska, B.; Miazga, A.; Cofta, S.; Szczepaniak-Chicheł, L.; Trafas, T.; Krasiński, Z.; Pawlaczyk-Gabriel, K.; Tykarski, A. Effect of eplerenone on the severity of obstructive sleep apnea and arterial stiffness in patients with resistant arterial hypertension. *Pol. Arch. Med. Wewn.* **2016**, *126*, 330–339. [CrossRef] [PubMed]
45. Dobrowolski, P.; Kołodziejczyk-Kruk, S.; Warchoł-Celińska, E.; Kabat, M.; Ambroziak, U.; Wróbel, A.; Piekarczyk, P.; Ostrowska, A.; Januszewicz, M.; Śliwiński, P.; et al. Primary aldosteronism is highly prevalent in patients with moderate to severe obstructive sleep apnea. *J. Clin. Sleep Med.* **2021**, *17*, 629–637. [CrossRef]
46. Wang, Y.; Li, C.X.; Lin, Y.N.; Zhang, L.Y.; Li, S.Q.; Zhang, L.; Yan, Y.R.; Lu, F.Y.; Li, N.; Li, Q.Y. The Role of Aldosterone in OSA and OSA-Related Hypertension. *Front. Endocrinol.* **2022**, *12*, 801689. [CrossRef] [PubMed]
47. Bucca, C.B.; Brussino, L.; Battisti, A.; Mutani, R.; Rolla, G.; Mangiardi, L.; Cicolin, A. Diuretics in obstructive sleep apnea with diastolic heart failure. *Chest* **2007**, *132*, 440–446. [CrossRef]
48. Kario, K.; Weber, M.; Ferrannini, E. Nocturnal hypertension in diabetes: Potential target of sodium/glucose cotransporter 2 (SGLT2) inhibition. *J. Clin. Hypertens.* **2018**, *20*, 424–428. [CrossRef]
49. Liu, L.; Cao, Q.; Guo, Z.; Dai, Q. Continuous positive airway pressure in patients with obstructive sleep apnea and resistant hypertension: A meta-analysis of randomized controlled trials. *J. Clin. Hypertens.* **2016**, *18*, 153–158. [CrossRef]
50. Pengo, M.F.; Soranna, D.; Giontella, A.; Perger, E.; Mattaliano, P.; Schwarz, E.I.; Lombardi, C.; Bilo, G.; Zambon, A.; Steier, J.; et al. Obstructive sleep apnoea treatment and blood pressure: Which phenotypes predict a response? A systematic review and meta-analysis. *Eur. Respir. J.* **2020**, *55*, 1901945. [CrossRef]
51. Bratton, D.J.; Gaisl, T.; Wons, A.M.; Kohler, M. CPAP vs mandibular advancement devices and blood pressure in patients with obstructive sleep apnea. A systematic review and meta-analysis. *JAMA* **2015**, *314*, 2280–2293. [CrossRef]
52. Iftikhar, I.H.; Hays, E.R.; Iverson, M.A.; Magalang, U.J.; Maas, A.K. Effect of oral appliances on blood pressure in obstructive sleep apnea: A systematic review and meta-analysis. *J. Clin. Sleep Med.* **2013**, *9*, 165–174. [CrossRef] [PubMed]

53. Schein, A.S.; Kerkhoff, A.C.; Coronel, C.C.; Plentz, R.D.; Sbruzzi, G. Continuous positive airway pressure reduces blood pressure in patients with obstructive sleep apnea; a systematic review and meta-analysis with 1000 patients. *J. Hypertens.* **2014**, *32*, 1762–1773. [CrossRef] [PubMed]
54. Fava, C.; Dorigoni, S.; Dalle Vedove, F.; Danese, E.; Montagnana, M.; Guidi, G.C.; Narkiewicz, K.; Minuz, P. Effect of CPAP on blood pressure in patients with OSA/hypopnea: A systematic review and meta-analysis. *Chest* **2014**, *145*, 762–771. [CrossRef] [PubMed]
55. Labarca, G.; Schmidt, A.; Dreyse, J.; Jorquera, J.; Enos, D.; Torres, G.; Barbe, F. Efficacy of continuous positive airway pressure (CPAP) in patients with obstructive sleep apnea (OSA) and resistant hypertension (RH): Systematic review and meta-analysis. *Sleep Med. Rev.* **2021**, *58*, 101446. [CrossRef]
56. Shang, W.; Zhang, Y.; Liu, L.; Chen, F.; Wang, G.; Han, D. Benefits of continuous positive airway pressure on blood pressure in patients with hypertension and obstructive sleep apnea: A meta-analysis. *Hypertens. Res.* **2022**, *45*, 1802–1813. [CrossRef] [PubMed]
57. Law, M.R.; Morris, J.K.; Wald, N.J. Use of blood pressure lowering drugs in the prevention of cardiovascular disease: Meta-analysis of 147 randomised trials in the context of expectations from prospective epidemiological studies. *BMJ* **2009**, *338*, b1665. [CrossRef]
58. Peker, Y.; Balcan, B. Cardiovascular outcomes of continuous positive airway pressure therapy for obstructive sleep apnea. *J. Thorac. Dis.* **2018**, *10* (Suppl. 34), S4262–S4279. [CrossRef]
59. Haentjens, P.; Van Meerhaeghe, A.; Moscariello, A.; De Weerdt, S.; Poppe, K.; Dupont, A.; Velkeniers, B. The impact of continuous positive airway pressure on blood pressure in patients with obstructive sleep apnea syndrome: Evidence from a meta-analysis of placebo-controlled randomized trials. *Arch. Intern. Med.* **2007**, *167*, 757–764. [CrossRef]
60. Muxfeldt, E.S.; Margallo, V.; Costa, L.M.; Guimarães, G.; Cavalcante, A.H.; Azevedo, J.C.; de Souza, F.; Cardoso, C.R.L.; Salles, G.F. Effects of continuous positive airway pressure treatment on clinic and ambulatory blood pressures in patients with obstructive sleep apnea and resistant hypertension: A randomized controlled trial. *Hypertension* **2015**, *65*, 736–742. [CrossRef]
61. Salman, L.A.; Shulman, R.; Cohen, J.B. Obstructive Sleep Apnea, Hypertension, and Cardiovascular Risk: Epidemiology, Pathophysiology, and Management. *Curr. Cardiol. Rep.* **2020**, *22*, 6. [CrossRef] [PubMed]
62. Kartali, N.; Daskalopoulou, E.; Geleris, P.; Chatzipantazi, S.; Tziomalos, K.; Vlachogiannis, E.; Karagiannis, A. The effect of continuous positive airway pressure therapy on blood pressure and arterial stiffness in hypertensive patients with obstructive sleep apnea. *Sleep Breath* **2014**, *18*, 635–640. [CrossRef] [PubMed]
63. Hoyos, C.M.; Yee, B.J.; Wong, K.K.; Grunstein, R.R.; Phillips, C.L. Treatment of Sleep Apnea with CPAP Lowers Central and Peripheral Blood Pressure Independent of the Time-of-Day: A Randomized Controlled Study. *Am. J. Hypertens.* **2015**, *28*, 1222–1228. [CrossRef] [PubMed]
64. Yang, M.C.; Huang, Y.C.; Lan, C.C.; Wu, Y.K.; Huang, K.F. Beneficial Effects of Long-Term CPAP Treatment on Sleep Quality and Blood Pressure in Adherent Subjects with Obstructive Sleep Apnea. *Respir. Care* **2015**, *60*, 1810–1818. [CrossRef]
65. Campos-Rodriguez, F.; Perez-Ronchel, J.; Grilo-Reina, A.; Lima-Alvarez, J.; Benitez, M.A.; Almeida-Gonzalez, C. Long-term effect of continuous positive airway pressure on BP in patients with hypertension and sleep apnea. *Chest* **2007**, *132*, 1847–1852. [CrossRef]
66. Chen, Q.; Cheng, Y.B.; Shen, M.; Yin, B.; Yi, H.-H.; Feng, J.; Li, M.; Li, Q.-Y.; Li, Y.; Wang, J.-G. A randomized controlled trial on ambulatory blood pressure lowering effect of CPAP in patients with obstructive sleep apnea and nocturnal hypertension. *Blood Press.* **2020**, *29*, 21–30. [CrossRef]
67. Sapiña-Beltrán, E.; Torres, G.; Benítez, I.; Santamaría-Martos, F.; Durán-Cantolla, J.; Egea, C.; Sánchez-de-la-Torre, M.; Barbé, F.; Dalmases, M.; on behalf of the Spanish Sleep and Breathing Group. Differential blood pressure response to continuous positive airway pressure treatment according to the circadian pattern in hypertensive patients with obstructive sleep apnoea. *Eur. Respir. J.* **2019**, *54*, 1900098. [CrossRef]
68. Lui, M.M.; Tse, H.F.; Lam, D.C.; Lau, K.K.; Chan, C.W.; Ip, M.S. Continuous positive airway pressure improves blood pressure and serum cardiovascular biomarkers in obstructive sleep apnoea and hypertension. *Eur. Respir. J.* **2021**, *58*, 2003687. [CrossRef]
69. Baran, R.; Grimm, D.; Infanger, M.; Wehland, M. The Effect of Continuous Positive Airway Pressure Therapy on Obstructive Sleep Apnea-Related Hypertension. *Int. J. Mol. Sci.* **2021**, *22*, 2300. [CrossRef]
70. Thunström, E.; Manhem, K.; Rosengren, A.; Peker, Y. Blood Pressure Response to Losartan and Continuous Positive Airway Pressure in Hypertension and Obstructive Sleep Apnea. *Am. J. Respir. Crit. Care Med.* **2016**, *193*, 310–320. [CrossRef]
71. Martínez-García, M.A.; Capote, F.; Campos-Rodríguez, F.; Lloberes, P.; Díaz de Atauri, M.J.; Somoza, M.; Masa, J.F.; González, M.; Sacristán, L.; Barbé, F.; et al. Spanish Sleep Network. Effect of CPAP on blood pressure in patients with obstructive sleep apnea and resistant hypertension: The HIPARCO randomized clinical trial. *JAMA* **2013**, *310*, 2407–2415. [CrossRef] [PubMed]
72. Javaheri, S.; Barbe, F.; Campos-Rodriguez, F.; Dempsey, J.A.; Khayat, R.; Javaheri, S.; Malhotra, A.; Martinez-Garcia, M.A.; Mehra, R.; Pack, A.I.; et al. Sleep apnea: Types, mechanisms, and clinical cardiovascular consequences. *J. Am. Coll. Cardiol.* **2017**, *69*, 841–858. [CrossRef] [PubMed]
73. Lozano, L.; Tovar, J.L.; Sampol, G.; Romero, O.; Jurado, M.J.; Segarra, A.; Espinel, E.; Ríos, J.; Untoria, M.D.; Lloberes, P. Continuous positive airway pressure treatment in sleep apnea patients with resistant hypertension: A randomized, controlled trial. *J. Hypertens.* **2010**, *28*, 2161–2168. [CrossRef]

74. Colantonio, L.; Booth, J.; Bress, A.; Whelton, P.K.; Shimbo, D.; Levitan, E.B.; Howard, G.; Safford, M.M.; Muntner, P. 2017 ACC/AHA Blood Pressure Treatment Guideline Recommendations and Cardiovascular Risk. *J. Am. Coll. Cardiol.* **2018**, *72*, 1187–1197. [CrossRef] [PubMed]
75. Fehrm, J.; Friberg, D.; Bring, J.; Browaldh, N. Blood pressure after modified uvulopalatopharyngoplasty: Results from the SKUP3 randomized controlled trial. *Sleep Med.* **2017**, *34*, 156–161. [CrossRef] [PubMed]
76. Barbe, F.; Duran-Cantolla, J.; Sanchez-de-la-Torre, M.; Martinez-Alonso, M.; Carmona, C.; Barcelo, A.; Chiner, E.; Masa, J.F.; Gonzalez, M.; Marín, J.M.; et al. Effect of continuous positive airway pressure on the incidence of hypertension and cardiovascular events in nonsleepy patients with obstructive sleep apnea: A randomized controlled trial. *JAMA* **2012**, *307*, 2161–2168. [CrossRef]
77. Lin, Y.-C.; Chen, C.-T.; Chao, P.-Z.; Chen, P.-Y.; Liu, W.-T.; Tsao, S.-T.; Lin, S.-F.; Bai, C.-H. Prevention of Incident Hypertension in Patients with Obstructive Sleep Apnea Treated with Uvulopalatopharyngoplasty or Continuous Positive Airway Pressure: A Cohort Study. *Front. Surg.* **2022**, *9*, 818591. [CrossRef]
78. Wang, D.; Gao, S.F.; Chen, J.; Hua, H.T.; Ma, Y.X.; Liu, Y.H.; Gao, C.B. The long-term impact of expansion sphincter pharyngoplasty treatment on blood pressure control and health-related quality of life in patients with obstructive sleep apnea and hypertension. *Sleep Breath* **2021**, *25*, 2155–2162. [CrossRef]
79. Daniels, F.; De Freitas, S.; Smyth, A.; Garvey, J.; Judge, C.; Gilmartin, J.J.; Sharif, F. Effects of renal sympathetic denervation on blood pressure, sleep apnoea severity and metabolic indices: A prospective cohort study. *Sleep Med.* **2017**, *30*, 180–184. [CrossRef]
80. Warchol-Celinska, E.; Prejbisz, A.; Kadziela, J.; Florczak, E.; Januszewicz, M.; Michalowska, I.; Dobrowolski, P.; Kabat, M.; Sliwinski, P.; Klisiewicz, A.; et al. Renal denervation in resistant hypertension and obstructive sleep apnea: Randomized proof-of-concept phase II trial. *Hypertension* **2018**, *72*, 381–390. [CrossRef]

Disclaimer/Publisher's Note: The statements, opinions and data contained in all publications are solely those of the individual author(s) and contributor(s) and not of MDPI and/or the editor(s). MDPI and/or the editor(s) disclaim responsibility for any injury to people or property resulting from any ideas, methods, instructions or products referred to in the content.

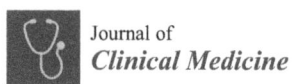

Article

The Effect of Pharyngeal Surgery on Positive Airway Pressure Therapy in Obstructive Sleep Apnea: A Meta-Analysis

Ki Hwan Kwak [1], Young Jeong Lee [2], Jae Yong Lee [2], Jae Hoon Cho [3,*,†] and Ji Ho Choi [2,*,†]

1. Department of Otorhinolaryngology-Head and Neck Surgery, Gumi Hospital, Soonchunhyang University College of Medicine, 179, 1gongdan-ro, Gumi 39371, Korea
2. Department of Otorhinolaryngology-Head and Neck Surgery, Bucheon Hospital, Soonchunhyang University College of Medicine, 170, Jomaru-ro, Bucheon 14584, Korea
3. Department of Otorhinolaryngology-Head and Neck Surgery, Konkuk University School of Medicine, 120-1, Neungdong-ro, Gwangjin-gu, Seoul 05030, Korea
* Correspondence: jaehoon@kuh.ac.kr (J.H.C.); handsomemd@hanmail.net (J.H.C.); Tel.: +82-2-2030-7667 (J.H.C.); +82-32-621-5015 (J.H.C.); Fax: +82-2-2030-5299 (J.H.C.); +82-32-621-5016 (J.H.C.)
† These authors contributed equally to this work and should be considered co-corresponding authors.

Abstract: There is controversy about the effect of pharyngeal surgery for obstructive sleep apnea (OSA) on positive airway pressure (PAP) adherence, and the related results of meta-analysis have not yet been available. Therefore, the purpose of this meta-analysis was to assess the effect of pharyngeal OSA surgery on PAP therapy parameters such as optimal pressure levels and usage time. We selected studies investigating optimal PAP levels or usage time before and after pharyngeal OSA surgery, regardless of the study design. Pharyngeal OSA surgery included uvulopalatopharyngoplasty and its variants, tonsillectomy, Pillar implants, radiofrequency ablation, tongue base surgery and its variants, and genioglossus advancement. Studies in which isolated nasal surgery was performed were excluded. The random-effects model was used due to significant heterogeneity among the studies. Nine studies were included in the meta-analysis of optimal PAP levels, and five studies in the meta-analysis of PAP usage time. After pharyngeal OSA surgery, the summed optimal PAP level was significantly decreased (standardized mean difference (SMD), −1.113; 95% confidence interval (CI), −1.667 to −0.559)), and the summed usage time of PAP was significantly increased (SMD, 0.794; 95% CI, 0.259 to 1.329). This study illustrated that pharyngeal OSA surgery lowered optimal PAP levels and enhanced PAP usage time. The results of the meta-analysis contribute to our understanding of the role of pharyngeal OSA surgery in patients with PAP intolerance.

Keywords: continuous positive airway pressure; pharynx; sleep apnea; obstructive

1. Introduction

Obstructive sleep apnea (OSA) is a widely prevalent disease characterized by repetitive obstruction of the upper airway, particularly the pharynx, during sleep [1]. Repeated upper airway collapse induces various pathophysiologic conditions, including a hyperactive sympathetic nervous system, intrathoracic pressure swings, sleep fragmentation, intermittent hypoxia, and hypercapnia [2]. These detrimental phenomena may lead to diverse symptoms and critical complications such as excessive daytime sleepiness, impaired concentration, memory loss, impotence, systemic hypertension, diabetes, stroke, decreased quality of life, and an elevated risk of traffic accidents [3]. Therefore, when OSA is suspected, prompt diagnosis and proper therapy are necessary to prevent or manage OSA-related consequences. The treatment options for OSA consist of several methods, including positive airway pressure (PAP), surgical modifications of the upper airway, oral appliances, weight control, and positional therapy [4]. Ultimately, among these therapeutic options, the most appropriate treatment is carried out by considering the patient's information, such as anatomical structures, polysomnographic results, and treatment preferences [5].

PAP therapy to prevent upper airway obstruction during sleep by providing a pneumatic splint in patients with OSA was first reported by Sullivan et al. [6] in 1981. According to the American Academy of Sleep Medicine (AASM) guidelines, PAP is commonly recommended for the management of patients with OSA, especially moderate-to-severe types and mild-type with comorbidities or significant symptoms [2,7]. The effectiveness of PAP for OSA treatment has been proven through many clinical studies. Compared to no treatment, PAP showed substantial favorable effects in varied aspects, such as excessive daytime sleepiness, diminished sleep-related quality of life, and comorbid systemic hypertension [8–10]. To fully achieve the effect of PAP therapy in patients with OSA, an optimal pressure level suitable for the patient's condition and sufficient usage time play important roles [11].

Surgical modification or reconstruction of the upper airway is usually performed to improve OSA by increasing muscle tension and/or widening the airway space [12]. According to the upper airway anatomy, various surgical techniques for OSA can be classified into nasal surgery (e.g., turbinate surgery, septoplasty, and endoscopic sinus surgery), nasopharyngeal surgery (e.g., nasopharyngeal mass removal and adenoidectomy), oropharyngeal surgery (e.g., uvulopalatopharyngoplasty [UPPP] and its variants, Pillar implants, and tonsillectomy), and hypopharyngeal surgery (e.g., genioglossus advancement and tongue base reduction) [13]. Of these, one or more appropriate surgical techniques are selected and implemented based on the surgical indication and the patient's anatomical structure.

Some clinical studies have reported that surgical management influenced PAP therapy such as optimal levels and the duration of use [14,15]. Two recent meta-analyses demonstrated that surgical modifications of the upper airway were associated with decreases in optimal PAP levels and improvement in PAP adherence [16,17]. However, one study evaluated the effect of nasal surgery alone on PAP treatment, and the other study investigated the effect of upper airway surgery, including isolated nasal surgery and pharyngeal surgery, on PAP management [16,17]. Furthermore, there is controversy about the effect of pharyngeal OSA surgery on PAP adherence [18]. Therefore, the goal of this study was to ascertain the effect of pharyngeal OSA surgery on PAP therapy, such as optimal pressure levels and the duration of use.

2. Materials and Methods

2.1. Search Strategy

We performed a comprehensive literature search on the effect of pharyngeal surgery on PAP therapy, including optimal pressure levels and usage time in OSA, using PubMed, SCOPUS, EMBASE, and the Cochrane Library. The keywords included "obstructive sleep apnea," "sleep-disordered breathing," "surgery (surgical treatment)," and "continuous positive airway pressure." The search was conducted on 19 June 2021.

2.2. Eligibility Criteria and Study Selection

The studies selected in this review were original articles investigating PAP therapy (optimal pressure levels and/or compliance) before and after pharyngeal OSA surgery, regardless of the study design, which included randomized controlled trials, prospective (non-randomized), and retrospective studies. Studies in which pharyngeal OSA surgery with or without nasal surgery was performed were included. However, studies in which nasal surgery alone was performed were excluded. In addition, studies were excluded if PAP therapy data, such as optimal pressure and/or compliance, were not clearly provided before and after surgery or if they lacked the data necessary for meta-analysis. Pharyngeal OSA surgery included tonsillectomy, UPPP and its variants, Pillar implants, tongue base surgery and its variants, genioglossus advancement, and radiofrequency ablation.

After two reviewers independently screened all titles and abstracts for candidate papers, we excluded clinical studies that were ineligible or irrelevant. There were no language restrictions in any articles reviewed in this study. We thoroughly reviewed the finally selected studies.

2.3. Data Extraction

We extracted data from the finally selected articles based on standardized forms. The data collected included the study design, the total number of subjects, age (years), sex (male:female), body mass index (kg/m^2), the apnea-hypopnea index (AHI; events/h), surgical procedures, PAP therapy-related outcome measures, optimal pressure level (cm H$_2$O), and usage time (h/night).

2.4. Quality Assessment

The risk of bias was assessed by using the STROBE tool (https://www.strobe-statement.org/, accessed on 26 September 2022). Five domains of bias, including selection, measuring exposure and outcome, controlling confound, sources of bias, and statistical method, were categorized as low, high, or unclear risk. The total quality of each study was defined as good, fair, or low. Two reviewers assessed the risk of bias in each included study independently, and disagreements were resolved by discussion with the other authors.

2.5. Statistical Analysis

The optimal levels and PAP usage time before and after pharyngeal OSA surgery were compared. For this, we collected the mean and standard deviation (SD) values of optimal levels and the usage time of PAP before and after pharyngeal surgery from the relevant studies. Heterogeneity was calculated with Cochran's Q and I^2 tests. The I^2 test describes the rate of variation across studies because of heterogeneity rather than chance and ranges from 0 (no heterogeneity) to 100 (maximum heterogeneity). All results are reported with 95% confidence intervals (CIs), and all p-values were two-tailed. When significant heterogeneity among the outcomes was found ($I^2 > 50$), the random-effects model according to DerSimonian and Laird was used. This model assumes that the true treatment effects in the individual studies may be different from one another and that they are normally distributed. If the heterogeneity was not large ($I^2 < 50$), we planned to analyze it with a fixed-effect model. However, the effect model was not used due to the large heterogeneity of all results. We used a funnel plot and Egger's test simultaneously to detect publication bias. Analyses were performed using Comprehensive Meta-Analysis V2 software (Biostat, Englewood, NJ, USA).

3. Results

Figure 1 shows a flow diagram of the literature selection. After screening for relevance, 19 studies that investigated PAP therapy data, such as optimal pressure levels and/or usage time before and after surgery, were retrieved for further review [14,15,18–37]. We excluded eight studies evaluating the effect of nasal surgery alone on PAP therapy [14,19–25]. Two other studies were excluded due to the lack of data required for meta-analysis [15,18]. Finally, nine eligible studies were included in the meta-analysis (nine studies for optimal pressure levels and five studies for usage time) [26–34]. Table 1 presents the characteristics of the studies that met the inclusion criteria. Table 2 summarizes the comparison of PAP therapy, including optimal pressure and usage time before and after pharyngeal OSA surgery. All studies were judged to be fair for the risk of bias by combining judgments in the five domains.

Table 1. Characteristics of the included studies.

References	Year	Level of Evidence (Study Design)	Total No. of Subjects	Age (Years)	Sex (M:F)	BMI (kg/m^2)	AHI (Events/Hour)	Surgical Procedures	PAP Therapy Related Outcomes Measures
Zonato et al. [26]	2006	Level IV (retrospective)	17	49.0 ± 9.0	16:1	30.0 ± 4.0	38.0 ± 19.0	Tonsillectomy ± nasal surgery	Optimal PAP level
Nakata et al. [27]	2006	Level II-2 (prospective)	30	33.2 ± 6.8	28:2	30.7 ± 6.0	69.0 ± 28.4	Tonsillectomy	Optimal PAP level

Table 1. Cont.

References	Year	Level of Evidence (Study Design)	Total No. of Subjects	Age (Years)	Sex (M:F)	BMI (kg/m^2)	AHI (Events/Hour)	Surgical Procedures	PAP Therapy Related Outcomes Measures
Lin et al. [28]	2008	Level IV (retrospective)	16			34.1 ± 4.7	65.2 ± 49.2	Site-specific upper airway surgery (UPPP, pillar palatoplasty, GA, HMA, and repose tongue suspension)	Optimal PAP level PAP usage time
Khan et al. [29]	2009	Level IV (retrospective)	63	42.1 ± 13.9	51:12	34.9 ± 7.2	62.0 ± 35.4	UPPP ± tongue base surgery ± nasal surgery	Optimal PAP level
Friedman et al. [30]	2009	Level IV (retrospective)	52	43.1 ± 9.1	42:10	31.2 ± 5.0	63.2 ± 22.0	Multi-level surgery (UPPP, RFBOT, and nasal surgery)	Optimal PAP level PAP usage time
Bertoletti et al. [31]	2009	Level II-2 (prospective)	21	49.6 ± 11.2	16:5	31.4 ± 3.2	41.1 ± 5.8	Pillar palatal implants	Optimal PAP level PAP usage time
Gillespie et al. [32]	2011	Level I (RCT)	26	52.3 ± 10.3	22:4	34.7 ± 5.0	42.0 ± 21.0	Pillar palatal implants	Optimal PAP level PAP usage time
Turhan et al. [33]	2015	Level II-2 (prospective)	31	48 (31–66)	27:4	31.0 ± 2.4	44.7 ± 17.1	Modified tongue base suspension	Optimal PAP level PAP usage time
Azbay et al. [34]	2016	Level IV (retrospective)	67	47.0 ± 9.8	59:8	31.6 ± 4.2	45.0 ± 19.8	Modified UPPP + septoplasty ± modified tongue base suspension	Optimal PAP level

RCT, randomized controlled trial; M, male; F, female; BMI, body mass index; AHI, apnea-hypopnea index; UPPP, uvulopalatopharyngoplasty; GA, genioglossus advancement; HMA, hyoid myotomy and advancement; RFBOT, radiofrequency base of tongue reduction; PAP, positive airway pressure.

Table 2. Effects of pharyngeal obstructive sleep apnea surgery on positive airway pressure therapy, including optimal pressure and usage time.

References	Year	Final No. of Patients	Preoperative Optimal Pressure (cmH$_2$O)	Postoperative Optimal Pressure (cmH$_2$O)	p Value	Final No. of Patients	Preoperative Usage Time (Hours/Night)	Postoperative Usage Time (Hours/Night)	p Value
Zonato et al. [26]	2006	4	13.8 ± 1.5	10.4 ± 2.0	<0.05				
Nakata et al. [27]	2006	5	13.6 ± 2.5	10.6 ± 1.3	<0.05				
Lin et al. [28]	2008	12	11.5 ± 3.7	9.4 ± 2.6	<0.05	16	4.1 ± 2.4	5.5 ± 2.5	<0.05
Khan et al. [29]	2009	27	9.7 ± 3.0	8.3 ± 2.4	<0.05				
Friedman et al. [30]	2009	52	10.6 ± 2.1	9.8 ± 2.1	<0.05	49	0.02 ± 0.14	3.2 ± 2.6	<0.001
Bertoletti et al. [31]	2009	21	11.2 ± 1.6	9.3 ± 2.5	<0.05	21	5.7 ± 0.9	6.3 ± 0.6	<0.05
Gillespie et al. [32]	2011	26	10.9 ± 2.7	10.3 ± 2.4	NS	26	6.0 ± 2.5	6.0 ± 2.4	NS
Turhan et al. [33]	2015	31	12.6 ± 1.6	8.0 ± 1.8	<0.001	31	5.3 ± 0.8	6.5 ± 0.9	<0.001
Azbay et al. [34]	2016	67	11.8 ± 1.4	9.0 ± 1.2	<0.001				

NS, not significant.

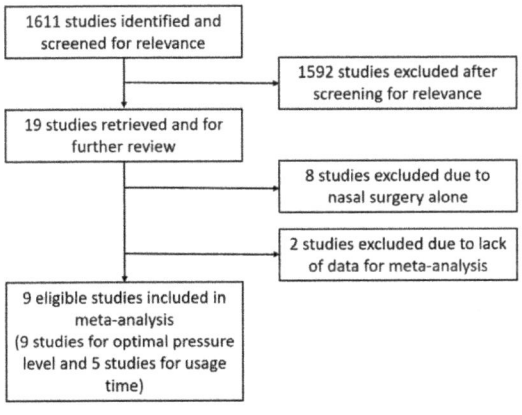

Figure 1. Flow diagram of the literature selection.

3.1. Optimal PAP Level before and after Pharyngeal OSA Surgery

As heterogeneity was present among the studies (Q-value, 28.7; $p < 0.001$; I^2, 86.1), a random-effects model was used. Figure 2 shows the forest plot for the effects of pharyngeal OSA surgery on optimal PAP levels. The summed optimal PAP level was significantly lower after pharyngeal OSA surgery than before surgery (standardized mean difference (SMD), −1.113; 95% CI, −1.667 to −0.559) [26–34]. Although the funnel plot looks slightly asymmetrical, we thought there was no publication bias because the Egger test p-value was 0.182 (Figure 3).

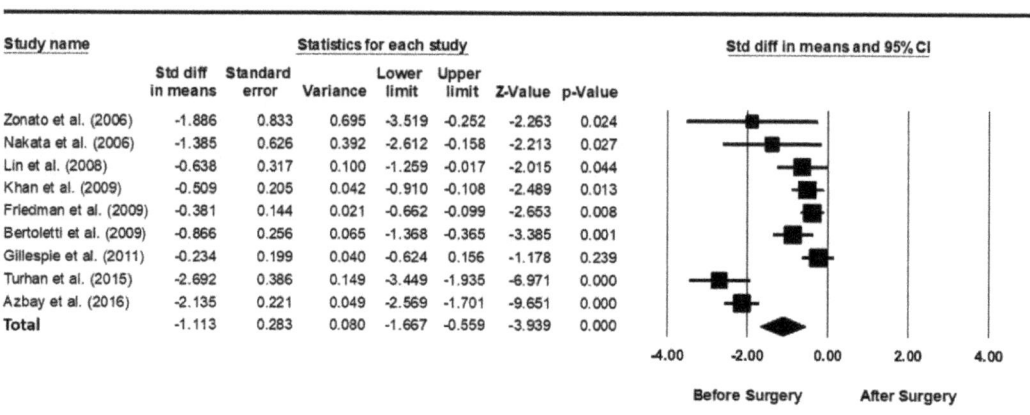

Figure 2. Forest plot for the effects of pharyngeal obstructive sleep apnea surgery on the optimal positive airway pressure level. The summed optimal PAP level was significantly lower after pharyngeal OSA surgery than before surgery. Std diff, standardized difference; CI, confidence interval [26–34].

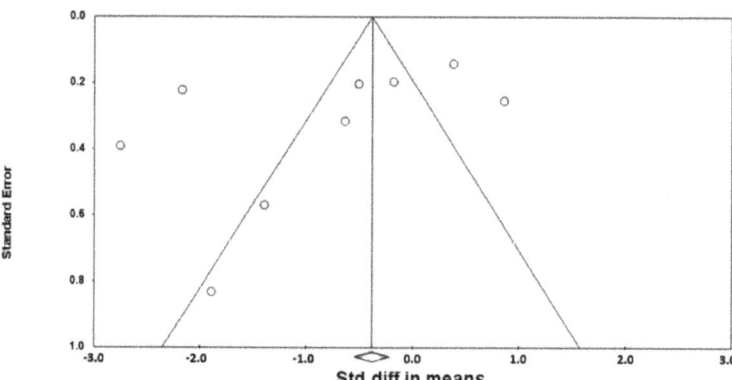

Figure 3. Funnel plot for the effects of pharyngeal obstructive sleep apnea surgery on the optimal positive airway pressure level. There was no publication bias (the Egger test p-value = 0.182). Std diff, standardized difference.

3.2. Usage Time of PAP before and after Pharyngeal OSA Surgery

As heterogeneity was present among the studies (Q-value, 28.7; $p < 0.001$; I^2, 86.1), a random-effects model was used. Figure 4 shows the forest plot for the effects of pharyngeal OSA surgery on usage time. The summed usage time of PAP increased significantly after pharyngeal OSA surgery compared to before surgery (SMD, 0.794; 95% CI, 0.259 to 1.329) [28,31–33]. The funnel plot looks symmetrical, and the Egger test p-value was 0.792, indicating no publication bias (Figure 5).

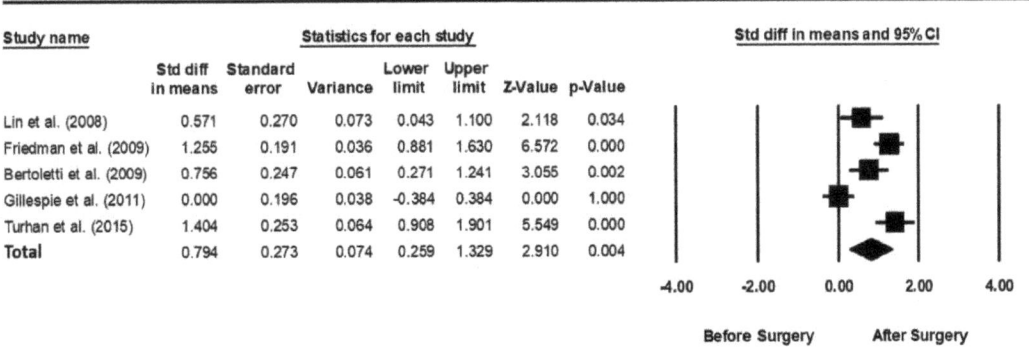

Figure 4. Forest plot for the effects of pharyngeal obstructive sleep apnea surgery on positive airway pressure usage time. The summed usage time of PAP increased significantly after pharyngeal OSA surgery compared to before surgery. Std diff, standardized difference; CI, confidence interval [28,30–33].

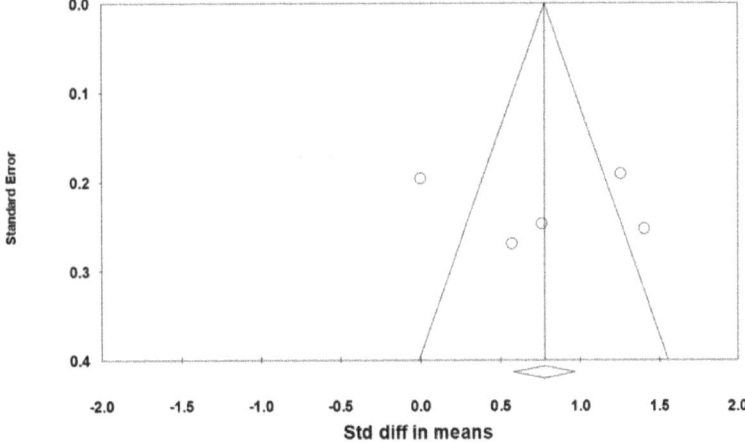

Figure 5. Funnel plot for the effects of pharyngeal obstructive sleep apnea surgery on positive airway pressure usage time. There was no publication bias (the Egger test p-value = 0.792). Std diff, standardized difference.

4. Discussion

There are several surgical indications for managing OSA [2,5]. Surgical modifications of the upper airway are usually performed for the purpose of directly improving respiratory disturbances during sleep. In addition, surgical therapy can be carried out as adjunctive management to alleviate the intolerance of other OSA treatments, such as PAP therapy. This study was designed to determine the effect of pharyngeal OSA surgery on PAP therapy, including optimal pressure levels, and compliance based on a meta-analysis. The results of the study demonstrated that optimal PAP levels decreased, and PAP usage time increased in patients with OSA after pharyngeal surgery.

Surgical outcomes may vary in patients with OSA depending upon the type of surgical procedure [35]. The results of numerous clinical studies have shown that isolated nasal surgery improved excessive daytime sleepiness and sleep-disordered breathing, such as snoring [36]. In contrast, whether nasal surgery alone statistically decreases the AHI is controversial [36,37]. A recent meta-analysis showed that isolated nasal surgery significantly improved the AHI in patients with OSA, but the alleviation of AHI was only slightly significant [37]. The outcomes of pharyngeal surgery for OSA are somewhat different from those of nasal surgery alone. For example, UPPP, one of the most representative pharyngeal surgeries, has been reported to have a surgical success rate of 35% to 70% when conducted randomly in patients with OSA [38,39]. According to our recent study assessing the AHI reduction ratio after oropharyngeal OSA surgery, such as UPPP, the postoperative AHI decreased by 30.4% to 74.1% based on an anatomy-based staging system [40]. The results of the study indicated that two different types of surgery, nasal surgery and pharyngeal surgery, had a similar effect on PAP treatment in patients with OSA despite different surgical sites and effects.

This meta-analysis comparing changes in optimal PAP levels before and after pharyngeal OSA surgery confirmed that the optimal pressure levels decreased from a mean ± standard error (SE) of 11.6 ± 0.4 to 9.3 ± 0.3 cm H_2O. These outcomes are quite similar to earlier meta-analyses reports that isolated nasal surgery or upper airway surgery influenced optimal PAP levels in patients with OSA [16,17]. Camacho et al. [16] investigated the effect of nasal surgery alone on optimal PAP levels using meta-analysis. In their study, isolated nasal surgery included septoplasty, turbinoplasty, septoturbinoplasty, septorhinoplasty, and endoscopic sinus surgery [16]. The results of the meta-analysis of seven eligible studies established that the optimal pressure levels (mean ± SD) diminished from 11.6 ± 2.2 to 9.5 ± 2.0 cm H_2O after nasal surgery alone [16]. Ayers et al. [17] evaluated the effect of upper airway surgery for OSA on optimal PAP levels based on a meta-analysis. In their meta-analysis of 11 eligible studies, upper airway surgery included isolated nasal surgery and various other types of pharyngeal surgery [17]. They found that the optimal pressure level reduced from a mean of 10.8 to 9.4 cm H_2O in patients with OSA after upper airway surgery [17]. Although these two previous meta-analyses demonstrated that diverse surgical treatments play an important role in decreasing optimal PAP levels, the effect of pharyngeal OSA surgery on optimal pressure levels was not verified.

There are various PAP-related adverse effects, including mouth dryness, unintentional mask removal, skin irritation, air or mouth leak, pressure intolerance, mask claustrophobia, aerophagia (bloating), and nasal symptoms [11]. If these side effects are not addressed, PAP adherence could inevitably decrease. In particular, nasal obstruction or congestion leads to discomfort for patients with OSA because the nose is where the air generated from the PAP device comes into direct contact for the first time. A patient's discomfort during PAP therapy can cause mouth leaks or unintentional mask removal, which diminishes PAP usage time [11]. There are two main methods to alleviate nasal obstructions, medical and surgical therapy. In general, surgical treatment is considered when medical management, including nasal irrigation, topical spray, and medication, is not effective. It is well-recognized that PAP adherence is improved in patients with OSA after nasal surgery alone [16]. Poirier et al. [25] examined the hypothesis that isolated nasal surgery enhanced PAP adherence in PAP-intolerant OSA patients with nasal obstructions and found that PAP usage time improved significantly from a mean ± SD of 0.5 ± 0.7 to 5.0 ± 2.4 h per night ($n = 16$) after nasal surgery (e.g., septoplasty and turbinoplasty) alone. In addition, the outcomes of the meta-analysis from four eligible papers demonstrated that PAP usage time increased by 0.62 h per night with a 95% CI of 0.22 to 1.01 after upper airway surgery, including isolated nasal surgery [17]. However, the effect of pharyngeal surgery on PAP adherence in patients with OSA has not yet been demonstrated based on a meta-analysis. Moreover, it has been argued that pharyngeal surgery such as UPPP may be associated with decreased PAP adherence [18]. This study found that PAP usage time increased from a mean ± SE of 4.2 ± 1.7 to 5.5 ± 0.5 h per night, comparing changes between preoperative and postoperative PAP usage. As a result, pharyngeal OSA surgery can indirectly enhance PAP adherence, as well as directly alleviate objective respiratory parameters, such as AHI, and subjective symptoms, such as excessive daytime sleepiness.

This meta-analysis had several limitations. There were few clinical studies with high-quality evidence in the analysis. Only one randomized controlled trial, three prospective studies, and five retrospective studies were included in the final analysis. Clinical investigations related to surgery have difficulties planning high-level evidence-based designs due to the nature of surgery. Nevertheless, further high-quality evidence studies are required. The study had heterogeneity in many aspects including the study design, sample size, differences in the surgical procedures, and characteristics of the populations. The results should be interpreted cautiously because the studies included in this meta-analysis were relatively small.

5. Conclusions

This meta-analysis demonstrated that pharyngeal surgery in patients with OSA decreased optimal PAP levels and increased PAP usage time. OSA should be regarded as a chronic disorder requiring long-term and comprehensive treatment. Although PAP is the main therapy for OSA, some patients with OSA are intolerant of PAP or fail PAP treatment. In these cases, pharyngeal OSA surgery can be considered an adjunct therapy to increase PAP adherence, even in patients who are not expected to be cured by surgery. The results of the study contribute to our understanding of the role of pharyngeal OSA surgery in PAP-intolerant patients.

Author Contributions: Conceptualization, K.H.K., J.H.C. (Jae Hoon Cho) and J.H.C. (Ji Ho Choi); methodology, K.H.K. and J.H.C. (Jae Hoon Cho); formal analysis, K.H.K. and J.H.C. (Jae Hoon Cho); investigation, K.H.K., Y.J.L. and J.H.C. (Ji Ho Choi); writing—original draft preparation, K.H.K. and J.H.C. (Ji Ho Choi); writing—review and editing, K.H.K., J.Y.L., J.H.C. (Jae Hoon Cho) and J.H.C. (Ji Ho Choi); supervision, J.H.C. (Jae Hoon Cho) and J.H.C. (Ji Ho Choi). All authors have read and agreed to the published version of the manuscript.

Funding: This study was supported by the Soonchunhyang University Research Fund.

Institutional Review Board Statement: Not applicable.

Informed Consent Statement: Not applicable.

Data Availability Statement: The datasets used and/or analyzed during the current study available from the corresponding author on request.

Conflicts of Interest: The authors declare no conflict of interest.

References

1. Guilleminault, C.; Tilkian, A.; Dement, W.C. The sleep apnea syndromes. *Annu. Rev. Med.* **1976**, *27*, 465–484. [CrossRef]
2. Epstein, L.J.; Kristo, D.; Strollo, P.J., Jr.; Friedman, N.; Malhotra, A.; Patil, S.P.; Ramar, K.; Rogers, R.; Schwab, R.J.; Weaver, E.M.; et al. Clinical guideline for the evaluation, management and long-term care of obstructive sleep apnea in adults. *J. Clin. Sleep Med.* **2009**, *5*, 263–276. [PubMed]
3. American Academy of Sleep Medicine. *International Classification of Sleep Disorders*; American Academy of Sleep Medicine: Darien, IL, USA, 2014.
4. Gottlieb, D.J.; Punjabi, N.M. Diagnosis and Management of Obstructive Sleep Apnea: A Review. *JAMA* **2020**, *323*, 1389–1400. [CrossRef] [PubMed]
5. Choi, J.H. Treatments for adult obstructive sleep apnea. *Sleep Med. Res.* **2021**, *12*, 9–14. [CrossRef]
6. Sullivan, C.E.; Issa, F.G.; Berthon-Jones, M.; Eves, L. Reversal of obstructive sleep apnoea by continuous positive airway pressure applied through the nares. *Lancet* **1981**, *1*, 862–865. [CrossRef]
7. Kushida, C.A.; Littner, M.R.; Hirshkowitz, M.; Morgenthaler, T.I.; Alessi, C.A.; Bailey, D.; Boehlecke, B.; Brown, T.M.; Coleman, J., Jr.; Friedman, L.; et al. Practice parameters for the use of continuous and bilevel positive airway pressure devices to treat adult patients with sleep-related breathing disorders. *Sleep* **2006**, *29*, 375–380. [CrossRef] [PubMed]
8. Ballester, E.; Badia, J.R.; Hernández, L.; Carrasco, E.; de Pablo, J.; Fornas, C.; Rodriguez-Roisin, R.; Montserrat, J.M. Evidence of the effectiveness of continuous positive airway pressure in the treatment of sleep apnea/hypopnea syndrome. *Am. J. Respir. Crit. Care Med.* **1999**, *159*, 495–501. [CrossRef]
9. Jenkinson, C.; Davies, R.J.; Mullins, R.; Stradling, J.R. Comparison of therapeutic and subtherapeutic nasal continuous positive airway pressure for obstructive sleep apnoea: A randomised prospective parallel trial. *Lancet* **1999**, *353*, 2100–2105. [CrossRef]
10. Becker, H.F.; Jerrentrup, A.; Ploch, T.; Grote, L.; Penzel, T.; Sullivan, C.E.; Peter, J.H. Effect of nasal continuous positive airway pressure treatment on blood pressure in patients with obstructive sleep apnea. *Circulation* **2003**, *107*, 68–73. [CrossRef]
11. Kakkar, R.K.; Berry, R.B. Positive airway pressure treatment for obstructive sleep apnea. *Chest* **2007**, *132*, 1057–1072. [CrossRef]
12. Liu, S.Y.; Riley, R.W.; Yu, M.S. Surgical Algorithm for Obstructive Sleep Apnea: An Update. *Clin. Exp. Otorhinolaryngol.* **2020**, *13*, 215–224. [PubMed]

13. Smith, D.F.; Cohen, A.P.; Ishman, S.L. Surgical management of OSA in adults. *Chest* **2015**, *147*, 1681–1690. [CrossRef] [PubMed]
14. Reilly, E.K.; Boon, M.S.; Vimawala, S.; Chitguppi, C.; Patel, J.; Murphy, K.; Doghramji, K.; Nyquist, G.G.; Rosen, M.R.; Rabinowitz, M.R.; et al. Tolerance of Continuous Positive Airway Pressure After Sinonasal Surgery. *Laryngoscope* **2021**, *131*, E1013–E1018. [PubMed]
15. Chandrashekariah, R.; Shaman, Z.; Auckley, D. Impact of upper airway surgery on CPAP compliance in difficult-to-manage obstructive sleep apnea. *Arch. Otolaryngol. Head Neck Surg.* **2008**, *134*, 926–930. [CrossRef] [PubMed]
16. Camacho, M.; Riaz, M.; Capasso, R.; Ruoff, C.M.; Guilleminault, C.; Kushida, C.A.; Certal, V. The effect of nasal surgery on continuous positive airway pressure device use and therapeutic treatment pressures: A systematic review and meta-analysis. *Sleep* **2015**, *38*, 279–286.
17. Ayers, C.M.; Lohia, S.; Nguyen, S.A.; Gillespie, M.B. The Effect of Upper Airway Surgery on Continuous Positive Airway Pressure Levels and Adherence: A Systematic Review and Meta-Analysis. *ORL J. Otorhinolaryngol. Relat. Spec.* **2016**, *78*, 119–125. [CrossRef]
18. Han, F.; Song, W.; Li, J.; Zhang, L.; Dong, X.; He, Q. Influence of UPPP surgery on tolerance to subsequent continuous positive airway pressure in patients with OSAHS. *Sleep Breath.* **2006**, *10*, 37–42.
19. Mayer-Brix, J.; Müller-Marschhausen, U.; Becker, H.; Peter, J.H. How frequent are pathologic ENT findings in patients with obstructive sleep apnea syndrome? *HNO* **1989**, *37*, 511–516.
20. Friedman, M.; Tanyeri, H.; Lim, J.W.; Landsberg, R.; Vaidyanathan, K.; Caldarelli, D. Effect of improved nasal breathing on obstructive sleep apnea. *Otolaryngol. Head Neck Surg.* **2000**, *122*, 71–74. [CrossRef]
21. Dorn, M.; Pirsig, W.; Verse, T. Postoperative management following rhinosurgery interventions in severe obstructive sleep apnea. A pilot study. *HNO* **2001**, *49*, 642–645.
22. Nowak, C.; Bourgin, P.; Portier, F.; Genty, E.; Escourrou, P.; Bobin, S. Nasal obstruction and compliance to nasal positive airway pressure. *Ann. Otolaryngol. Chir. Cervicofac.* **2003**, *120*, 161–166. [PubMed]
23. Nakata, S.; Noda, A.; Yagi, H.; Yanagi, E.; Mimura, T.; Okada, T.; Misawa, H.; Nakashima, T. Nasal resistance for determinant factor of nasal surgery in CPAP failure patients with obstructive sleep apnea syndrome. *Rhinology* **2005**, *43*, 296–299. [PubMed]
24. Sufioğlu, M.; Ozmen, O.A.; Kasapoglu, F.; Demir, U.L.; Ursavas, A.; Erişen, L.; Onart, S. The efficacy of nasal surgery in obstructive sleep apnea syndrome: A prospective clinical study. *Eur. Arch. Otorhinolaryngol.* **2012**, *269*, 487–494. [CrossRef] [PubMed]
25. Poirier, J.; George, C.; Rotenberg, B. The effect of nasal surgery on nasal continuous positive airway pressure compliance. *Laryngoscope* **2014**, *124*, 317–319. [CrossRef]
26. Zonato, A.I.; Bittencourt, L.R.; Martinho, F.L.; Gregório, L.C.; Tufik, S. Upper airway surgery: The effect on nasal continuous positive airway pressure titration on obstructive sleep apnea patients. *Eur. Arch. Otorhinolaryngol.* **2006**, *263*, 481–486. [CrossRef]
27. Nakata, S.; Noda, A.; Yanagi, E.; Suzuki, K.; Yamamoto, H.; Nakashima, T. Tonsil size and body mass index are important factors for efficacy of simple tonsillectomy in obstructive sleep apnoea syndrome. *Clin. Otolaryngol.* **2006**, *31*, 41–45. [CrossRef]
28. Lin, H.S.; Toma, R.; Glavin, C.; Toma, M.; Badr, M.S.; Rowley, J.A. Tolerance of positive airway pressure following site-specific surgery of upper airway. *Open Sleep J.* **2008**, *1*, 34–39.
29. Khan, A.; Ramar, K.; Maddirala, S.; Friedman, O.; Pallanch, J.F.; Olson, E.J. Uvulopalatopharyngoplasty in the management of obstructive sleep apnea: The mayo clinic experience. *Mayo Clin. Proc.* **2009**, *84*, 795–800.
30. Friedman, M.; Soans, R.; Joseph, N.; Kakodkar, S.; Friedman, J. The effect of multilevel upper airway surgery on continuous positive airway pressure therapy in obstructive sleep apnea/hypopnea syndrome. *Laryngoscope* **2009**, *119*, 193–196. [CrossRef]
31. Bertoletti, F.; Indelicato, A.; Banfi, P.; Capolunghi, B. Sleep apnoea/hypopnoea syndrome: Combination therapy with the Pillar palatal implant technique and continuous positive airway pressure (CPAP). A preliminary report. *B-ENT* **2009**, *5*, 251–257.
32. Gillespie, M.B.; Wylie, P.E.; Lee-Chiong, T.; Rapoport, D.M. Effect of palatal implants on continuous positive airway pressure and compliance. *Otolaryngol. Head Neck Surg.* **2011**, *144*, 230–236. [CrossRef] [PubMed]
33. Turhan, M.; Bostanci, A.; Akdag, M. The impact of modified tongue base suspension on CPAP levels in patients with severe OSA. *Eur. Arch. Otorhinolaryngol.* **2015**, *272*, 995–1000. [CrossRef] [PubMed]
34. Azbay, S.; Bostanci, A.; Aysun, Y.; Turhan, M. The influence of multilevel upper airway surgery on CPAP tolerance in non-responders to obstructive sleep apnea surgery. *Eur. Arch. Otorhinolaryngol.* **2016**, *273*, 2813–2818. [CrossRef] [PubMed]
35. Caples, S.M.; Rowley, J.A.; Prinsell, J.R.; Pallanch, J.F.; Elamin, M.B.; Katz, S.G.; Harwick, J.D. Surgical modifications of the upper airway for obstructive sleep apnea in adults: A systematic review and meta-analysis. *Sleep* **2010**, *33*, 1396–1407. [CrossRef] [PubMed]
36. Li, H.Y.; Wang, P.C.; Chen, Y.P.; Lee, L.A.; Fang, T.J.; Lin, H.C. Critical appraisal and meta-analysis of nasal surgery for obstructive sleep apnea. *Am. J. Rhinol. Allergy* **2011**, *25*, 45–49. [CrossRef]
37. Wu, J.; Zhao, G.; Li, Y.; Zang, H.; Wang, T.; Wang, D.; Han, D. Apnea-hypopnea index decreased significantly after nasal surgery for obstructive sleep apnea: A meta-analysis. *Medicine* **2017**, *96*, e6008. [CrossRef]
38. Millman, R.P.; Carlisle, C.C.; Rosenberg, C.; Kahn, D.; McRae, R.; Kramer, N.R. Simple predictors of uvulopalatopharyngoplasty outcome in the treatment of obstructive sleep apnea. *Chest* **2000**, *118*, 1025–1030. [CrossRef]
39. Wilhelmsson, B.; Tegelberg, A.; Walker-Engström, M.L.; Ringqvist, M.; Andersson, L.; Krekmanov, L.; Ringqvist, I. A prospective randomized study of a dental appliance compared with uvulopalatopharyngoplasty in the treatment of obstructive sleep apnoea. *Acta Otolaryngol.* **1999**, *119*, 503–509.
40. Choi, J.H.; Lee, J.Y.; Cha, J.; Kim, K.; Hong, S.N.; Lee, S.H. Predictive models of objective oropharyngeal OSA surgery outcomes: Success rate and AHI reduction ratio. *PLoS ONE* **2017**, *12*, e0185201.

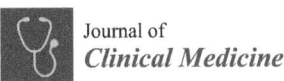

Systematic Review

Maxillomandibular Advancement and Upper Airway Stimulation for Treatment of Obstructive Sleep Apnea: A Systematic Review

Ning Zhou [1,2,3,*,†], Jean-Pierre T. F. Ho [1,2,4,†], René Spijker [5,6], Ghizlane Aarab [3], Nico de Vries [3,7,8], Madeline J. L. Ravesloot [7] and Jan de Lange [1,2]

1. Department of Oral and Maxillofacial Surgery, Amsterdam UMC, University of Amsterdam, Meibergdreef 9, 1105 AZ Amsterdam, The Netherlands
2. Academic Centre for Dentistry Amsterdam (ACTA), University of Amsterdam and Vrije Universiteit Amsterdam, 1081 LA Amsterdam, The Netherlands
3. Department of Orofacial Pain and Dysfunction, Academic Centre for Dentistry Amsterdam (ACTA), University of Amsterdam and Vrije Universiteit Amsterdam, 1081 LA Amsterdam, The Netherlands
4. Department of Oral and Maxillofacial Surgery, Northwest Clinics, 1815 JD Alkmaar, The Netherlands
5. Medical Library, Amsterdam UMC, University of Amsterdam, 1105 AZ Amsterdam, The Netherlands
6. Cochrane Netherlands, Julius Center for Health Sciences and Primary Care, University Medical Center Utrecht, 3584 CG Utrecht, The Netherlands
7. Department of Otorhinolaryngology—Head and Neck Surgery, OLVG, 1061 AE Amsterdam, The Netherlands
8. Department of Otorhinolaryngology—Head and Neck Surgery, Antwerp University Hospital (UZA), 2650 Edegem, Antwerp, Belgium
* Correspondence: n.zhou@amsterdamumc.nl
† These authors contributed equally to this work.

Abstract: This systematic review aimed to comparatively evaluate the efficacy and safety of maxillomandibular advancement (MMA) and upper airway stimulation (UAS) in obstructive sleep apnea (OSA) treatment. A MEDLINE and Embase database search of articles on MMA and/or UAS for OSA was conducted. Twenty-one MMA studies and nine UAS studies were included. All the MMA studies demonstrated a reduction in apnea hypopnea index (AHI) postoperatively, and success rates ranged from 41.1% to 100%. Ten MMA studies reported pre- and postoperative Epworth sleepiness scale (ESS), and all but one study demonstrated a reduction in ESS. In the UAS studies, all but one demonstrated a reduction in AHI, and success rates ranged from 26.7% to 77.8%. In the eight UAS studies reporting pre- and postoperative ESS, an ESS reduction was demonstrated. No studies reported any deaths related to MMA or UAS. The most common postoperative complications after MMA and UAS were facial paresthesia in the mandibular area and discomfort due to electrical stimulation, respectively. This systematic review suggests that both MMA and UAS are effective and generally safe therapies for OSA. However, due to the limitations of the included studies, there is no evidence yet to directly compare these two procedures in OSA treatment.

Keywords: obstructive sleep apnea; therapy; maxillomandibular surgery; hypoglossal nerve; systematic review

1. Introduction

Obstructive sleep apnea (OSA) is a prevalent sleep-related breathing disorder characterized by recurrent upper airway obstruction during sleep [1], and its overall prevalence ranges from 9% to 38% in the general adult population [2]. OSA is associated with considerable health risks, such as cardiovascular and cerebrovascular disease [3,4]. Continuous positive airway pressure (CPAP) is accepted as the first-line therapy for moderate to severe OSA, but poor compliance and suboptimal use of CPAP drive OSA patients to seek alternative therapies, including other non-invasive therapies and surgical treatment [5,6].

Moderate-to-severe OSA is usually caused by multilevel obstructions of the upper airway, which highlights the need for surgical therapies able to resolve multilevel upper airway collapse [7]. One such therapy that has existed for many decades is maxillomandibular advancement (MMA) [8,9]. MMA is a multilevel skeletal surgery in which the maxilla and mandible are advanced by a combination of a Le Fort I osteotomy of the maxilla and a bilateral sagittal split osteotomy of the mandible [8,9]. By expanding the skeletal framework attached with the pharyngeal soft tissues, MMA enlarges the velo-orohypopharyngeal airway [10] and increases the tension of the pharyngeal soft tissues, decreasing the collapsibility of the upper airway [11]. MMA is currently considered as the most effective surgical treatment modality for moderate-to-severe OSA in adults aside from tracheostomy.

A more contemporary therapy is hypoglossal nerve stimulation (HNS), which works by electrically stimulating the branches of the hypoglossal nerves that innervate muscles responsible for protruding the tongue and thus maintaining upper airway patency during sleep [12]. Currently, there are three different systems for HNS therapy, including the Aura6000 Targeted Hypoglossal Neurostimulation system (LivaNova PLC, London, England, UK), the GenioTM system (Nyxoah SA, Mont-Saint-Guibert, Belgium), and the Inspire II upper airway stimulation (UAS) system (Inspire Medical Systems, Maple Grove, MN, USA) [13]. Given that the Inspire UAS system is the most widely used system having Food and Drug Administration (FDA) approval for clinical use [14], this review only focused on UAS therapy (Inspire® system). Over the past decade, UAS has emerged as an effective therapy and therefore has become an increasingly popular treatment option for moderate-to-severe OSA [15,16].

Currently, the main indications for MMA are moderate-to-severe OSA, and mild OSA in patients presenting with a dentofacial deformity [17]. UAS therapy is generally indicated for patients with the following characteristics: moderate-to-severe OSA (apnea hypopnea index (AHI) 15–65 events/h with <25% central or mixed apneas), positive airway pressure (PAP) therapy failure, and absence of complete concentric velum collapse (CCCp) on drug-induced sleep endoscopy (DISE) [18]. When no generally accepted indicative results are found during clinical, laboratory, or endoscopic examinations (e.g., significant skeletal-dental deformity, AHI > 65 events/h, CCCp on DISE), patients with moderate-to-severe OSA may be expected to benefit from MMA as well as UAS therapy. Although MMA and UAS have both demonstrated efficacy and safety for patients, there is a paucity of evidence on comparison of these two treatment options [17].

Therefore, the purpose of this systematic review is to comprehensively evaluate and compare the efficacy of MMA and UAS for moderate-to-severe OSA through the assessment of AHI and Epworth sleepiness score (ESS) as primary outcomes. Secondly, the postoperative complications of these two therapies were investigated.

2. Materials and Methods

This systematic review was performed in accordance with the preferred reporting items for systematic review and meta-analysis (PRISMA) statement [19]. The protocol for this systematic review was registered at PROSPERO (PROSPERO ID: CRD42021261394; https://www.crd.york.ac.uk/prospero/display_record.php?RecordID=261394 (accessed on 14 November 2022)).

2.1. Selection Criteria

The inclusion criteria were: (1) adult patients (> 18 years old) with moderate-to-severe OSA diagnosed by polysomnography (PSG; AHI ≥ 15 events/h); (2) patients who underwent MMA or UAS for OSA; (3) studies that reported pre- and postoperative PSG data; (4) studies with a follow-up ≥ 6 months; (5) study designs: randomized controlled trials (RCTs), quasi-experimental studies, and cohort studies; and (6) English language.

The exclusion criteria were: (1) sample size < 10 patients; (2) patients who underwent other adjunctive surgical procedures (e.g., uvulopalatopharyngoplasty) at the time of MMA or UAS; and (3) preliminary studies in which the findings had been nested in other studies with larger sample size and/or longer follow-up.

2.2. Literature Search

A literature search was performed with the help of an information specialist (RS) using MEDLINE and Embase databases on 14 December 2021. Search terms and search strategies used for each database are available in Supplementary Materials (Table S1 (a)).

2.3. Study Selection

After removal of duplicate articles, the remaining results were screened based on title and abstract by two independent reviewers (NZ and JH). The full texts of potentially relevant articles were retrieved and further evaluated by NZ and JH independently for compliance of studies with the eligibility criteria. Discrepancies were resolved by discussion. Reference lists of eligible studies were checked for additional studies.

2.4. Data Extraction

The extracted data included article title, year of publication, first author, study design, specific surgical technique, length of follow-up, sample size, age, gender, body mass index (BMI), preoperative and postoperative PSG data (AHI, respiratory disturbance index (RDI), and oxygen desaturation index (ODI)), preoperative and postoperative ESS score, preoperative and postoperative data on quality of life (QoL), surgical success rate and cure rate, and postoperative complications. According to the accordion severity grading system of surgical complications [20], the postoperative complications were classified as major or minor depending on the needs for endoscopic or interventional radiologic procedures or reoperation as well as failure of one or more organ systems.

Data were extracted by NZ and JH independently. Discrepancies were resolved through discussion. If RDI was reported by a study, it would be extracted as AHI, since these two respiratory parameters have been consolidated based on the 2013 American Academy of Sleep Medicine's manual for the scoring of sleep and associated events [21]. If there were multiple follow-up data in a study, the data with longest follow-up time were included. Surgical success was defined as "a postoperative AHI < 20 and at least 50% reduction in AHI after surgery" [22], and surgical cure was defined as "a postoperative AHI < 5" [23].

2.5. Quality Assessment

Methodologic quality assessment of each study was performed by NZ and JH independently, and any discrepancies were resolved by discussion.

The Methodological Index for Non-Randomized Studies (MINORS) quality assessment tool, a validated tool for the methodological assessment of non-randomized surgical studies [24], was used to assess the methodological quality of the included studies. The MINORS tool is composed of eight items applicable to all non-randomized studies and four additional items specifically for comparative studies. Each item was scored as 0 (not reported), 1 (reported but inadequate), or 2 (reported and adequate), giving a global ideal score of 24 for comparative studies and 16 for non-comparative studies. For comparative studies, the categorizations are as follows: 0–6, very low quality; 7–10, low quality; 11–15 fair quality; and ≥ 16, high quality. For non-comparative studies, the categorizations are as follows: 0–4, very low quality; 5–7, low quality; 8–12, fair quality; and ≥ 13, high quality [25].

2.6. Statistical Analysis

The collected parameters (age, BMI, AHI, ODI, and ESS) were pooled by weighted average and weighted standard deviation [26]. When there were RCTs or comparative studies between MMA and UAS, meta-analyses were performed to compare the overall effect of MMA and UAS in treating OSA. Heterogeneity of the studies was assessed using the I^2 statistic with a cutoff of 25% (low), 50% (moderate) and 75% (high) [27]. When moderate-to-high heterogeneity was present, a random effects model was adopted; otherwise, a fixed effects model was used. Because some patients may report multiple complications, the complication rate of each study was calculated by dividing the number of events by the number of patients.

3. Results

3.1. Search Results

The flow diagram of study selection progress is summarized in Figure 1. A total of 2952 studies were screened after deduplication, and 212 were retrieved for full-text review.

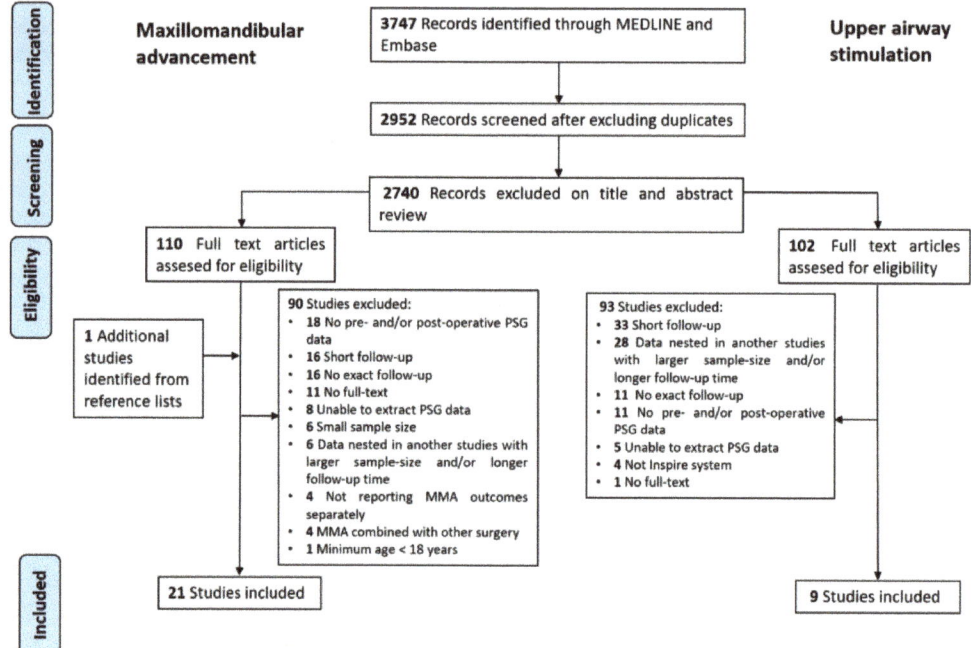

Figure 1. PRISMA flow diagram of the study selection process.

MMA group. Twenty-one studies [11,28–47] were identified, producing a pooled data set of 581 patients (male 78.5%) with a weighted age of 42.2 ± 11.5 years and a weighted BMI of 28.1 ± 6.4 kg/m². The mean follow-up period from surgery to final postoperative PSG was 25.9 months (range, 6 months–12.5 years). One study [39] was excluded from the analyses for clinical efficacy because the data of a subset of the patients with a longer follow-up period were nested in another included study [38]. The characteristics of these studies are shown in Table 1.

UAS group. In total, nine studies [15,48–55] were identified, yielding 1029 patients (male 96.2%) with a weighted age of 55.1 ± 10.1 years and a weighted BMI of 29.1 ± 4.2 kg/m². The mean follow-up period was 18.8 months (range, 6 months–5 years). The characteristics are summarized in Table 2.

Because there was no RCT or comparative study of MMA and UAS in treating OSA, a meta-analysis could not be performed to compare their overall effect sizes on OSA.

Table 1. Characteristics of studies on maxillomandibular advancement.

Study	Design	N	Age (Years) (Mean ± SD)	% Male	Degree of Advancement (mm) (Mean ± SD) Max	Degree of Advancement (mm) (Mean ± SD) Mand	Follow-Up (Mean ± SD)	BMI (Mean ± SD) Pre-op	BMI (Mean ± SD) Post-op	AHI (Mean ± SD) Pre-op	AHI (Mean ± SD) Post-op	ODI (Mean ± SD) Pre-op	ODI (Mean ± SD) Post-op	ESS (Mean ± SD) Pre-op	ESS (Mean ± SD) Post-op	% Success	% Cure
Bettega et al., 2000 [28]	Retro	20	44.4 ± 10.6	90	11.8 ± 0.5	11.8 ± 0.5	6 m	26.9 ± 4.3	25.4 ± 3.3	59.3 ± 29.0	11.1 ± 8.9					75 [c]	
Bianchi et al., 2014 [29]	Retro	10	45 ± 14	100	10	10	6 m			56.8 ± 5.2	12.3 ± 5.5						
Boyd et al., 2015 [30]	Pro	14			7.0 ± 2.3	9.2 ± 3.3	6.6 ± 2.8 y			50.0 ± 20.0	8.0 ± 10.7						
Conradt et al., 1997 [31]	Retro	15	44 ± 12	93.3			>2 y	28.3 ± 3.4		51.4 ± 16.9	8.5 ± 9.4						
Gerbino et al., 2014 [32]	Pro	10	44.9		9.2 ± 1.2	10.4 ± 2.2	6 m	31.6 ± 5.5	28 ± 1.4	69.8 ± 35.2	17.3 ± 16.7	59.5 ± 5.3	9.1 ± 8			80 [d]	
Goh et al., 2003 [33]	Pro	11	42.8 ± 8.2	100	10	10	7.7 m	29.4 ± 4.6	27.2 ± 3.3	70.7 ± 15.9	11.4 ± 7.4					81.8	
Goodday et al., 2016 [34]	Retro	13	37.8 ± 8.6	84.6			9.6 m	38.8 ± 10.9	37.3 ± 8.0	117.9 ± 9.2	16.1 ± 26.2			12.9 ± 5.5	5.0 ± 4.1 [b]	76.9	46.2
Hsieh et al., 2014 [35]	Pro	16	33 ± 7.9	75			12 ± 8 m	22 ± 3.3		35.7 ± 18	4.8 ± 4.4					100	
Kastoer et al., 2019 [36]	Retro	14	51.1 ± 7.3	57.1			6 m	25.7 ± 3.7		40.2 ± 25.6	9.9 ± 7.2	13.5 ± 18.6	4.0 ± 3.5	13 ± 6	9 ± 7		
Li et al., 1999 [39]	Retro	175	43.5 ± 11.5	83			6 m			72.3 ± 26.7 [a]	7.2 ± 7.5 [a]					95 [e]	
Li et al., 2000 [38]	Retro	40	45.6 ± 20.7	82.5	10.8 ± 2.7	10.8 ± 2.7	4.2 ± 2.7 y	31.4 ± 6.7	32.2 ± 6.3	71.2 ± 27.0 [a]	7.6 ± 5.1 [a]					90 [e]	
Li et al., 2001 [40]	Retro	52	46.6 ± 6.7	82.7	10.5 ± 1.5		6 m	32.0 ± 6.0		61.6 ± 23.9 [a]	9.2 ± 8 [a]					90 [f]	
Li et al., 2002 [37]	Pro	12	47.3 ± 9.8	75	10.5 ± 1.2	10.5 ± 1.2	6 m	33.5 ± 6.2	32.3 ± 4.1	75.3 ± 26.4 [a]	10.4 ± 10.8 [a]					83.3 [f]	
Liao et al., 2015 [41]	Pro	20	33.4 ± 6.5	85			14 ± 9.3 m	22.4 ± 3.4		41.6 ± 19.2	5.3 ± 4			11.9 ± 7.3	7 ± 3	100 [c]	
Lin et al., 2020 [42]	Pro	53	35.7 ± 11.7	75.7	4.3 ± 2.9	13.3 ± 3.8	24 m	24.8 ± 3.3	23.9 ± 4.7	34.8 ± 26.0	7.4 ± 6.7	38.7 ± 30.3	8.1 ± 9.2	10.8 ± 5	10.2 ± 5.1		67.9
Liu et al., 2016 [11]	Retro	20	44 ± 12	85	7 ± 1.4		6 m	27 ± 4.6	27.4 ± 4.6	53.6 ± 26.6	9.5 ± 7.4			17.0 ± 4.8	5.7 ± 2.7	90	50
Rubio-Bueno et al., 2017 [43]	Pro	34	40.8 ± 13.9	41.2	4.9 ± 3.2	10.4 ± 3.9	6 m	27.6 ± 4.5	25.5 ± 4.3	38.3 ± 10.7	6.5 ± 4.3	34.7 ± 12.5	5.4 ± 4.1	17.4 ± 5.4	0.8 ± 1.4	100	52.9
Veys et al., 2017 [44]	Pro	10	44.7 ± 9.5	80	4.8 ± 2.8	8.3 ± 2.3	6 m			26.8 ± 12.7	12.3 ± 14.4			14.1 ± 5.9	5.7 ± 3.0	70	40
Vicini et al., 2010 [45]	RCT	25	49.1 ± 9.1	92	11	11	13 ± 2.5 m	32.7 ± 5.8	31.4 ± 6.5	56.8 ± 16.5	8.1 ± 7			11.6 ± 2.8	7.7 ± 1.3	88	36

Table 1. Cont.

Study	Design	N	% Male	Age (Years) (Mean ± SD)	Degree of Advancement (mm) (Mean ± SD)		Follow-Up (Mean ± SD)	BMI (Mean ± SD)		AHI (Mean ± SD)		ODI (Mean ± SD)		ESS (Mean ± SD)		% Success	% Cure
					Max	Mand		Pre-op	Post-op	Pre-op	Post-op	Pre-op	Post-op	Pre-op	Post-op		
Vigneron et al., 2017 [46]	Retro	29		40.7 ± 12.6	8.4 ± 4.1	11.7 ± 5.1	12.5 ± 3.5 y	24.6 ± 4		56.6 ± 24	25.5 ± 20.6				7.5 ± 4.7	41.4	
Wu et al., 2019 [47]	Retro	28	53.6	37.2 ± 11.8	2.0 ± 3.1	8.8 ± 3.7	>1 y	24.2 ± 5.1		59.3 ± 14.5	10.9 ± 3.3			12.8 ± 2.8	6.9 ± 2.5	85.7	46.4

AHI, apnea–hypopnea index (events/h); BMI, body mass index (kg/m^2); ESS, Epworth sleepiness scale; m, months; Max, maxilla; Mand, mandible; N, number of patients; ODI, oxygen desaturation index (events/h); post-op, postoperative; pre-op, preoperative; pro, prospective; RCT, randomized controlled trial; retro, retrospective; y, years. [a] An AHI < 15/h with ≥ 50% reduction in postoperative AHI. [b] The number of patients was 9. [c] This study defined surgical success as an AHI < 15/h with ≥ 50% reduction in postoperative AHI. [d] This study did not define the criteria of surgical success. [e] This study defined surgical success as an RDI < 15/h with ≥ 50% reduction in postoperative RDI. [f] This study defined surgical success as a postoperative RDI < 20/h.

Table 2. Characteristics of studies on upper airway stimulation.

Study	Design	N	Age (Years) (Mean ± SD)	% Male	Follow-Up (Month)	BMI (Mean ± SD)		AHI (Mean ± SD)		ODI (Mean ± SD)		ESS (Mean ± SD)		% Success	% Cure
						Pre-op	Post-op	Pre-op	Post-op	Pre-op	Post-op	Pre-op	Post-op		
Bachour et al., 2021 [55]	Retro	15	52.9 ± 6.6	86.7	18 ± 9.6	29.1 ± 3.3	30.1 ± 4.5	33.0 ± 16.5	36.5 ± 23.8	25.3 ± 18.3	30.3 ± 21.1	11.5 ± 3.8	8.1 ± 4.5	26.7	6.7
Heiser et al., 2017 [48]	Pro	20	57 ± 12	100	12	28.1 ± 13.1		28.9 ± 7.6	6.6 ± 5.1						
Philip et al., 2018 [49]	Pro	10	52.0 ± 9.4	100	6	28.8 ± 3.3		46.7 ± 12.2	14.5 ± 8.9	38.1 ± 21.1	10.5 ± 9.9	15.9 ± 3.5	10.0 ± 6.1	77.8	33.3
Steffen et al., 2019 [50]	Retro	18	51.5		24	27.9 ± 4.5	28.0 ± 4.7	26.3 ± 10.6	10.4 ± 10.1	12.8 ± 10.2	10.1 ± 12.0	12.7 ± 5.2	5.1 ± 3.8		
Steffen et al., 2020 [51]	Pro	38	58.0 ± 10.0	97.4	36	29.1 ± 3.9	28.6 ± 3.3	30.0 ± 13.7	13.1 ± 14.1	25.8 ± 16.7	11.6 ± 14.0	12.1 ± 5.8	6.0 ± 3.2	62	35
Suurna et al., 2021 [54]	Pro	782			14.3 ± 7.0	29.2 ± 4		35.8 ± 15.0	14.5 ± 14.9			11.4 ± 5.5	7.1 ± 4.6	69.7	
Van de Heyning et al., 2012 [52]	Pro	28	55.1 ± 9.2	96.4	6	29.5 ± 2.5		42.3 ± 16.4	32.6 ± 29.1	30.7 ± 21.6	26.7 ± 27.0	11.0 ± 5.0	7.6 ± 4.3	50	
Vanderveken et al., 2013 [53]	Retro	21	55 ± 11	95.2	6	28 ± 2		38.5 ± 11.8	20.3 ± 20.6			8.2 ± 5.0 [a]	6.4 ± 4.3 [a]	62	
Woodson et al., 2018 [15]	Pro	97	54.4 ± 10.3		60	28.6 ± 2.5		30.4 ± 9.4 [b]	12.4 ± 16.3	27.2 ± 10.0 [b]	9.9 ± 14.5	11.3 ± 5.2	6.9 ± 4.7 [c]	74.6 [b]	44

AHI, apnea–hypopnea index (events/h); BMI, body mass index (kg/m^2); ESS, Epworth sleepiness scale; N, number of patients; ODI, oxygen desaturation index (events/h); post-op, post-operative; pre-op, pre-operative; pro, prospective; retro, retrospective. [a] The number of patients was 18. [b] The number of patients was 71. [c] The number of patients was 92.

3.2. Quality Assessment

MMA group. One of the included studies was an RCT of MMA and autotitrating positive airway pressure (APAP), one was a retrospective quasi-experimental study, ten were prospective cohort studies, and nine were retrospective cohort studies. As only the MMA cohort of the RCT was included in the analyses, after omitting the unrequired APAP cohort, this study was regarded as a single-arm trial. The quality of the RCT was therefore assessed using the MINORS tool as per the other included studies. Of these studies, three studies were classified as "high quality", and the others were classified as "fair quality" (Supplementary Table S2 (a)).

UAS group. Six prospective studies and three retrospective studies were included. Of these, one study was classified as "high quality" and eight studies as "fair quality" (Supplementary Table S2 (b)).

3.3. Respiratory Parameters

MMA group. Fifteen MMA studies [11,28–31,33–37,41,42,44,45,47] reported a significant reduction in AHI postoperatively ($p < 0.05$). The others [32,38,40,43,46] reported an AHI reduction but did not report a p value. All the studies [11,28–38,40–47], totaling 446 patients, demonstrated a weighted baseline AHI of 54.6 ± 27.4/h and a weighted postoperative AHI of 10.1 ± 10.8/h.

Of four studies [11,32,36,43] (n = 78) reporting pre- and postoperative ODI, two demonstrated a significant reduction in ODI after MMA ($p < 0.05$), and the other two also reported an ODI reduction but without a p value. The weighted pre- and postoperative ODIs were 35.1 ± 22.8/h and 6.3 ± 6.4/h, respectively.

UAS group. Of the selected studies, the study by Bachour et al. [55] did not show a significant reduction in AHI postoperatively. Five studies [48–51,54] demonstrated a significant reduction in AHI postoperatively ($p < 0.05$), and three studies [15,52,53] showed an AHI reduction but did not report a p value. The weighted pre- and postoperative AHIs in 1003 patients were 35.2 ± 14.7/h and 15.0 ± 16.1/h, respectively.

Of six studies [15,49–52,55] reporting pre- and postoperative ODI, the study by Bachour et al. [55] did not find a significant improvement in ODI postoperatively, while the others [15,49–52] reported a reduction in ODI after surgery, of which two studies did not report a p value. The weighted pre- and postoperative ODIs were 26.5 ± 16.0/h and 14.6 ± 18.5/h (n = 180), respectively.

3.4. Subjective Parameters

MMA group. Of nine studies [11,34,36,41–45,47] (n = 217) reporting pre- and postoperative ESS, the study from Lin et al. did not show an improvement in ESS after MMA, one study demonstrated a reduction in ESS but without a p value, and the others reported a significant reduction in ESS ($p < 0.05$). The weighted pre- and postoperative ESS values were 13.1 ± 5.5 and 6.7 ± 4.8, respectively.

Three studies [30,42,44] assessed pre- and postoperative QoL. Boyd et al. found that after MMA, there was a significant improvement in the Functional Outcomes of Sleep Questionnaire (FOSQ) ($p < 0.05$) [30]. Veys et al. assessed the subjective outcome of MMA using the OSA QoL questionnaire. They found that there was an improvement in all of the following six symptoms after MMA—daytime sleepiness, snoring, concentration, waking up at night, headache, and high blood pressure—while the influence of MMA on nocturia and sexual activity was variable [44]. Lin et al. found that there was no significant improvement in Short Form-36 quality of life (SF-36) after MMA [42].

UAS group. Of eight studies [15,49–55] reporting pre- and postoperative ESS, seven demonstrated a significant reduction in ESS postoperatively ($p < 0.05$), and one reported a ESS reduction but did not report a p value. The weighted pre- and postoperative ESS values were 11.4 ± 5.4 (n = 1006) and 7.0 ± 4.6 (n = 1001), respectively.

Two studies reported pre- and post-UAS FOSQ scores. The STAR trial cohort demonstrated an increase in FOSQ score five years after surgery (14.3 ± 3.3 to 18.0 ± 2.2). Van de Heyning et al. also found a significant improvement in FOSQ score postoperatively (89.1 ± 23.5 to 100.8 ± 16.9, $p < 0.05$).

3.5. Surgical Success and Cure

MMA group. Surgical success rate of MMA was available in 15 studies [11,28,32–35,37,38,40,41,43–47] and ranged from 41.1% to 100%. Surgical cure rate of MMA was reported in seven studies [11,34,42–45,47] and ranged from 36% to 67.9%.

UAS group. Surgical success rate of UAS was available in six studies [15,50–52,54,55], ranging from 26.5% to 77.8%. Surgical cure rate was reported in four studies [15,50,51,55] and ranged from 6.7% to 44%.

3.6. Long-Term Follow-Up Outcomes

MMA group. Five studies [30,31,38,42,46] reported long-term follow-up (≥2 years) data in 151 patients with weighted baseline AHI of 51.7 ± 28.2/h. At a mean follow-up of 5.0 years, the weighted postoperative AHI was 11.1 ± 13.0/h. Only one study [42], with 53 patients, reported long-term follow-up ESS (10.8 ± 5.0 to 10.2 ± 5.1, $p > 0.05$). Boyd et al. [30] reported a long-term improvement in FOSQ score after MMA. Surgical success rate was reported in two studies [38,46] (90% and 41.4%, respectively), and surgical cure rate was only available in one study [42] (67.9%).

UAS group. Three studies [15,50,51] reported long-term follow-up (≥2 years) data in 127 patients with weighted baseline AHI of 29.7 ± 11.0/h. At a mean follow-up of 4.2 years, the weighted postoperative AHI was 12.3 ± 14.8/h. These three studies [15,50,51] also reported a long-term improvement in ODI and ESS after UAS therapy. One study [15] reported a long-term (five years follow-up) improvement in FOSQ score. Surgical success and cure rates were reported in all three studies [15,50,51] (success rate: 77.8%, 71.1%, and 74.6%, respectively; cure rate: 33.3%, 35%, and 44%, respectively).

3.7. Safety

There were no studies reporting any deaths related to MMA or UAS surgery.

MMA group. Of the included studies, 10 reported participants' complications after MMA (n = 428) [28,30,33,39,42–47]. The rate of major complication ranged from 0 to 18%. Five studies reported the major compilations after MMA, which included reoperations for removal of osteosynthesis screws and plates (n = 8) [30,33,46], reoperations for maxillary non-union (n = 2) [28,46], and acute dyspnea (n = 1) [45].

The most common minor complication reported was facial paresthesia caused by the impairment of inferior alveolar nerve [30,33,39,43,45–47]. Four studies [39,45–47] reported both the rates of transient and persistent paresthesia in mandibular area, which were 100% and 13% (n = 175), 100% and 28% (n = 25), 90% and 60% (n = 34), and 32% and 0% (n = 28), respectively. Additionally, one study [43] (n = 34) reported only the rate of transient paresthesia in mandibular area—75%; one study [33] (n = 11) reported only the rate of the persistent symptom—27%. In the long-term follow-up study from Boyd et al. [30] (n = 30), although no patients exhibited such facial anesthesia as measured objectively, 40% of patients subjectively perceived a decrease in sensation. Facial paresthesia in the infraorbital area was reported by two studies [45,46]. In the study by Vicini et al. [45] (n = 25), the rates of transient and persistent paresthesia in infraorbital area were 100% and 4%, respectively; in the study by Vigneron et al. [46] (n = 34), they were 37% and 30%, respectively.

Excluding facial paresthesia, the other reported minor complications consisted of developed malocclusion [30,45–47] (n = 13), temporomandibular disorders [46,47] (n = 11), local infection [28,30,47] (n = 6), minor postoperative wound pain [33] (n = 2), and others (n = 5) [28,44,47]. Of ten studies [28,30,32,41–47] that investigated patients' perception of their facial appearance after MMA, two studies [30,46] reported that there were 13% (4/30) and 15% (5/34) patients who perceived worsening of their facial appearance after MMA, respectively; the others [28,32,41–45,47] reported that the perception of facial appearance was positive or neutral in all the patients after MMA.

UAS group. Of the five studies reporting patients' complications (n = 2051) [15,49,51,52,54], the rate of serious device-related adverse events range from 0 to 7%. Four studies [15,51,52,54] reported a total of 50 serious device-related adverse events requiring surgical repositioning or replacement of the neurostimulator or implanted leads. In addition, in the study from Suurna et al. [54] (n = 1849), 0.4% of the patients reported serious intraoperative adverse events, including but not limited to hematoma (n = 8), infection (n = 2), extra implant procedure (n = 1), intraoperative arrest (n = 1), and pneumothorax (n = 1).

Since one study [54] did not report the count of minor complications, the safety outcomes of a subset of the study population (ADHERE cohort) reported in a previous study [56] were used to analyze the minor complication rate. In that study [56], the rates of minor surgery-related and device-related complications 137 ± 77 days after UAS implant were 6% (18/313) and 22% (69/313), respectively; 386 ± 136 days after UAS implant were 4% (8/217) and 24% (53/217), respectively. In the STAR trial cohort [15] consisting of 126 participants, the rates of minor surgery-related and device-related complication were both 136% (171/126) at the first year; at the fifth year, they were decreased to 1% (1/126) and 16% (20/126), respectively. Van de Heyning et al. [52] reported only minor surgery-related adverse events in their population, which yielded a minor complication rate of 57% (16/28). Philip et al. [49] and Steffen et al. [51] did not report any minor complications in their study populations. The most common minor surgery-related and device-related complications were incision discomfort [15,51,56] and discomfort due to electrical stimulation [15,56], respectively.

4. Discussion

This is the first systematic review aiming to comparatively evaluate MMA and UAS therapy in treating OSA. We reviewed 21 studies on MMA and 9 studies on UAS in treating OSA. Due to the fact that there is no RCT or comparative study of MMA and UAS, a meta-analysis cannot be performed to directly compare these two interventions. Separate analyses of studies on MMA and UAS were utilized for this review. In this review, the trials for MMA tended to be published earlier than those for UAS. Therefore, for some patients in the UAS group, MMA could have been considered at first as an alternative therapy to CPAP and not been chosen. It should be noted that UAS therapy has stricter and clearer inclusion criteria (e.g., 15/h ≤ AHI ≤ 65 /h, absence of CCCp during DISE) [14,17] for patients, especially in comparison to MMA. There is therefore discrepancy of patients' baseline characteristics between the MMA cohort and UAS cohort. In this review, the MMA cohort has younger age and higher baseline AHI compared to the UAS cohort. Moreover, it is impossible for us to compare other patients' characteristics associated with OSA, such as the size of tongue, retrolingual space, and jaw position. To obtain definitive results on the comparison of MMA and UAS, future studies should include comparative studies of these two therapies where participants would have comparable baseline characteristics and be qualified for both therapies. Another point to be noted is that the variations in MMA surgeries are probably greater than in UAS as the training and the lineage of potential variations are much higher in MMA than in UAS.

4.1. Objective Outcomes

Based on the separate analysis of studies on MMA and UAS, we reported that these two procedures are both effective treatment modalities for OSA. However, compared to UAS, MMA seems to be more effective in treating OSA with a more significant decrease in AHI and higher success rate. Through different mechanisms, MMA and UAS have been proven to be able to address multiple sites of collapse simultaneously [11,36]. MMA enlarges the entire pharynx and reduces the collapsibility of the upper airway by advancing the maxillomandibular complex and anterior pharyngeal tissues attached to the maxilla, mandible, and hyoid bone [39]. The mechanism by which UAS resolves multilevel collapse, is enlargement of the retropalatal airway associated with tongue protrusion, which is so called "palatoglossus coupling" phenomenon [48]. Safiruddin et al. found that the retropalatal enlargement in response to UAS was statistically significant only in the responders, while the responders and non-responders had similar degrees of retrolingual opening to stimulation [57]. Therefore, we are of the opinion that the superiority of MMA over UAS in OSA treatment may be associated with the ability of MMA to enlarge the retropalatal airway more significantly. To improve patient selection for MMA and UAS, the mechanism of action of these two surgical procedures and the role of pathogenesis of OSA on the outcome of both surgeries require clarification in future studies.

4.2. Subjective Outcomes

It is interesting to note that several studies [42,55] reported a discordance between objective outcome measures (e.g., AHI) and patient-reported outcome measures, which highlights the importance of subjective outcome evaluation for OSA patients. In contrast to published ESS data, there is a scarcity of evidence related to other subjective outcomes of surgical treatment for OSA. Boyd et al. [30] evaluated the impact of MMA on quality of life (QoL) using the Functional Outcomes of Sleep Questionnaire (FOSQ). Two years after MMA, a significant improvement in mean FOSQ scores of 4.7 was observed. In a study by Woodson et al. [15], the improvements in mean FOSQ scores following UAS were 3.0 at 1 year and 3.7 at 5 years, respectively. In addition to daytime sleepiness and QoL, patient satisfaction—an important measure of therapy quality—should be noted when evaluating treatment options for OSA. Currently, only a few studies have evaluated patient satisfaction with MMA or UAS for the management of OSA [56,58–62]. In a study by Butterfield et al. [59], 95.5% of patients were satisfied with MMA surgery for OSA, 90.9% would repeat the procedure, and 86.4% would recommend MMA to others for OSA treatment. In the ADHERE registry, 94% of patients reported that they were satisfied with UAS therapy and would undergo UAS again, and 93% reported that they would recommend UAS to others [56]. According to the available evidence, both MMA and UAS could significantly improve the perception for OSA patients with high levels of patient satisfaction. However, the comparison of improvement in patient-perceived measures between the two therapies must be addressed in future studies.

4.3. Long-Term Outcomes

The long-term follow-up period of the included MMA studies ranges from 2 years to 12.5 years. Because of the small sample size, one study by Pottel et al. [63] reporting the longest follow-up result of MMA was excluded. In that study, the short term (within 2 years) success rate was 66.67% (8/12), and the long-term (median 19 years; range 14–20 years) success rate of MMA was 44.44% (4/9). Of the nine patients who attended long-term re-evaluation, the median ages at the time of MMA surgery and re-evaluation were 43 years (range 34–63 years) and 62 years (range 49–82 years), respectively. At the long-term follow up, two of the six patients who were initially successfully treated by MMA had relapse of OSA with AHI comparable to preoperative values. Both patients had significant weight gain (+4.1 and +7.9 kg/m^2). In a study of 29 OSA patients treated by MMA, Vigneron et al. [46] concluded that the success rate was 85.7% in the immediate postoperative period and 41.1% at 12.5 years. Additionally, they concluded that the good candidates for long-term success of MMA were the young patients (<45 years old) with BMI < 25 kg/m^2, AHI < 45/h, SNB angle < 75°, narrow retrolingual space (<8 mm), preoperative orthodontics, and without co-morbidity. It has been suggested that long-term failure of MMA might be attributed to weight gain [38,63,64], skeletal relapse [64], and ageing [63]. Given that UAS is an innovative therapy for OSA from the last decade, the longest follow-up period of the UAS studies was 5 years, from the STAR trial [15]. The success rates of UAS in the STAR trial cohort were 66% (83/126), 74% (73/98), and 75% (53/71) at 1, 3, and 5 years, respectively. In UAS therapy for OSA treatment, patients' adherence is necessary to guarantee clinical efficacy [65]. The STAR trial revealed a high adherence to UAS therapy in the long-term, with a patient-self-reported nightly device use of 80% at 5 years, which might partially explain the stability of treatment effect. In addition, lower baseline ODI was found to be predictive of 5-year response to UAS therapy. It is therefore concluded that both MMA and UAS were relatively stable treatments for patients with moderate-to-severe OSA. In order to maintain clinical efficacy, more effort is needed to provide continuous follow-up for OSA patients and to ascertain the factors associated with long-term stability of outcomes.

4.4. Safety

In terms of treatment safety, this systematic review revealed that both MMA and UAS were generally safe surgical procedures for OSA, with relatively low rates of major complication. In the included MMA studies, all but one of the major complications were reoperation for removal of hardware. Age has been shown to be a risk factor for increased need for hardware removal [66]. In addition, Passeri et al. found that patients who were active smokers or had a history of smoking had higher risk of complications, which included removal of hardware [67]. The most common minor complication of MMA detailed in the literature was paresthesia of the lower lip and chin. It has been suggested that age at the time of surgery and addition of a genioplasty increase the risk of facial paresthesia, and a large degree of advancement further increases the risk in older patients [68,69]. In the STAR cohort (n = 126), the rates of major complication requiring device explanation, reposition, or replacement were 4% at 4 years and 9.5% at 5 years, indicating that the reoperations after UAS may occur more often during the late time frame. The STAR cohort also suggested that the majority of minor complications after UAS were gradually resolved. Notably, Withrow et al. evaluated the impact of age on safety of UAS and found no significant difference between younger and older cohorts in complication rates [70]. Current evidence suggests that both MMA and UAS appear to be safe approaches in OSA treatment, and compared to MMA, treating OSA with UAS may lead to fewer complications for older patients.

4.5. Clinical Relevance

In patients with moderate to severe OSA and failure of CPAP treatment, a portion of them could qualify for both MMA and UAS therapy. Current evidence shows that MMA may have superior efficacy in OSA treatment. However, MMA is a more invasive intervention, exposing patients to longer recovery time and higher risk of postoperative complications. Overnight admission to the intensive care unit is required for OSA patients following MMA surgery, and the length of hospitalization after MMA reported previously ranged from <2 days to 5–8 days [69]. Additionally, MMA surgery often involves time-consuming preoperative and/or postoperative orthodontic work. One notable potential problem with MMA has been the accompanying alteration in facial appearance; however, most patients undergoing MMA for OSA view the change in facial appearance as neutral or even positive [30,32,46]. In comparison to MMA, UAS surgery is less invasive and more patient-friendly and does not require extended recovery. The majority of patients are discharged the same day or one day after UAS surgery [71]. In addition to the information regarding treatment efficacy and safety, the cost of treatment options is important in assisting decision-making in OSA treatment. It has been indicated that UAS is cost-effective, with a lifetime incremental cost effectiveness ratio (ICER) of USD 39,471 per quality-adjusted life year (QALY) in the United States healthcare system [72] and EUR 44,446 per QALY in a European setting [73]. However, to our knowledge, no study has assessed the cost-effectiveness of MMA, which precludes the comparison of cost-effectiveness between these two therapies. Hence, to further assist decision-making in OSA treatment, there is a need to assess and compare the costs and cost-effectiveness of each intervention.

Since the primary target patient population differs between MMA and UAS, these two procedures are usually not put on par in the current practice guidelines. In the current Stanford protocol, UAS and MMA are considered phase I and phase II surgical procedures, respectively [74]. It has been proposed that these two procedures might be considered as complementary therapies [17]. For example, UAS may be considered when a patient fails to respond to MMA or for a patient with relapse of OSA after previously successful MMA [75]. It is interesting to note that in a recent study [76], Sarber et al. evaluated the efficacy of UAS therapy in 18 OSA patients who did not meet all FDA criteria for UAS and found promising treatment outcomes. They suggested that future studies must consider the expansion of current FDA criteria for UAS, particularly in BMI and AHI criteria. Thus, to optimize surgical outcomes, reduce rates of mortality and morbidity, and improve quality of life and other subjective outcomes, further investigation is essential to clarify indications of each therapy for OSA.

In addition to MMA and UAS, there are other evidence-based therapeutic options for OSA, which include behavioral strategies (e.g., weight loss), medical therapy (e.g., CPAP), other surgical options, and adjuvant therapy (e.g., pharyngeal muscle training) [77,78]. Of the non-CPAP therapies for OSA, more invasive procedures, such as MMA, are not well accepted. Oral appliances offer a non-invasive option for managing OSA, the most common of which are mandibular advancement devices (MADs). MADs modify the position of the jaw, the tongue, and other supporting structures of the upper airway, thereby increasing upper airway volume and preventing collapse of the upper airway [79]. MADs are recommended as a first-line therapy for mild-to-moderate OSA and for severe OSA after CPAP failure, intolerance, or refusal [80]. Growing evidence suggests that MADs could achieve favorable outcomes regardless of the severity of OSA [81,82].

In the era of precision medicine, the interconnected risk factors for OSA must be considered in order to achieve precision medicine in OSA [78]. The combined modern therapies for OSA must be adjusted continuously in respect to recent scientific research in order to deliver the best results for patients, emphasizing their quality of life in addition to medical care. Therefore, any of the therapies may either have an important role as monotherapy in the treatment of OSA or could be used in combination with the other therapies. The greater the complexity of a clinical case, the greater the need for multidisciplinary collaboration.

4.6. Limitations

There are several limitations of the present review. Firstly, because of the inherent difficulty of randomizing patients to different surgical interventions or sham surgery [83], except for one RCT and one quasi-experimental trial, all the included studies were cohort studies, the majority of which demonstrated fair quality according to the MINORS tool. Due to the lack of RCT and comparative studies of MMA and UAS for OSA, a meta-analysis cannot be performed to directly compare these two procedures. Additionally, meta-analyses were not conducted to separately assess overall effect sizes of MMA and UAS therapy on OSA, as mean and SD of the difference between pre- and postoperative measures were absent in majority of the selected studies. In this review, we performed separate analyses for MMA and UAS studies, combined with noticeable differences between the two cohorts in age and OSA severity, which prevented us from generating a solid conclusion on the comparison of these two procedures. Due to the fact that some patients may fall between two stools, comparison of the two procedures is important. Future studies should include quasiexperimental trials and comparative cohort studies comparing MMA and UAS to better clarify which modality is superior in OSA treatment. These studies can be part of a future large international consortium, which is more likely to generate solid conclusions. Secondly, due to the implemented inclusion criteria, which included the presence of both preoperative and postoperative PSG data, some well-conducted studies reporting on only subjective outcomes and/or safety were excluded for this study. Therefore, the present analysis of subjective outcomes and safety may not be entirely representative of the population undergoing MMA or UAS in the current literature. Lastly, our review is exclusively based on studies published in English, which can introduce a language bias [84].

5. Conclusions

The results presented in this review suggest that both MMA and UAS are effective and generally safe surgical treatment modalities for patients with moderate-to-severe OSA.

However, within the limitation of the selected studies, there is currently no evidence on the comparison of MMA and UAS in the treatment of OSA.

Supplementary Materials: The following supporting information can be downloaded at: https://www.mdpi.com/article/10.3390/jcm11226782/s1, Table S1: (a). Search strategy in MEDLINE database. (b) Search strategy in Embase database; Table S2: (a) Methodological appraisal of the individual studies according to MINORS assessment tool—maxillomandibular advancement surgery. (b) Methodological appraisal of the individual studies according to MINORS assessment tool—upper airway stimulation.

Funding: This research received no external funding.

Institutional Review Board Statement: Not applicable.

Informed Consent Statement: Not applicable.

Data Availability Statement: Not applicable.

Conflicts of Interest: Author G.A. receives research grants from Sunstar Suisse SA and Vivisol-ResMed and is an unpaid member of the academic advisory board for Oral Function (Sunstar Suisse SA); author N.d.V is member of the Medical Advisory Board of NightBalance and consultant to Philips Healthcare, Inspire, and Nyxoah; the other authors declare they have no conflicts of interest. The funders had no role in the design of the study; in the collection, analysis, or interpretation of data; in the writing of the manuscript; or in the decision to publish the results.

References

1. Jordan, A.S.; McSharry, D.G.; Malhotra, A. Adult obstructive sleep apnoea. *Lancet* **2014**, *383*, 736–747. [CrossRef]
2. Senaratna, C.V.; Perret, J.L.; Lodge, C.J.; Lowe, A.J.; Campbell, B.E.; Matheson, M.C.; Hamilton, G.S.; Dharmage, S.C. Prevalence of obstructive sleep apnea in the general population: A systematic review. *Sleep Med. Rev.* **2017**, *34*, 70–81. [CrossRef] [PubMed]
3. Bagai, K. Obstructive sleep apnea, stroke, and cardiovascular diseases. *Neurologist* **2010**, *16*, 329–339. [CrossRef] [PubMed]
4. Knauert, M.; Naik, S.; Gillespie, M.B.; Kryger, M. Clinical consequences and economic costs of untreated obstructive sleep apnea syndrome. *World J. Otorhinolaryngol. Head Neck Surg.* **2015**, *1*, 17–27. [CrossRef]
5. Gottlieb, D.J.; Punjabi, N.M. Diagnosis and Management of Obstructive Sleep Apnea: A Review. *JAMA* **2020**, *323*, 1389–1400. [CrossRef]
6. Rotenberg, B.W.; Vicini, C.; Pang, E.B.; Pang, K.P. Reconsidering first-line treatment for obstructive sleep apnea: A systematic review of the literature. *J. Otolaryngol. Head Neck Surg.* **2016**, *45*, 23. [CrossRef]
7. Sharifian, M.R.; Zarrinkamar, M.; Alimardani, M.S.; Bakhshaee, M.; Asadpour, H.; Morovatdar, N.; Amini, M. Drug Induced Sleep Endoscopy in Obstructive Sleep Apnea. *Tanaffos* **2018**, *17*, 122–126.
8. Li, K.K. Surgical management of obstructive sleep apnea. *Clin. Chest Med.* **2003**, *24*, 365–370. [CrossRef]
9. Riley, R.W.; Powell, N.B.; Guilleminault, C.; Nino-Murcia, G. Maxillary, mandibular, and hyoid advancement: An alternative to tracheostomy in obstructive sleep apnea syndrome. *Otolaryngol. Head Neck Surg.* **1986**, *94*, 584–588. [CrossRef]
10. Gokce, S.M.; Gorgulu, S.; Gokce, H.S.; Bengi, A.O.; Karacayli, U.; Ors, F. Evaluation of pharyngeal airway space changes after bimaxillary orthognathic surgery with a 3-dimensional simulation and modeling program. *Am. J. Orthod. Dentofac. Orthop.* **2014**, *146*, 477–492. [CrossRef]
11. Liu, S.Y.; Huon, L.K.; Iwasaki, T.; Yoon, A.; Riley, R.; Powell, N.; Torre, C.; Capasso, R. Efficacy of Maxillomandibular Advancement Examined with Drug-Induced Sleep Endoscopy and Computational Fluid Dynamics Airflow Modeling. *Otolaryngol. Head Neck Surg.* **2016**, *154*, 189–195. [CrossRef] [PubMed]
12. Strollo, P.J.; Soose, R.J.; Maurer, J.T.; de Vries, N.; Cornelius, J.; Froymovich, O.; Hanson, R.D.; Padhya, T.A.; Steward, D.L.; Gillespie, M.B.; et al. Upper-Airway Stimulation for Obstructive Sleep Apnea. *N. Engl. J. Med.* **2014**, *370*, 139–149. [CrossRef] [PubMed]
13. Steffen, A.; Heiser, C.; Galetke, W.; Herkenrath, S.D.; Maurer, J.T.; Günther, E.; Stuck, B.A.; Woehrle, H.; Löhler, J.; Randerath, W. Hypoglossal nerve stimulation for obstructive sleep apnea: Updated position paper of the German Society of Oto-Rhino-Laryngology, Head and Neck Surgery. *Eur. Arch. Oto-Rhino-Laryngol.* **2022**, *279*, 61–66. [CrossRef]
14. Vanderveken, O.M.; Beyers, J.; Op de Beeck, S.; Dieltjens, M.; Willemen, M.; Verbraecken, J.A.; De Backer, W.A.; Van de Heyning, P.H. Development of a Clinical Pathway and Technical Aspects of Upper Airway Stimulation Therapy for Obstructive Sleep Apnea. *Front. Neurosci.* **2017**, *11*, 523. [CrossRef]
15. Woodson, B.T.; Strohl, K.P.; Soose, R.J.; Gillespie, M.B.; Maurer, J.T.; de Vries, N.; Padhya, T.A.; Badr, M.S.; Lin, H.S.; Vanderveken, O.M.; et al. Upper Airway Stimulation for Obstructive Sleep Apnea: 5-Year Outcomes. *Otolaryngol. Head Neck Surg.* **2018**, *159*, 194–202. [CrossRef] [PubMed]
16. Dedhia, R.C.; Strollo, P.J.; Soose, R.J. Upper Airway Stimulation for Obstructive Sleep Apnea: Past, Present, and Future. *Sleep* **2015**, *38*, 899–906. [CrossRef]

17. Yu, M.S.; Ibrahim, B.; Riley, R.W.; Liu, S.Y. Maxillomandibular Advancement and Upper Airway Stimulation: Extrapharyngeal Surgery for Obstructive Sleep Apnea. *Clin. Exp. Otorhinolaryngol.* **2020**, *13*, 225–233. [CrossRef]
18. Mashaqi, S.; Patel, S.I.; Combs, D.; Estep, L.; Helmick, S.; Machamer, J.; Parthasarathy, S. The Hypoglossal Nerve Stimulation as a Novel Therapy for Treating Obstructive Sleep Apnea—A Literature Review. *Int. J. Environ. Res. Public Health* **2021**, *18*, 1642. [CrossRef]
19. Page, M.J.; McKenzie, J.E.; Bossuyt, P.M.; Boutron, I.; Hoffmann, T.C.; Mulrow, C.D.; Shamseer, L.; Tetzlaff, J.M.; Akl, E.A.; Brennan, S.E.; et al. The PRISMA 2020 Statement: An Updated Guideline for Reporting Systematic Reviews. *BMJ* **2021**, *372*, n160. [CrossRef]
20. Strasberg, S.M.; Linehan, D.C.; Hawkins, W.G. The accordion severity grading system of surgical complications. *Ann. Surg.* **2009**, *250*, 177–186. [CrossRef]
21. Berry, R.B.; Brooks, R.; Gamaldo, C.E.; Harding, S.M.; Lloyd, R.M.; Marcus, C.L.; Vaughn, B.V. *The AASM Manual for the Scoring of Sleep and Associated Events: Rules, Terminology and Technical Specifications, Version 2.0.2*; American Academy of Sleep Medicine: Darien, IL, USA, 2013.
22. Sher, A.E.; Schechtman, K.B.; Piccirillo, J.F. The efficacy of surgical modifications of the upper airway in adults with obstructive sleep apnea syndrome. *Sleep* **1996**, *19*, 156–177. [CrossRef] [PubMed]
23. Elshaug, A.G.; Moss, J.R.; Southcott, A.M.; Hiller, J.E. Redefining success in airway surgery for obstructive sleep apnea: A meta analysis and synthesis of the evidence. *Sleep* **2007**, *30*, 461–467. [CrossRef] [PubMed]
24. Slim, K.; Nini, E.; Forestier, D.; Kwiatkowski, F.; Panis, Y.; Chipponi, J. Methodological index for non-randomized studies (minors): Development and validation of a new instrument. *ANZ J. Surg.* **2003**, *73*, 712–716. [CrossRef] [PubMed]
25. Shah, A.; Memon, M.; Kay, J.; Wood, T.J.; Tushinski, D.M.; Khanna, V. Preoperative Patient Factors Affecting Length of Stay following Total Knee Arthroplasty: A Systematic Review and Meta-Analysis. *J. Arthroplast.* **2019**, *34*, 2124–2165. [CrossRef] [PubMed]
26. Altman, D.G.; Machin, D.; Bryant, T.N.; Gardner, M.J. *Statistics with Confidence: Confidence Intervals and Statistical Guidelines*, 2nd ed.; BMJ Books: London, UK, 2000; p. 254.
27. Higgins, J.P.; Thompson, S.G.; Deeks, J.J.; Altman, D.G. Measuring inconsistency in meta-analyses. *BMJ* **2003**, *327*, 557–560. [CrossRef] [PubMed]
28. Bettega, G.; Pepin, J.L.; Veale, D.; Deschaux, C.; Raphael, B.; Levy, P. Obstructive sleep apnea syndrome. fifty-one consecutive patients treated by maxillofacial surgery. *Am. J. Respir. Crit. Care Med.* **2000**, *162*, 641–649. [CrossRef]
29. Bianchi, A.; Betti, E.; Tarsitano, A.; Morselli-Labate, A.M.; Lancellotti, L.; Marchetti, C. Volumetric three-dimensional computed tomographic evaluation of the upper airway in patients with obstructive sleep apnoea syndrome treated by maxillomandibular advancement. *Br. J. Oral Maxillofac. Surg.* **2014**, *52*, 831–837. [CrossRef]
30. Boyd, S.B.; Walters, A.S.; Waite, P.; Harding, S.M.; Song, Y. Long-Term Effectiveness and Safety of Maxillomandibular Advancement for Treatment of Obstructive Sleep Apnea. *J. Clin. Sleep Med.* **2015**, *11*, 699–708. [CrossRef]
31. Conradt, R.; Hochban, W.; Brandenburg, U.; Heitmann, J.; Peter, J.H. Long-term follow-up after surgical treatment of obstructive sleep apnoea by maxillomandibular advancement. *Eur. Respir. J.* **1997**, *10*, 123–128. [CrossRef]
32. Gerbino, G.; Bianchi, F.A.; Verzé, L.; Ramieri, G. Soft tissue changes after maxillo-mandibular advancement in OSAS patients: A three-dimensional study. *J. Cranio-Maxillofac. Surg.* **2014**, *42*, 66–72. [CrossRef]
33. Goh, Y.H.; Lim, K.A. Modified maxillomandibular advancement for the treatment of obstructive sleep apnea: A preliminary report. *Laryngoscope* **2003**, *113*, 1577–1582. [CrossRef] [PubMed]
34. Goodday, R.H.; Bourque, S.E.; Edwards, P.B. Objective and Subjective Outcomes Following Maxillomandibular Advancement Surgery for Treatment of Patients With Extremely Severe Obstructive Sleep Apnea (Apnea-Hypopnea Index >100). *J. Oral Maxillofac. Surg.* **2016**, *74*, 583–589. [CrossRef] [PubMed]
35. Hsieh, Y.J.; Liao, Y.F.; Chen, N.H.; Chen, Y.R. Changes in the calibre of the upper airway and the surrounding structures after maxillomandibular advancement for obstructive sleep apnoea. *Br. J. Oral Maxillofac. Surg.* **2014**, *52*, 445–451. [CrossRef] [PubMed]
36. Kastoer, C.; Op de Beeck, S.; Dom, M.; Neirinckx, T.; Verbraecken, J.; Braem, M.J.; Van de Heyning, P.H.; Nadjmi, N.; Vanderveken, O.M. Drug-Induced Sleep Endoscopy Upper Airway Collapse Patterns and Maxillomandibular Advancement. *Laryngoscope* **2020**, *130*, E268–E274. [CrossRef]
37. Li, K.K.; Guilleminault, C.; Riley, R.W.; Powell, N.B. Obstructive sleep apnea and maxillomandibular advancement: An assessment of airway changes using radiographic and nasopharyngoscopic examinations. *J. Oral Maxillofac. Surg.* **2002**, *60*, 526–530; discussion 531. [CrossRef]
38. Li, K.K.; Powell, N.B.; Riley, R.W.; Troell, R.; Guilleminault, C. Long Term Results of Maxillomandibular Advancement Surgery. *Sleep Breath.* **2000**, *4*, 137–140. [CrossRef]
39. Li, K.K.; Riley, R.W.; Powell, N.B.; Troell, R.; Guilleminault, C. Overview of phase II surgery for obstructive sleep apnea syndrome. *Ear Nose Throat J.* **1999**, *78*, 851, 854–857. [CrossRef]
40. Li, K.K.; Troell, R.J.; Riley, R.W.; Powell, N.B.; Koester, U.; Guilleminault, C. Uvulopalatopharyngoplasty, maxillomandibular advancement, and the velopharynx. *Laryngoscope* **2001**, *111*, 1075–1078. [CrossRef]
41. Liao, Y.F.; Chiu, Y.T.; Lin, C.H.; Chen, Y.A.; Chen, N.H.; Chen, Y.R. Modified maxillomandibular advancement for obstructive sleep apnoea: Towards a better outcome for Asians. *Int. J. Oral Maxillofac. Surg.* **2015**, *44*, 189–194. [CrossRef]

42. Lin, C.H.; Chin, W.C.; Huang, Y.S.; Wang, P.F.; Li, K.K.; Pirelli, P.; Chen, Y.H.; Guilleminault, C. Objective and subjective long term outcome of maxillomandibular advancement in obstructive sleep apnea. *Sleep Med.* **2020**, *74*, 289–296. [CrossRef]
43. Rubio-Bueno, P.; Landete, P.; Ardanza, B.; Vazquez, L.; Soriano, J.B.; Wix, R.; Capote, A.; Zamora, E.; Ancochea, J.; Naval-Gías, L. Maxillomandibular advancement as the initial treatment of obstructive sleep apnoea: Is the mandibular occlusal plane the key? *Int. J. Oral Maxillofac. Surg.* **2017**, *46*, 1363–1371. [CrossRef] [PubMed]
44. Veys, B.; Pottel, L.; Mollemans, W.; Abeloos, J.; Swennen, G.; Neyt, N. Three-dimensional volumetric changes in the upper airway after maxillomandibular advancement in obstructive sleep apnoea patients and the impact on quality of life. *Int. J. Oral Maxillofac. Surg.* **2017**, *46*, 1525–1532. [CrossRef] [PubMed]
45. Vicini, C.; Dallan, I.; Campanini, A.; De Vito, A.; Barbanti, F.; Giorgiomarrano, G.; Bosi, M.; Plazzi, G.; Provini, F.; Lugaresi, E. Surgery vs ventilation in adult severe obstructive sleep apnea syndrome. *Am. J. Otolaryngol.* **2010**, *31*, 14–20. [CrossRef] [PubMed]
46. Vigneron, A.; Tamisier, R.; Orset, E.; Pepin, J.L.; Bettega, G. Maxillomandibular advancement for obstructive sleep apnea syndrome treatment: Long-term results. *J. Cranio-Maxillofac. Surg.* **2017**, *45*, 183–191. [CrossRef] [PubMed]
47. Wu, Q.; Wang, Y.; Wang, P.; Xiang, Z.; Ye, B.; Li, J. The inverted-L ramus osteotomy versus sagittal split ramus osteotomy in maxillomandibular advancement for the treatment of obstructive sleep apnea patients: A retrospective study. *J. Cranio-Maxillofac. Surg.* **2019**, *47*, 1839–1847. [CrossRef]
48. Heiser, C.; Edenharter, G.; Bas, M.; Wirth, M.; Hofauer, B. Palatoglossus coupling in selective upper airway stimulation. *Laryngoscope* **2017**, *127*, E378–E383. [CrossRef]
49. Philip, P.; Heiser, C.; Bioulac, S.; Altena, E.; Penchet, G.; Cuny, E.; Hofauer, B.; Monteyrol, P.J.; Micoulaud-Franchi, J.A. Hypoglossal nerve stimulation on sleep and level of alertness in OSA: A preliminary study. *Neurology* **2018**, *91*, e615–e619. [CrossRef]
50. Steffen, A.; Abrams, N.; Suurna, M.V.; Wollenberg, B.; Hasselbacher, K. Upper-Airway Stimulation Before, After, or Without Uvulopalatopharyngoplasty: A Two-Year Perspective. *Laryngoscope* **2019**, *129*, 514–518. [CrossRef]
51. Steffen, A.; Sommer, U.J.; Maurer, J.T.; Abrams, N.; Hofauer, B.; Heiser, C. Long-term follow-up of the German post-market study for upper airway stimulation for obstructive sleep apnea. *Sleep Breath.* **2020**, *24*, 979–984. [CrossRef]
52. Van de Heyning, P.H.; Badr, M.S.; Baskin, J.Z.; Cramer Bornemann, M.A.; De Backer, W.A.; Dotan, Y.; Hohenhorst, W.; Knaack, L.; Lin, H.S.; Maurer, J.T.; et al. Implanted upper airway stimulation device for obstructive sleep apnea. *Laryngoscope* **2012**, *122*, 1626–1633. [CrossRef]
53. Vanderveken, O.M.; Maurer, J.T.; Hohenhorst, W.; Hamans, E.; Lin, H.S.; Vroegop, A.V.; Anders, C.; de Vries, N.; Van de Heyning, P.H. Evaluation of drug-induced sleep endoscopy as a patient selection tool for implanted upper airway stimulation for obstructive sleep apnea. *J. Clin. Sleep Med.* **2013**, *9*, 433–438. [CrossRef] [PubMed]
54. Suurna, M.V.; Steffen, A.; Boon, M.; Chio, E.; Copper, M.; Patil, R.D.; Green, K.; Hanson, R.; Heiser, C.; Huntley, C.; et al. Impact of Body Mass Index and Discomfort on Upper Airway Stimulation: ADHERE Registry 2020 Update. *Laryngoscope* **2021**, *131*, 2616–2624. [CrossRef] [PubMed]
55. Bachour, A.; Bäck, L.; Pietarinen, P. No changes in nocturnal respiration with hypoglossal neurostimulation therapy for obstructive sleep apnoea. *Clin. Respir. J.* **2021**, *15*, 329–335. [CrossRef] [PubMed]
56. Heiser, C.; Steffen, A.; Boon, M.; Hofauer, B.; Doghramji, K.; Maurer, J.T.; Sommer, J.U.; Soose, R.; Strollo, P.J., Jr.; Schwab, R.; et al. Post-approval upper airway stimulation predictors of treatment effectiveness in the ADHERE registry. *Eur. Respir. J.* **2019**, *53*, 1801405. [CrossRef]
57. Safiruddin, F.; Vanderveken, O.M.; de Vries, N.; Maurer, J.T.; Lee, K.; Ni, Q.; Strohl, K.P. Effect of upper-airway stimulation for obstructive sleep apnoea on airway dimensions. *Eur. Respir. J.* **2015**, *45*, 129–138. [CrossRef]
58. Li, K.K.; Riley, R.W.; Powell, N.B.; Gervacio, L.; Troell, R.J.; Guilleminault, C. Obstructive sleep apnea surgery: Patient perspective and polysomnographic results. *Otolaryngol. Head Neck Surg.* **2000**, *123*, 572–575. [CrossRef]
59. Butterfield, K.J.; Marks, P.L.; McLean, L.; Newton, J. Quality of life assessment after maxillomandibular advancement surgery for obstructive sleep apnea. *J. Oral Maxillofac. Surg.* **2016**, *74*, 1228–1237. [CrossRef]
60. Beranger, T.; Garreau, E.; Ferri, J.; Raoul, G. Morphological impact on patients of maxillomandibular advancement surgery for the treatment of obstructive sleep apnea-hypopnea syndrome. *Int. Orthod.* **2017**, *15*, 40–53. [CrossRef]
61. Cillo, J.E.; Robertson, N.; Dattilo, D.J. Maxillomandibular Advancement for Obstructive Sleep Apnea Is Associated With Very Long-Term Overall Sleep-Related Quality-of-Life Improvement. *J. Oral Maxillofac. Surg.* **2020**, *78*, 109–117. [CrossRef]
62. Mehra, R.; Steffen, A.; Heiser, C.; Hofauer, B.; Withrow, K.; Doghramji, K.; Boon, M.; Huntley, C.; Soose, R.J.; Stevens, S.; et al. Upper Airway Stimulation versus Untreated Comparators in Positive Airway Pressure Treatment-Refractory Obstructive Sleep Apnea. *Ann. Am. Thorac. Soc.* **2020**, *17*, 1610–1619. [CrossRef]
63. Pottel, L.; Neyt, N.; Hertegonne, K.; Pevernagie, D.; Veys, B.; Abeloos, J.; De Clercq, C. Long-term quality of life outcomes of maxillomandibular advancement osteotomy in patients with obstructive sleep apnoea syndrome. *Int. J. Oral Maxillofac. Surg.* **2019**, *48*, 332–340. [CrossRef]
64. Riley, R.W.; Powell, N.B.; Li, K.K.; Troell, R.J.; Guilleminault, C. Surgery and obstructive sleep apnea: Long-term clinical outcomes. *Otolaryngol. Head Neck Surg.* **2000**, *122*, 415–421. [CrossRef] [PubMed]
65. Hofauer, B.; Steffen, A.; Knopf, A.; Hasselbacher, K.; Heiser, C. Patient experience with upper airway stimulation in the treatment of obstructive sleep apnea. *Sleep Breath.* **2019**, *23*, 235–241. [CrossRef] [PubMed]
66. Peacock, Z.S.; Lee, C.C.; Klein, K.P.; Kaban, L.B. Orthognathic surgery in patients over 40 years of age: Indications and special considerations. *J. Oral Maxillofac. Surg.* **2014**, *72*, 1995–2004. [CrossRef] [PubMed]

67. Passeri, L.A.; Choi, J.G.; Kaban, L.B.; Lahey, E.T. Morbidity and Mortality Rates After Maxillomandibular Advancement for Treatment of Obstructive Sleep Apnea. *J. Oral Maxillofac. Surg.* **2016**, *74*, 2033–2043. [CrossRef]
68. Van Sickels, J.E.; Hatch, J.P.; Dolce, C.; Bays, R.A.; Rugh, J.D. Effects of age, amount of advancement, and genioplasty on neurosensory disturbance after a bilateral sagittal split osteotomy. *J. Oral Maxillofac. Surg.* **2002**, *60*, 1012–1017. [CrossRef]
69. Zhou, N.; Ho, J.P.T.F.; Huang, Z.; Spijker, R.; de Vries, N.; Aarab, G.; Lobbezoo, F.; Ravesloot, M.J.L.; de Lange, J. Maxillomandibular advancement versus multilevel surgery for treatment of obstructive sleep apnea: A systematic review and meta-analysis. *Sleep Med. Rev.* **2021**, *57*, 101471. [CrossRef]
70. Withrow, K.; Evans, S.; Harwick, J.; Kezirian, E.; Strollo, P. Upper Airway Stimulation Response in Older Adults with Moderate to Severe Obstructive Sleep Apnea. *Otolaryngol. Head Neck Surg.* **2019**, *161*, 714–719. [CrossRef]
71. Murphey, A.W.; Baker, A.B.; Soose, R.J.; Padyha, T.A.; Nguyen, S.A.; Xiao, C.C.; Gillespie, M.B. Upper airway stimulation for obstructive sleep apnea: The surgical learning curve. *Laryngoscope* **2016**, *126*, 501–506. [CrossRef]
72. Pietzsch, J.B.; Liu, S.; Garner, A.M.; Kezirian, E.J.; Strollo, P.J. Long-Term Cost-Effectiveness of Upper Airway Stimulation for the Treatment of Obstructive Sleep Apnea: A Model-Based Projection Based on the STAR Trial. *Sleep* **2015**, *38*, 735–744. [CrossRef]
73. Pietzsch, J.B.; Richter, A.-K.; Randerath, W.; Steffen, A.; Liu, S.; Geisler, B.P.; Wasem, J.; Biermann-Stallwitz, J. Clinical and economic benefits of upper airway stimulation for obstructive sleep apnea in a European setting. *Respiration* **2019**, *98*, 38–47. [CrossRef] [PubMed]
74. Liu, S.Y.; Awad, M.; Riley, R.; Capasso, R. The Role of the Revised Stanford Protocol in Today's Precision Medicine. *Sleep Med. Clin.* **2019**, *14*, 99–107. [CrossRef] [PubMed]
75. Liu, S.Y.; Riley, R.W. Continuing the Original Stanford Sleep Surgery Protocol from Upper Airway Reconstruction to Upper Airway Stimulation: Our First Successful Case. *J. Oral Maxillofac. Surg.* **2017**, *75*, 1514–1518. [CrossRef]
76. Sarber, K.M.; Chang, K.W.; Ishman, S.L.; Epperson, M.V.; Dhanda Patil, R. Hypoglossal Nerve Stimulator Outcomes for Patients Outside the U.S. FDA Recommendations. *Laryngoscope* **2020**, *130*, 866–872. [CrossRef] [PubMed]
77. Trăistaru, T.; Pantea, M.; Țâncu, A.M.C.; Imre, M. Elements of Diagnosis and Non-surgical Treatment of Obstructive Sleep Apnea in Adults from the Dental Medicine Perspective. In *Sleep Medicine and the Evolution of Contemporary Sleep Pharmacotherapy*; Larrivee, D., Ed.; IntechOpen: London, UK, 2021.
78. Carberry, J.C.; Amatoury, J.; Eckert, D.J. Personalized Management Approach for OSA. *Chest* **2018**, *153*, 744–755. [CrossRef]
79. Chan, A.S.; Sutherland, K.; Schwab, R.J.; Zeng, B.; Petocz, P.; Lee, R.W.; Darendeliler, M.A.; Cistulli, P.A. The effect of mandibular advancement on upper airway structure in obstructive sleep apnoea. *Thorax* **2010**, *65*, 726–732. [CrossRef]
80. Ramar, K.; Dort, L.C.; Katz, S.G.; Lettieri, C.J.; Harrod, C.G.; Thomas, S.M.; Chervin, R.D. Clinical Practice Guideline for the Treatment of Obstructive Sleep Apnea and Snoring with Oral Appliance Therapy: An Update for 2015. *J. Clin. Sleep Med.* **2015**, *11*, 773–827. [CrossRef]
81. Lee, C.H.; Mo, J.H.; Choi, I.J.; Lee, H.J.; Seo, B.S.; Kim, D.Y.; Yun, P.Y.; Yoon, I.Y.; Won Lee, H.; Kim, J.W. The mandibular advancement device and patient selection in the treatment of obstructive sleep apnea. *Arch. Otolaryngol. Head Neck Surg.* **2009**, *135*, 439–444. [CrossRef]
82. Vecchierini, M.F.; Attali, V.; Collet, J.M.; d'Ortho, M.P.; Goutorbe, F.; Kerbrat, J.B.; Leger, D.; Lavergne, F.; Monaca, C.; Monteyrol, P.J.; et al. Mandibular advancement device use in obstructive sleep apnea: ORCADES study 5-year follow-up data. *J. Clin. Sleep Med.* **2021**, *17*, 1695–1705. [CrossRef]
83. Cook, J.A. The challenges faced in the design, conduct and analysis of surgical randomised controlled trials. *Trials* **2009**, *10*, 9. [CrossRef]
84. Higgins, J.P.; Thomas, J.; Chandler, J.; Cumpston, M.; Li, T.; Page, M.J.; Welch, V.A. *Cochrane Handbook for Systematic Reviews of Interventions*, 2nd ed.; John Wiley & Sons: Chichester, UK, 2019; pp. 182–183.

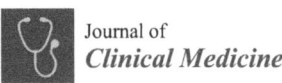

Review

Medical Treatment of Obstructive Sleep Apnea in Children

Almala Pinar Ergenekon [1], Yasemin Gokdemir [1] and Refika Ersu [2,*]

[1] Division of Pediatric Pulmonology, Marmara University, 34890 Istanbul, Turkey; drpergenekon@hotmail.com (A.P.E.); yasemingokdemir@yahoo.com.tr (Y.G.)
[2] Division of Respirology, Department of Pediatrics, Children's Hospital of Eastern Ontario, University of Ottawa, Ottawa, ON K1N 6N5, Canada
* Correspondence: rersu@yahoo.com

Abstract: Obstructive sleep apnea (OSA) is characterized by recurrent complete or partial obstruction of the upper airway. The prevalence is 1–4% in children aged between 2 and 8 years and rising due to the increase in obesity rates in children. Although persistent OSA following adenotonsillectomy is usually associated with obesity and underlying complex disorders, it can also affect otherwise healthy children. Medical treatment strategies are frequently required when adenotonsillectomy is not indicated in children with OSA or if OSA is persistent following adenotonsillectomy. Positive airway pressure treatment is a very effective modality for persistent OSA in childhood; however, adherence rates are low. The aim of this review article is to summarize medical treatment options for OSA in children.

Keywords: obstructive sleep apnea; persistent obstructive sleep apnea; children; medical treatment; PAP therapy; anti-inflammatory treatment; high flow nasal cannula

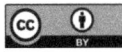

1. Introduction

Obstructive sleep apnea (OSA) is a syndrome involving upper airway dysfunction during sleep that is characterized by snoring and/or increased respiratory effort resulting from increased upper airway resistance and pharyngeal collapsibility [1–3]. It is estimated that 1–4% of children aged between 2 and 8 years have OSA. However, the prevalence may be as high as 80% in children with coexisting medical conditions, such as Trisomy 21 [4,5]. The prevalence of OSA is rising due to the increase in obesity rates in children [6].

Obstructive sleep apnea in children is caused by anatomic upper airway narrowing and/or increased upper airway collapsibility. Previous research showed that children with OSA had narrower pharyngeal airways when compared to control children during wakefulness, sedation, and paralysis. A smaller cranial base angle, longer lower facial height, mandibular retrognathia, a narrower dental arch, and various additional dental arch deformations, such as an anterior open bite, are cephalometric features that contribute to OSA. Children with OSA have dynamic inspiratory airway narrowing during tidal breathing in addition to the effect of increased soft tissue volumes on the static dimensions of the pharyngeal airway. The airway collapse can happen at different levels of the pharynx [7]. Drug-induced sleep endoscopy (DISE) refers to a flexible UA endoscopy performed during a sedative state that allows for a dynamic and three-dimensional evaluation of the entire upper airway. DISE helps to decide if there is a need for further surgical intervention other than adenotonsillectomy for treatment of OSA, specifically for post-adenotonsillectomy children, and what kind of intervention should be indicated for an individual patient, which may help to personalize treatment [8].

Depending on a child's craniofacial morphology, tonsillar and adenoidal growth, and body habitus, as well as whether rhinitis symptoms are present, childhood OSA may consist of various overlapping phenotypes. Additionally, children with the same severity of OSA have variable end-organ morbidity. Compared to nonobese children, who typically present with impaired growth and adenotonsillar hypertrophy between the ages of 2 and 8 years, obese children may present later with symptoms that are more similar to those of adult OSA, such as excessive daytime sleepiness [9,10]. The OSA phenotype in children with complex diseases is determined by anatomical and functional abnormalities that are specific to each underlying disorder, such as Down syndrome and Prader Willi syndrome. It is essential that clinicians consider the symptoms, physical examinations, the presence of risk factors, and signs of end-organ morbidity to diagnose patients and develop a personalized management strategy [11–13].

Snoring, observed apneas, and gasping sounds while sleeping are signs of OSA [1]. Overnight polysomnography (PSG) is used to confirm the OSA diagnosis and the obstructive apnea hypopnea index (oAHI) is the main parameter used to diagnose and define the severity of OSA. However, PSG is associated with a significant financial and healthcare burden and it would be ideal to have a simple, reliable method for identifying children at high risk for OSA. For the purpose of pediatric OSA screening, several questionnaires have been developed. Determining a highly sensitive and focused questionnaire that is simple for patients/parents to complete and for clinicians to assess, however, is still a difficulty, and the sensitivity and specificity of these questionnaires are low [14]. However, pediatric sleep questionnaires are widely used not only to identify children at risk for OSA but also to evaluate response to treatment [15].

Polygraphies are simpler to perform and produce respiratory data comparable to a PSG. Overnight home or hospital use of respiratory polygraphies in children is more common now, much like adult sleep services. According to recent research, respiratory polygraphy can be successfully used with 81–87% of pediatric patients when it has been set up at a medical facility [16]. A recent European Respiratory Society technical standards paper summarized current data on the use of polygraphy in children for diagnosis of sleep-disordered breathing [17].

Although it has limitations, overnight oximetry can be a valuable tool for identifying children with OSA and determining the most urgent treatment needs if polygraphy or PSG are not available. These studies can be performed at home or in the hospital. The use of an appropriate oximeter is essential for correctly interpreting data. Averaging time is a key setting for evaluation of the oximeter's diagnostic effectiveness. According to McGill's system of evaluation, indicators of moderate to severe OSA include at least three clusters of desaturation events and at least three SpO_2 drops below 90% in a nighttime oximetry recording [18]. Although this is not a very sensitive method of diagnosing OSA, it identifies children with moderate to severe disease successfully.

OSA is associated with cardiovascular morbidity and neurobehavioral impairments; therefore, it is important to diagnose and treat OSA in a timely manner [19–21]. Guidelines recommend treatment for children with an oAHI > 5 events/h and with an oAHI of 1–5 events/h in the presence of OSA morbidity or concomitant disease [22,23]. The objectives of OSA treatment in children are to reduce daytime symptoms, improve quality of life and sleep, and avoid short- and long-term consequences [24].

Even though the pathophysiology of pediatric OSA is heterogeneous, the overgrowth of the tonsils and adenoids, which restricts the upper airway during sleep, is the most frequent cause in children, even when associated obesity or complex disorders are present. Therefore, adenotonsillectomy (AT) is commonly the primary treatment option for children with OSA [1,25]. After surgery, OSA may relapse or persist in 21% to 73% of children [26,27]. Additional assessment and medical treatment strategies are frequently required when AT is not indicated or if there is persistent OSA after surgery, as well as when complex medical issues are present. The aim of this review is to summarize the current evidence for medical treatment of children with OSA (Table 1).

Table 1. Medical treatment modalities for obstructive sleep apnea in children.

	Indications and Benefits	Challenges
Anti-inflammatory treatment Nasal steroids/oral montelukast/oral steroids	Children with symptoms of allergic or non-allergic rhinitis may benefit. Anti-inflammatory medications may decrease the size of adenotonsillar tissue, leading to improvement in OSA.	Follow up is necessary Efficacy has to be evaluated due to variety in responses Nasal irritation and bleeding may occur with nasal steroids Montelukast can have adverse effects on behavior and mood
Antibiotics	Currently not recommended	Larger studies are needed to determine the role of antibiotics in the treatment of OSA
Positive airway pressure therapy	Children with moderate to severe OSA who are not candidates for surgery and children with persistent OSA after surgical intervention may benefit	Requires all-night and long-term use Low adherence rates It may be associated with midface hypoplasia
High-flow nasal cannula therapy	Children who cannot tolerate CPAP may benefit from HFNC treatment	Rarely covered by health insurance in many countries No home units recording adherence and no proper alarms
Positional therapy	Can be considered in children with persistent OSA Can be a simple, cheap, and low-risk treatment option	Requires all-night and chronic use Larger studies are needed to demonstrate its effectiveness No adherence data
Myofunctional therapy	Currently not routinely recommended	Requires training and daily exercises
Dental procedures	Recommended in children with narrow transversal maxillary arch, who collaborate in the expansion by turning screws to widen the airway and improve OSA	Effects not clear Long treatment duration Mostly not covered by insurance companies
Weight loss	Efficacious in treating OSA associated with obesity in children If medical treatment of obesity is not achieved, surgical options can be considered	Other treatment modalities should be initiated until enough weight loss has been achieved

2. Anti-Inflammatory Treatment (Nasal Steroids/Montelukast/Oral Steroids) and Antibiotics

Many studies have investigated the effectiveness of anti-inflammatory medications, such as nasal steroids (NSs) or leukotriene receptor antagonists (montelukast), in children with mild to severe OSA since the pathophysiology of the condition has a significant inflammatory component [28]. Research has shown that pediatric adenotonsillar tissues contain glucocorticoid receptors, and children with OSA have increased levels of these receptors [29]. Additionally, leukotriene receptors were found to be expressed in adenotonsillar tissue surgically removed from children with OSA [30]. Therefore, it is plausible that anti-inflammatory medications may decrease the size of adenotonsillar tissue, leading to improvements in OSA.

The aim of NS use is to decrease the volume of adenoids via suppression of inflammation when adenotonsillectomy is contraindicated or in children with mild OSA [1]. A partial reduction in adenoidal hypertrophy has been observed with the administration of NSs for 4 to 6 weeks [31,32]. Sixty-two children underwent a double blind, randomized, controlled study comparing nasal budesonide with a placebo. Following a 6-week treatment with nasal budesonide, the oAHI decreased from 3.7 ± 0.3 to 1.3 ± 0.2 events/h in children with mild OSA. On the other hand, in the placebo group, the oAHI increased from 2.9 ± 0.4 to 4.0 ± 0.4 events/h ($p < 0.0001$). Significant changes were seen in sleep macroarchitecture, such as sleep latency and the percentages of total sleep time spent in slow-wave sleep and rapid-eye-movement sleep ($p < 0.05$). Additionally, there was a long-lasting effect 8 weeks after the end of the treatment [32].

A recent double blind, randomized, controlled trial of NSs for the treatment of OSA in children included 134 children aged 5 to 12 years. Patients were randomized 2:1 to receive 3 months of NSs or a placebo. NS or placebo treatments for 9 months were then randomly reassigned to the children in the NS group. Changes in the oAHI at 3 months (median: −1.72 (interquartile range (IQR): −3.91 to 1.92) events/h) and 12 months (median: −1.2 (IQR: −4.22 to 1.71) events/h) were not different between the two groups ($p = 0.7$). OSA symptoms and neurobehavioral outcomes at 3 and 12 months were also similar between groups. Although there was a statistically significant decrease in the oAHI (7.2 (3.62 to 9.88) events/h to 3.7 (1.56 to 6.4) events/h, $p = 0.39$) in 38 children who received NSs for 12 months, this was not clinically significant [33]. Nasal irritation and bleeding are the two most common adverse effects of NSs. If NSs are administered for a prolonged period, there may be an increased risk of adrenal gland and growth suppression [34].

Gozal et al. included 64 children in a randomized, controlled study evaluating the effect of montelukast therapy. Of the 64 participants, 57 (89.0%) completed the 16-week trial with montelukast or a placebo, and among these, 42 were adherent to the assigned treatment (21 in the montelukast group and 21 in the placebo group). The study revealed that a 16-week treatment with montelukast significantly decreased the severity of OSA in children compared to the placebo. The AHI decreased from 9.2 ± 4.1 events/h to 4.2 ± 2.8 events/h ($p < 0.0001$) in the treatment group, whereas in the placebo group, the AHI increased from 8.2 ± 5.0 events/h to 8.7 ± 4.9 events/h. While 20 pediatric patients who received treatment (71.4%) experienced positive benefits, just 2 (6.9%) of the patients receiving the placebo showed decreases in the AHI ($p < 0.001$). Similarly, the 3% Oxygen Desaturation Index (number of 3% reductions in SpO_2 per hour of sleep) and arousal indices significantly improved in the treatment group, whereas no significant changes occurred in the placebo group [35].

According to a meta-analysis, five studies with 166 children that evaluated montelukast alone for pediatric OSA revealed a 55% improvement in the AHI (mean of 6.2 events/h pre-treatment vs. 2.8 events/h post-treatment), with improvement in the lowest oxygen saturation (LSAT) from 89.5% to 92.1%. Two studies with 502 children evaluating the effects of montelukast with NSs on pediatric OSA found a 70% improvement in the AHI (4.7 events/h pre-treatment vs. 1.4 events/h post-treatment), with an improvement in LSAT from 87.8% to 92.6% [36]. However, it should be noted that montelukast has significant adverse effects on mood and behavior, and the FDA has published a boxed warning for this medication [37]. Before initiation of treatment, clinicians should assess the risks and benefits and inform the families of these risks.

Since enlarged adenoids and tonsils are composed of hypertrophic lymphoid tissue, anti-inflammatory medications, such as systemic corticosteroids, have been evaluated for treatment of children with OSA. Evangelisti et al. evaluated the effect of systemic steroids in 28 children (mean age: 4.5 ± 1.8 years) with OSA. Fifteen children received oral betamethasone (0.1 mg/kg per day) in addition to NS therapy for 7 days in group one, while 13 children received NSs for 21 days in group two. The sleep clinical record score (12.6 ± 1.2 vs. 8.3 ± 1.1, $p = 0.0001$), oxygen desaturation index (11.7 vs. 3.0, $p < 0.0001$), oxygen desaturation time < 90% (1.75 vs. 0.0, $p < 0.0001$), oxygen desaturation events < 90% (25.5 vs. 1.0 $p < 0.0001$), and mean (95.3 ± 1.1 vs. $97.0 \pm 0.8\%$, $p = 0.0001$) and minimum SpO_2 (78.8 ± 6.3 vs. 89.2 ± 4.2, $p = 0.001$) improved in children treated with NSs and oral betamethasone. The authors recommended the use of systemic steroids as a bridging therapy prior to AT therapy in children with severe OSA [38].

Various microorganisms have been isolated from patients with chronic tonsillar hypertrophy. There has been limited research supporting the use of broad-spectrum antibiotics to treat pediatric OSA. In a study involving 22 children with OSA and adenotonsillar hypertrophy, researchers divided the patients into two groups. The first group, consisting of

11 children, received 30 days of azithromycin therapy, and the second group of 11 children received 30 days of placebo treatment. The AHI decreased by -0.97 ± 2.09 events/h in the azithromycin group but increased by 3.41 ± 3.01 events/h in the placebo group ($p = 0.23$). The baseline and maximum end-tidal carbon dioxide pressure, the baseline and LSAT, and the number of pathological central apneas did not change significantly. The authors concluded that broad-spectrum antibiotic therapy may not be an appropriate alternative to surgery and that larger studies are needed to determine the role of antibiotics in the treatment of OSA [39].

A paranasal sinus infection that lasts for more than three months is referred to as chronic sinusitis. Children with chronic sinusitis may have biofilms in their nasopharynx that serve as long-term reservoirs for bacteria that are resistant to common antibiotics. A previous study revealed that extensive biofilm formations on the adenoids of children with chronic sinusitis and those with obstructive sleep apnea raise the possibility that the generation of biofilms may be a virulence factor for the organisms that cause the disease [40]. Despite the fact that broad-spectrum oral antibiotics are frequently used to treat infections, chronic rhinosinusitis may not respond to antibiotic therapy with a permanent or sustained improvement. There is currently no agreement on the optimal treatment duration, organism coverage, or antibiotics due to the large range of aerobic and anaerobic organisms cultivated from the paranasal sinuses. However, high-dose antibiotics are typically used for a minimum of three weeks, whereas adenoidectomy can mechanically eliminate infection [40].

3. Positive Airway Pressure

It is important to consider that residual OSA may remain even after surgical intervention, especially in children with complex disorders, such as Trisomy 21, Prader–Willi syndrome, or obesity [27,41]. Children who are not candidates for surgery, most children with cranio-facial anomalies, and children with persistent OSA after adenotonsillectomy are usually started on positive airway pressure (PAP) therapy. A study by Kearney et al. found that the majority of adolescents with obesity (74%) had severe OSA (AHI $\geq$ 10 events/h) with a mean baseline AHI of 33.9 events/h. After AT, the AHI levels in the obese and control groups both showed clinically significant improvements with median changes of 18.3 events/h ($p < 0.001$) and 14.6 events/h ($p < 0.001$), respectively. A total of 48% of the obese adolescent patients had an AHI < 5 events/h on postoperative PSGs. However, compared to patients who were not obese, adolescents with obesity were seven times more likely to have moderate or severe persistent OSA (AHI > 5 events/h) after AT ($p = 0.001$). Adolescents with obesity had a considerably higher requirement for post-AT PAP therapy (37.1% of patients required PAP, $p < 0.001$) [42].

A device that can produce various levels of PAP, expressed in centimeters of water pressure, is used for PAP therapy. By using a pneumatic splint for the soft tissues of the upper airway, PAP treatment sustains airway stability throughout the breathing cycle [1]. It aims to regulate sleep architecture, increase sleep quality, and alleviate daytime symptoms caused by inadequate sleep.

A mask known as an interface connects the patient to the PAP treatment device. Finding an interface with a good fit that ensures comfort and optimal air leakage for the patient is crucial. However, there are no standards for choosing the right interface. Age and facial morphology are the most important factors when choosing an interface. This can be difficult, particularly for infants and children with asymmetry or facial deformity. Each interface has an intentional leak built in to avoid carbon dioxide rebreathing. An interface should have a good seal, minimal resistance to airflow, low dead space volume, and the optimal unintended leakage. Children can use nasal pillows and nasal and oronasal masks as interfaces for PAP therapy. Nasal masks are commonly preferred, as oronasal masks carry the risk of aspiration. Since nasal pillows fit right into the nares, they may be a good option for teens and are well tolerated. Children with OSA should be evaluated for nasal obstruction before initiating PAP therapy. If soft tissue obstruction is noted, medical treatment, such as NSs or montelukast, should be considered [35,36,43]. Improving nasal breathing can enhance the efficiency and tolerability of PAP therapy [44,45]. The nose and mouth are both covered by an oronasal interface. There are challenges when using an oronasal mask. The pressure from the mask on the jaw may produce posterior displacement and exacerbate the obstruction of the upper airway. Furthermore, if the child has muscle weakness or is young and unable to remove the mask in cases of vomiting, there is a danger of aspiration. Patients tend to tolerate the mask less well and are more likely to feel claustrophobic [46]. Furthermore, oronasal masks with the same pressure were not as effective as nasal masks in a study that evaluated adults with OSA using DISE [47]. However, there are limited data regarding the performance of interfaces in children [48]. In a study by Ramirez et al., no differences were detected in PAP adherence, correction of nocturnal gas exchange abnormalities, or leak values with the usage of nasal and oronasal masks in a retrospective analysis of 62 children (>2 years of age) [49].

The eyes, nose, and mouth are covered with a full-face mask. The pressure points for this contact are farther away than with normal interfaces, which is a benefit. Skin erythema and midface hypoplasia are mostly avoided. Given the significant dead space, patients should be clinically evaluated while using this mask to confirm that CO_2 is not being re-breathed, especially in younger children. Additionally, if there is a risk of aspiration or if the child has increased oral secretions, full face masks should be avoided to prevent aspiration. These masks are mostly used in acute care of children with respiratory failure.

PAP therapy can be administered as continuous positive airway pressure (CPAP) or bi-level positive airway pressure (BPAP). CPAP prevents the collapse of the upper airway by continuously applying pressure at one level throughout the breathing cycle. It does not assist with the inspiration of the patient but improves gas exchange and oxygenation by increasing functional residual capacity [50]. BPAP provides assistance during inspiration by delivering cycling pressure. The ventilator's high airflow rate augments the patient's efforts to inhale. Therefore, it should be administered in accordance with the patient's breathing efforts. The three main objectives of inspiratory positive airway pressure (IPAP) are to decrease the work of breathing, the respiratory rate, and $PaCO_2$. The main objectives of the expiratory positive airway pressure (EPAP) are to increase oxygenation, decrease intrinsic PEEP, and remove upper airway obstruction. If the child needs a high expiratory pressure and cannot tolerate CPAP or has substantial hypoventilation that does not improve with CPAP use, BPAP can be used to treat OSA [51].

In BPAP devices, four different modes can be provided [46]. The mode of therapy is chosen depending on the patient's breathing pattern and the underlying disorder. The spontaneous BPAP mode (BPAP-S) is used for children who are intolerant of CPAP at high pressures due to discomfort at exhalation. In this mode, each breath is started by the patient, higher inspiratory pressure and lower expiratory pressure are used, and there is no back-up rate. The spontaneous-timed BPAP mode (BPAP-ST) is used for children who present with mixed apnea, CPAP emergent central apnea, or persistent hypoventilation following resolution of OSA with CPAP. In this mode, a back-up rate, which is usually 2–4 breaths lower than the patient's own respiratory rate, is employed [52]. The patient initiates the breaths and the device only delivers a breath when the patient's spontaneous respiratory rate drops below the pre-set back-up rate. In the pressure control mode, there is a set inspiratory time for both ventilator and spontaneous breaths. In the timed mode, which is rarely used in children, the device controls the patient's breathing rate and inspiratory times regardless of the patient effort. PAP treatment has been linked to significant clinical advantages, such as decreased risk of cardiovascular disease and reduction in insulin resistance [53–55].

A novel mode of ventilation known as the volume-assured pressure support (VAPS) BPAP mode provides automatically titrating pressure support that is designed to achieve a tidal volume goal. It has been shown to be useful for children with obesity hypoventilation syndrome and congenital central hypoventilation syndrome [52].

A titration sleep study with PAP titration usually precedes the beginning of PAP therapy. In order to prevent respiratory events and improve gas exchange, pressure/mode modifications are implemented during the sleep study. The goals for PAP titration include <2 obstructive apneas per hour, $ETCO_2 < 55$ mmHg and not greater than 50 mmHg for >10 min, $SpO_2 \geq 94\%$, and minimal paradoxical breathing and flow limitation [51]. Additionally, there are auto-adjusting CPAP/BPAP devices that utilize a unique algorithm. These devices might be useful when the severity of OSA is dependent on body posture and/or sleep stage [56]. CPAP titration with an auto-CPAP device in the home environment can be considered for children when access to a sleep laboratory is limited [57].

After initiation of PAP therapy, regular follow-up is necessary to ensure adequate therapy as the efficacy of PAP therapy is limited by low adherence. In children, physical discomfort and/or fear of the device may cause low adherence. Usage in the first week of treatment may predict longer-term use, and monitoring adherence in the first week of treatment and intervening in cases of low adherence may improve long-term CPAP use [58]. The largest PAP adherence analysis of pediatric patients with OSA was published in 2020 [59]. A total of 20,553 patients with a mean age of 13 years met the eligibility criteria and had accessible data. Based on 90 days of monitoring data, 12,699 patients (61%) used PAP continuously. However, only 46.3% of the cohort met the Centers for Medicare and Medicaid Services' adherence requirements after 90 days. This adherence was poorer than that shown in the results from studies using similar methodologies to measure adherence in adults. Additionally, this study suggested that children between the ages of 4 and 6 years and adolescents between the ages of 15 and 18 years might require more assistance than other age groups, necessitating age-specific behavioral interventions. As children spend more hours in sleep, using adult criteria for adherence may not be sufficient to prevent adverse consequences in children with OSA.

Developmental delay, female gender, and younger age are associated with better PAP compliance [60,61]. A recent study compared the efficacy and challenges of PAP therapy adherence in infants and school-aged children with OSA [62]. A total of 41 infants and 109 school-aged children were included in the study. After PAP titration, infants' oAHI levels decreased on average by 92.1%, while school-aged children's oAHI levels decreased on average by 93.4% (0 = 0.67). The same types of challenges for adherence were reported in infants and school-aged children, with behavioral issues being the most prevalent in both populations. Another study included 137 typically developing (TD) children and 103 children with developmental disabilities (DDs). At 3 and 6 months, the percentage of nights when devices were used was significantly higher for children with DDs ($p = 0.01$, $p = 0.003$, respectively). Hours of usage on nights when the devices were used at three and six months were similar between groups (DD group = 5.0, TD group = 4.6, $p = 0.71$; DD group = 6.4, TD group = 5.7, $p = 0.34$, respectively). Higher PAP was strongly predictive for hours of usage in both groups at 6 months, while higher median neighborhood income and titration at or before 6 months were significantly predictive of percentage of nights when devices were used [63].

In addition to the assistance provided by medical staff, the patient's environment and family at home are crucial for adherence. Marcus et al. found a high drop-out rate (35%), consistently low overnight use duration (5.3 h/night), and significant over-reporting of compliance by families in research on PAP adherence in children [64]. Another study on PAP compliance among pediatric patients revealed that <60% of patients adhered to recommended schedules ranging from 4.0 to 5.2 h per night [60]. Facemask discomfort contributed to low compliance. Teenagers' adherence to PAP therapy can be encouraged by support groups, phone applications, behavioral therapy, and motivational interviewing methods [65]. A systematic review showed that children with caregiver support had significantly longer CPAP use per night (by 86.60 min) and significantly higher percentages of CPAP usage for more than 4 h/night (by 18.10%) than those without caregiver support. Although data showing better compliance with BPAP mostly come from studies on adults, there is some evidence that supports this in children as well. When compared to those who received CPAP therapy, children who received BPAP therapy had an 18.17 times higher likelihood of having good PAP adherence [66]. Adherence to CPAP or BPAP therapy should be monitored by using the device software [67].

Although adverse effects of PAP therapy are mostly minor, it is important to address these issues to improve adherence. Air leaks frequently cause discomfort. Abdominal distension, oronasal dryness, eye irritation, and pressure sores on the nasal bridge caused by the masks may be seen in children. It is often recommended to use a humidifier to reduce discomfort caused by cold, dry air. Additionally, the midface may flatten as a result of the mask's continuous pressure on the growing facial tissues [68]. It is very important to make sure that the mask fits gently on the face rather than being firmly fixed to reduce the impact on the midface.

4. High-Flow Nasal Cannula Therapy

High-flow nasal cannula (HFNC) treatment has been used to treat neonates with respiratory distress linked to prematurity in neonatal intensive care units with varying but generally positive effects, including decreased effort in breathing and lower rates of respiratory failure [69,70]. HFNC therapy delivers humidified and heated air at a high flow rate via nasal prongs. Continuous positive pressure is produced in the airways by the HFNC, and oxygen is continuously pushed into the upper airways at a rate that is higher than the typical inspiratory flow rate (approximately 4–7 cm H_2O at maximal flow rates), preventing upper airway collapse [71–73].

Children with OSA who cannot tolerate the CPAP masks may benefit from HFNC treatment [74]. Pediatric OSA has been successfully treated with high-flow heated, humidified nasal air [28,75–77]. Ten children (1–18 years) with obstructive sleep apnea determined to be CPAP-intolerant by their caregivers were included in a study by Hawkins et al. High-flow humidified room air was initially delivered at rates of 5 to 15 L/min with pediatric or adult-sized cannulas and then gradually increased. If hypoxemia or desaturations persisted at the maximum rate of room air, oxygen was added. This study showed that HFNCs can successfully treat moderate to severe obstructive sleep apnea in CPAP-intolerant children (the oAHI improved from 11.1 to 2.1 events/h, $p = 0.002$; the obstructive hypopnea index improved from 9.9 to 0.5 events/h, $p = 0.002$) [78].

A total of 22 patients (mean age: 12.8 months) who had persistent OSA after adenotonsillectomy with CPAP intolerance, whose caregivers refused to use CPAP, or who were not good surgical candidates were included in a retrospective study. The HFNC titration study was performed an average of 128 days after the diagnostic sleep study. The oAHI decreased from 28.9 to 2.6 events/h, the oAI decreased from 14.4 to 0.4 events/h, and the OHI decreased from 14.5 to 2.2 events/h. In this study, HFNCs not only improved sleep parameters but were also well tolerated. The majority of patients adhered to their HFNC therapy throughout a 12-month period of home use. Cannula dislodgement was the most common complication of home HFNC therapy, as observed in 12 patients (63%). The authors suggested that HFNCs could be used as a temporary bridge therapy to treat OSA before surgery or an alternative long-term treatment [79]. Although HFNC use at home is currently limited and costly, use of HFNCs for OSA at home may become an option in the near future.

5. Positional Therapy

In positional OSA (POSA), the OSA occurs mostly while sleeping in the supine position, and this is known to affect 19–58% of children with OSA [80,81]. Obese children may have more profound upper airway obstruction during supine sleep, as greater fat deposition in the pharyngeal region results in a smaller upper airway [82]. POSA occurs when the supine AHI is at least two times higher than the non-supine AHI [80]. Decreased craniofacial volume, decreased lung volume, and the inability of the airway dilator muscles to prevent airway collapse during an occlusion may occur in the supine position [83–85]. A study by Selvadurai et al. evaluated 112 obese children with PSG, and 43 (38%) children had

OSA. Among those with OSA, 25 (58%) had POSA (mean age: 14.6 ± 2.3 years; mean body mass index: 37.7 ± 7.6 kg/m2; 68% male) and 18 (42%) had non-POSA (mean age: 13.9 ± 2.8 years; mean body mass index: 37.9 ± 7.2 kg/m2; 78% male). Among those with POSA, 13 (52%) had mild OSA, 7 (28%) had moderate OSA, and 5 (20%) had severe OSA. There were no significant differences in age, sex, or anthropometric measures between the POSA and non-POSA groups. However, older children were more likely to have POSA; 88% of the children with POSA were 12 years or older ($p = 0.41$) [81].

The capacity to sustain comfortable non-supine sleep is a requirement for positional therapy (PT) in children. A belt worn around the chest with pillows on the back to stop children from adopting the supine posture may be an effective treatment option for POSA. For children with persistent OSA, PT can be a simple, cheap, and low-risk treatment option. Children between the ages of 4 and 18 years with POSA who had a baseline PSG and a second PSG to assess the effectiveness of a positional device were included in a study by Xiao et al. [83]. The median body mass index z-score was 1.6. Compared to the baseline data, PSG results obtained while using a positional device showed reductions in the median oAHI (15.2 vs. 6.7 events/h, respectively; $p = 0.004$) and in the percentage of total sleep time in supine position (54.4 vs. 4.2 h, respectively; $p = 0.04$) [86]. More studies are needed but, considering the cost effectiveness and non-invasive nature of this treatment, positional therapy may be a viable option for children with POSA.

6. Myofunctional Therapy

Persistent oral breathing during sleep may affect the strength of the tongue and orofacial muscles, leading to abnormal airway development and OSA [39]. Myofunctional therapy (MT) is based on isotonic and isometric exercises that enhance the orofacial tissues' coordination and strength [87]. MT involves multiple tongue, soft palate, and facial muscle exercises. Daily practice of these exercises strengthens the orofacial muscles. A study by Villa et al. revealed that MT improved tongue tone and decreased respiratory symptoms and oral breathing during sleep in all 36 children with sleep-disorder breathing [88]. Another investigation on children with mild persistent OSA revealed that MT decreased OSA severity in 14 children after 2 months compared to 13 controls (decrease in oAHI of 58% in the MT group vs. 6.9% in the control group; $p = 0.004$). However, more studies are needed with children before MT can be widely used.

7. Dental Procedures

Although it has been suggested that a subset of craniofacial characteristics, including increased facial height, retrognathia, and a higher mandibular angle, may be more frequently present in children with OSA, a recent meta-analysis of nine studies revealed that, although a certain subgroup of pediatric OSA patients showed higher rates of specific craniofacial characteristics, this was not consistent across studies [89]. The authors concluded that there is insufficient evidence to report a link between pediatric cases of OSA and craniofacial morphology [90].

Rapid maxillary expansion (RME) is a type of orthodontic treatment that widens the hard palate by expanding the airway using a dental device, beginning around age four and continuing until the midpalatal suture fuses in adolescence [8]. According to the results of a meta-analysis, improvements in AHI and lowest oxygen saturation levels were observed in children who underwent RME treatment, particularly at short-term (3-year) follow-up [91]. Thirty children with OSA were included in a study by Hoxha et al.; fifteen were enrolled as the control group, while fifteen received semi-rapid maxillary expansion (SRME) orthodontic treatment for 5 months. In addition to respiratory parameters, the pharyngeal area, dental arch, postero-anterior widths, and OSA biomarker levels (ORM2, FABP4, perlecan, gelsolin, KLK1, and uric acid) in serum and urine were measured. The AHI decreased from 2.5 to 1.79 events/h (28% decrease, $p < 0.05$) after a 5-month treatment period, while it decreased from 2.67 to 1.8 events/h (33% decrease, $p < 0.05$) in the control group [92]. A recent systematic review compared the effect of RME to watchful waiting or alternative therapies for pediatric OSA and included five trials. Only one randomized clinical trial compared RME with watchful waiting. The other four studies (three of them were non-randomized) compared RME with the gold-standard therapy AT. There was no evidence that RME treatment significantly outperformed watchful waiting in patients with pediatric OSA in this systematic review. It was concluded that the non-homogeneous distribution of confounders and inadequate designs made comparisons between treatment alternatives difficult. Further studies are needed to compare the effect of RME to that of watchful waiting [93].

8. Weight Loss

Obesity is a risk factor for developing OSA [94]. OSA has been diagnosed in 13–59% of obese children [95]. A total of 139 children with a median age of 4.5 years were included in a study where 25 of the children were overweight and 21 were obese. The study revealed that, regardless of age or prior upper airway surgery, a one-unit increase in BMI z-score was associated with 67% increased odds of circumferential collapse during drug-induced sleep endoscopy (DISE). The authors reported that this circumferential pattern may be less sensitive to AT and that nonsurgical treatments, such as CPAP and weight loss, may be necessary in these patients. Other treatment approaches should be started until enough weight loss has been achieved since this treatment modality requires a motivated patient and family and the process might be slow [1]. The success rates and cure rates of DISE-directed treatment were similar in children who were normal weight, overweight, and obese [96].

In a study of 339 obese children with a median age of 15.4 years, after an average 32% decrease in BMI z-score, 80% of the children showed improved sleep-disordered breathing [97]. Ten studies conducted on participants with an age range of 10–19 years were included in a meta-analysis that evaluated the prevalence and severity of OSA in obese children, as well as the impact of weight loss strategies. There was an improvement in OSA prevalence post-intervention, and OSA was cured in 46.2–79.7% of the participants. The meta-analysis showed significant reductions in the AHI (effect size: -0.51, 95%CI -0.94 to -0.08, $p = 0.019$) and oxygen desaturation index (effect size: -0.28, 95%CI = -0.50 to -0.05, $p = 0.016$). Seventy-five percent of the studies reported improved sleep duration in participants with OSA [98].

As management of childhood obesity with diet and exercise alone is challenging, several drugs (metformin, glucagon-like peptide-1 receptor agonists, and phentermine-topiramate) have been studied to treat pediatric obesity. Liraglutide and exenatide are the most commonly investigated medications in terms of weight loss in adults. A randomized, double-blind, placebo-controlled trial evaluated the efficacy and safety of subcutaneous liraglutide 3.0 mg as an addition to lifestyle therapy for weight management in adolescents with obesity. Individuals (age 12 to 18 years) with obesity and a poor response to lifestyle changes alone were included to the study. There were 126 participants in the placebo group and 125 in the liraglutide group. With an estimated difference of 0.22, liraglutide exceeded the placebo in terms of the BMI standard deviation score change from baseline at week 56. A decrease in BMI of at least 5% was seen in 43.3% of the liraglutide group and 18.5% of placebo group participants; a decrease in BMI of at least 10% was seen in 33% and 9% of participants, respectively [99].

The phentermine/topiramate extended-release capsule is a fixed-dose combination of phentermine and topiramate developed for the treatment of obesity, sleep apnea syndrome, and type 2 diabetes mellitus. The once-daily formulation of phentermine and topiramate is designed to combat obesity by decreasing appetite and increasing satiety. Phentermine/topiramate has received its first US approval for chronic weight management in pediatric patients aged ≥ 12 years with a BMI in the 95th percentile or greater for age and sex in combination with a low-calorie diet and increased physical activity. Clinical development of phentermine/topiramate for sleep apnea syndrome and type 2 diabetes in obese patients is ongoing in the US, and it may be a treatment option in children with OSA related to obesity in the future [100].

Bariatric surgery has been found to be beneficial in decreasing excess weight and alleviating comorbidities in adolescents with severe obesity. A retrospective study was conducted in adolescents with morbid obesity who underwent laparoscopic adjustable gastric band (LAGB) surgery between 1995 and 2018. Fifty-nine adolescents (mean age: 17.7 ± 1.5 years, mean BMI: 40.9 ± 6.4) were included in the study. Sixty-nine percent of the adolescents with morbid obesity who had OSA at baseline showed resolution of the OSA at one-year follow up after bariatric surgery (the mean BMI was lower at 34.4 ± 6.3 kg/m^2). In seven adolescents with OSA (mean age: 17.8 years), bariatric surgery reduced the oAHI from 13 ± 6.9 events/h to 4.5 ± 2.5 events/h ($p < 0.05$) at 3 weeks post-operatively [101]. However, it should be noted that there are limited data on the long-term efficacy and safety of bariatric surgery in adolescents.

Considering the significant effects of obesity on OSA and the poor response to adenotonsillectomy in children with obesity, weight loss should be part of the treatment plan for all children with obesity and OSA.

9. Hypoglossal Nerve Stimulation

The recurrent collapse of the upper airway during sleep is a hallmark of obstructive sleep apnea. The contraction of the upper airway dilator muscles maintains the patency of the upper airways. Although there are numerous muscles that dilate the upper airways, the most significant upper airway dilator muscle is the genioglossus muscle. The hypoglossal nerve innervates the genioglossus muscle, and hypoglossal nerve stimulation has been successfully used with adults with moderate to severe OSA who cannot tolerate CPAP therapy [102].

OSA is common in people with Down syndrome, with a prevalence of 55–97% and a high risk of persistent OSA following adenotonsillectomy, and this population usually have low adherence rates to CPAP therapy [103]. Therefore, hypoglossal nerve stimulation use may be helpful in children with Down syndrome and persistent OSA who have low adherence to CPAP therapy. In a meta-analysis of nine articles involving 106 adolescents with Down syndrome and OSA, there was an improvement in the AHI by at least 50% when patients were treated with hypoglossal nerve stimulation. Participants also showed improvements in the OSA-18 (a validated, disease-specific quality of life instrument for OSA) and in daytime sleepiness measured with Epworth Sleepiness Scale questionnaires [104].

A recent study investigated four participants who underwent hypoglossal nerve implantation by age 13 and completed at least 44 months of follow-up. Over the follow-up period, all four participants' AHI levels remained at least 50% lower than they were at baseline. Two participants had persistent, moderate OSA despite stimulation therapy. The other two participants achieved 100% reductions in AHI levels with stimulation therapy; when they underwent split-night sleep studies, the severe OSA persisted with the device turned off [105,106].

10. Novel Pharmacotherapeutics

A selective norepinephrine reuptake inhibitor, atomoxetine, has been used to treat both adults and children with attention deficit hyperactivity disorder. Raising the norepinephrine content in the brainstem during sleep could activate the upper airway motorneurons to levels equivalent to those reported during wakefulness. An in vitro experiment revealed that atomoxetine also blocks G-coupled inwardly rectifying potassium channels, which are important in pharyngeal hypotonia during sleep. Oxybutynin, an antimuscarinic with strong affinity for all muscarinic receptors, is used to treat overactive bladder. Acetylcholine affects the hypoglossal motor nucleus in a variety of ways, with muscarinic-mediated genioglossus suppression typically outweighing nicotinic stimulation. Muscarinic blockade may increase the concentration of acetylcholine for nicotinic receptors and decrease the inhibitory effect of acetylcholine on upper airway muscle tone during

REM sleep, collaborating with norepinephrine in the stimulation of upper airway dilator muscles. The hypoglossal motor nucleus expresses the inhibitory muscarinic receptor that oxybutynin antagonizes. This receptor is crucial for controlling the activity of the hypoglossal nerve [107,108]. Twenty adults (median age of 53 (46–58) years and BMI of 34.8 (30.0–40.2) kg/m^2) participated in a randomized, placebo-controlled, double-blind crossover trial that compared 80 mg of atomoxetine and 5 mg of oxybutynin (ato-oxy) given before sleep versus a placebo for one night. This combination therapy lowered the AHI by 63% (34–86%) from 28.5 (10.9–51.6) events/h to 7.5 (2.4–18.6) events/h ($p = 0.001$) and increased genioglossus muscle responsiveness [107]. A trial is currently being conducted to investigate the effectiveness and safety of treating persistent OSA in children with Down syndrome with atomoxetine and oxybutynin (NCT04115878).

In conclusion, although adenotonsillectomy remains the primary treatment for children with OSA, there are medical treatment options that can be considered. As we acquire increased understanding of the phenotypes and endotypes of OSA in children, it will be possible to use the existing and emerging therapies in an individualized fashion.

Author Contributions: A.P.E.: writing—original draft preparation; Y.G.: writing—original draft preparation, writing—review and editing, supervision; R.E.: writing—review and editing, project administration, supervision. All authors have read and agreed to the published version of the manuscript.

Funding: This research received no external funding.

Institutional Review Board Statement: Not applicable.

Informed Consent Statement: Not applicable.

Data Availability Statement: Data available in a publicly accessible repository.

Conflicts of Interest: The authors declare no conflict of interest.

Abbreviations

OSA	obstructive sleep apnea
AHI	apnea–hypopnea index
oAHI	obstructive apnea hypopnea index
AT	adenotonsillectomy
NCS	nasal corticosteroid
LSAT	lowest oxygen saturation
PAP	positive airway pressure
CPAP	continuous positive airway pressure
BPAP	bi-level positive airway pressure
BPAP-ST	spontaneous-timed BPAP mode
BPAP-S	spontaneous BPAP mode
IPAP	inspiratory positive airway pressure
EPAP	expiratory positive airway pressure
VAPS	volume-assured pressure support
HFNC	high-flow nasal cannula
POSA	positional OSA
PT	positional therapy
MT	myofunctional therapy
RME	rapid maxillary expansion
SRME	semi-rapid maxillary expansion
BMI	body mass index

References

1. Marcus, C.L.; Brooks, L.J.; Draper, K.A.; Gozal, D.; Halbower, A.C.; Jones, J.; Schechter, M.S.; Ward, S.D.; Sheldon, S.H.; Shiffman, R.N. Diagnosis and management of childhood obstructive sleep apnea syndrome. *Pediatrics* **2012**, *130*, 576–584. [CrossRef] [PubMed]
2. Javaheri, S.; Barbe, F.; Campos-Rodriguez, F.; Dempsey, J.A.; Khayat, R.; Javaheri, S.; Malhotra, A.; Martinez-Garcia, M.A.; Mehra, R.; Pack, A.I.; et al. Sleep Apnea: Types, Mechanisms, and Clinical Cardiovascular Consequences. *J. Am. Coll. Cardiol.* **2017**, *69*, 841–858. [CrossRef] [PubMed]
3. Kaditis, A.G.; Alvarez, M.L.A.; Boudewyns, A.; Alexopoulos, E.I.; Ersu, R.; Joosten, K.; Larramona, H.; Miano, S.; Narang, I.; Trang, H.; et al. Obstructive sleep disordered breathing in 2- to 18-year-old children: Diagnosis and management. *Eur. Respir. J.* **2015**, *47*, 69–94. [CrossRef]
4. Lumeng, J.C.; Chervin, R.D. Epidemiology of Pediatric Obstructive Sleep Apnea. *Proc. Am. Thorac. Soc.* **2008**, *5*, 242–252. [CrossRef] [PubMed]
5. Lee, C.-H.; Hsueh, W.-Y.; Lin, M.-T.; Kang, K.-T. Prevalence of Obstructive Sleep Apnea in Children With Down Syndrome: A Meta-Analysis. *J. Clin. Sleep Med.* **2018**, *14*, 867–875. [CrossRef] [PubMed]
6. Arens, R.; Muzumdar, H.; Wootton, D.M.; Sin, S.; Luo, H.; Yazdani, A.; McDonough, J.M.; Wagshul, M.E.; Isasi, C.R. Childhood obesity and obstructive sleep apnea syndrome. *J. Appl. Physiol.* **2010**, *108*, 436–444. [CrossRef] [PubMed]
7. Vos, W.G.; De Backer, W.A.; Verhulst, S.L. Correlation between the severity of sleep apnea and upper airway morphology in pediatric and adult patients. *Curr. Opin. Allergy Clin. Immunol.* **2010**, *10*, 26–33. [CrossRef]
8. Ersu, R.; Chen, M.L.; Ehsan, Z.; Ishman, S.L.; Redline, S.; Narang, I. Persistent obstructive sleep apnoea in children: Treatment options and management considerations. *Lancet Respir. Med.* **2022**, *11*, 283–296. [CrossRef]
9. Gozal, D.; Kheirandish-Gozal, L. Childhood obesity and sleep: Relatives, partners, or both a critical perspective on the evidence. *Ann. N. Y. Acad. Sci.* **2012**, *1264*, 135–141. [CrossRef]
10. Au, C.T.; Zhang, J.; Cheung, J.Y.F.; Chan, K.C.C.; Wing, Y.K.; Li, A.M. Familial aggregation and heritability of obstructive sleep apnea using children probands. *J. Clin. Sleep Med.* **2019**, *15*, 1561–1570. [CrossRef]
11. Kamal, M.; Tamana, S.K.; Smithson, L.; Ding, L.; Lau, A.; Chikuma, J.; Mariasine, J.; Lefebvre, D.L.; Subbarao, P.; Becker, A.B.; et al. Phenotypes of sleep-disordered breathing symptoms to two years of age based on age of onset and duration of symptoms. *Sleep Med.* **2018**, *48*, 93–100. [CrossRef] [PubMed]
12. Tan, H.; Kaditis, A.G. Phenotypic variance in pediatric obstructive sleep apnea. *Pediatr. Pulmonol.* **2021**, *56*, 1754–1762. [CrossRef] [PubMed]
13. Gaines, J.; Vgontzas, A.N.; Fernandez-Mendoza, J.; Bixler, E.O. Obstructive sleep apnea and the metabolic syndrome: The road to clinically-meaningful phenotyping, improved prognosis, and personalized treatment. *Sleep Med. Rev.* **2018**, *42*, 211–219. [CrossRef]
14. Abumuamar, A.M.; Chung, S.A.; Kadmon, G.; Shapiro, C.M. A comparison of two screening tools for paediatric obstructive sleep apnea. *J. Sleep Res.* **2017**, *27*, e12610. [CrossRef]
15. Pabary, R.; Goubau, C.; Russo, K.; Laverty, A.; Abel, F.; Samuels, M. Screening for sleep-disordered breathing with Pediatric Sleep Questionnaire in children with underlying conditions. *J. Sleep Res.* **2018**, *28*, e12826. [CrossRef]
16. Ioan, I.; Weick, D.; Schweitzer, C.; Guyon, A.; Coutier, L.; Franco, P. Feasibility of parent-attended ambulatory polysomnography in children with suspected obstructive sleep apnea. *J. Clin. Sleep Med.* **2020**, *16*, 1013–1019. [CrossRef] [PubMed]
17. Riha, R.L.; Celmina, M.; Cooper, B.; Hamutcu-Ersu, R.; Kaditis, A.; Morley, A.; Pataka, A.; Penzel, T.; Roberti, L.; Ruehland, W.; et al. ERS technical standards for using type III devices (limited channel studies) in the diagnosis of sleep disordered breathing in adults and children. *Eur. Respir. J.* **2023**, *61*, 2200422. [CrossRef] [PubMed]
18. Trucco, F.; Rosenthal, M.; Bush, A.; Tan, H.-L. The McGill score as a screening test for obstructive sleep disordered breathing in children with co-morbidities. *Sleep Med.* **2019**, *68*, 173–176. [CrossRef] [PubMed]
19. Hunter, S.J.; Gozal, D.; Smith, D.L.; Philby, M.F.; Kaylegian, J.; Kheirandish-Gozal, L. Effect of Sleep-disordered Breathing Severity on Cognitive Performance Measures in a Large Community Cohort of Young School-aged Children. *Am. J. Respir. Crit. Care Med.* **2016**, *194*, 739–747. [CrossRef]
20. Narang, I.; McCrindle, B.W.; Manlhiot, C.; Lu, Z.; Al-Saleh, S.; Birken, C.S.; Hamilton, J. Intermittent nocturnal hypoxia and metabolic risk in obese adolescents with obstructive sleep apnea. *Sleep Breath.* **2018**, *22*, 1037–1044. [CrossRef]
21. Baker-Smith, C.M.; Isaiah, A.; Melendres, M.C.; Mahgerefteh, J.; Lasso-Pirot, A.; Mayo, S.; Gooding, H.; Zachariah, J. Sleep-Disordered Breathing and Cardiovascular Disease in Children and Adolescents: A Scientific Statement From the American Heart Association. *J. Am. Heart Assoc.* **2021**, *10*, e022427. [CrossRef]
22. Accardo, J.A.; Shults, J.; Leonard, M.B.; Traylor, J.; Marcus, C.L. Differences in Overnight Polysomnography Scores Using the Adult and Pediatric Criteria for Respiratory Events in Adolescents. *Sleep* **2010**, *33*, 1333–1339. [CrossRef] [PubMed]
23. Berry, R.B.; Budhiraja, R.; Gottlieb, D.J.; Gozal, D.; Iber, C.; Kapur, V.K.; Marcus, C.L.; Mehra, R.; Parthasarathy, S.; Quan, S.F.; et al. Rules for Scoring Respiratory Events in Sleep: Update of the 2007 AASM Manual for the Scoring of Sleep and Associated Events. *J. Clin. Sleep Med.* **2012**, *8*, 597–619. [CrossRef] [PubMed]
24. Wang, J.J.; Imamura, T.; Lee, J.; Wright, M.; Goldman, R.D. Continuous positive airway pressure for obstructive sleep apnea in children. *Can. Fam. Physician* **2021**, *67*, 21–23. [CrossRef] [PubMed]

25. Mitchell, R.B.; Archer, S.M.; Ishman, S.L.; Rosenfeld, R.M.; Coles, S.; Finestone, S.A.; Friedman, N.R.; Giordano, T.; Hildrew, D.M.; Kim, T.W.; et al. Clinical Practice Guideline: Tonsillectomy in Children (Update). *Otolaryngol. Head Neck Surg.* **2019**, *160* (Suppl. S1), S1–S42. [CrossRef] [PubMed]
26. Redline, S.; Amin, R.; Beebe, D.; Chervin, R.D.; Garetz, S.L.; Giordani, B.; Marcus, C.L.; Moore, R.H.; Rosen, C.L.; Arens, R.; et al. The Childhood Adenotonsillectomy Trial (CHAT): Rationale, Design, and Challenges of a Randomized Controlled Trial Evaluating a Standard Surgical Procedure in a Pediatric Population. *Sleep* **2011**, *34*, 1509–1517. [CrossRef]
27. Bhattacharjee, R.; Kheirandish-Gozal, L.; Spruyt, K.; Mitchell, R.B.; Promchiarak, J.; Simakajornboon, N.; Kaditis, A.G.; Splaingard, D.; Splaingard, M.; Brooks, L.J.; et al. Adenotonsillectomy outcomes in treatment of obstructive sleep apnea in children: A multicenter retrospective study. *Am. J. Respir. Crit. Care Med.* **2010**, *182*, 676–683. [CrossRef]
28. Gozal, D.; Tan, H.-L.; Kheirandish-Gozal, L. Obstructive sleep apnea in children: A critical update. *Nat. Sci. Sleep* **2013**, *5*, 109–123. [CrossRef]
29. Goldbart, A.D.; Tal, A. Inflammation and sleep disordered breathing in children: A state-of-the-art review. *Pediatr Pulmonol.* **2008**, *43*, 1151–1160. [CrossRef]
30. Dayyat, E.; Serpero, L.D.; Kheirandish-Gozal, L.; Goldman, J.L.; Snow, A.; Bhattacharjee, R.; Gozal, D. Leukotriene Pathways and In Vitro Adenotonsillar Cell Proliferation in Children With Obstructive Sleep Apnea. *Chest* **2009**, *135*, 1142–1149. [CrossRef]
31. Berlucchi, M.; Salsi, D.; Valetti, L.; Parrinello, G.; Nicolai, P. The Role of Mometasone Furoate Aqueous Nasal Spray in the Treatment of Adenoidal Hypertrophy in the Pediatric Age Group: Preliminary Results of a Prospective, Randomized Study. *Pediatrics* **2007**, *119*, e1392–e1397. [CrossRef] [PubMed]
32. Kheirandish-Gozal, L.; Gozal, D. Intranasal Budesonide Treatment for Children With Mild Obstructive Sleep Apnea Syndrome. *Pediatrics* **2008**, *122*, e149–e155. [CrossRef] [PubMed]
33. Tapia, I.E.; Shults, J.; Cielo, C.M.; Kelly, A.B.; Elden, L.M.; Spergel, J.M.; Bradford, R.M.; Cornaglia, M.A.; Sterni, L.M.; Radcliffe, J. A Trial of Intranasal Corticosteroids to Treat Childhood OSA Syndrome. *Chest* **2022**, *162*, 899–919. [CrossRef] [PubMed]
34. Cielo, C.M.; Gungor, A. Treatment Options for Pediatric Obstructive Sleep Apnea. *Curr. Probl. Pediatr. Adolesc. Health Care* **2016**, *46*, 27–33. [CrossRef] [PubMed]
35. Kheirandish-Gozal, L.; Bandla, H.P.R.; Gozal, D. Montelukast for Children with Obstructive Sleep Apnea: Results of a Double-blind Randomized Placebo-controlled Trial. *Ann. Am. Thorac. Soc.* **2016**, *13*, 1736–1741. [CrossRef]
36. Liming, B.J.; Ryan, M.; Mack, D.; Ahmad, I.; Camacho, M. Montelukast and Nasal Corticosteroids to Treat Pediatric Obstructive Sleep Apnea: A Systematic Review and Meta-analysis. *Otolaryngol. Neck Surg.* **2018**, *160*, 594–602. [CrossRef]
37. Aschenbrenner, D.S. New Boxed Warning for Singulair. *AJN Am. J. Nurs.* **2020**, *120*, 27. [CrossRef]
38. Evangelisti, M.; Barreto, M.; Di Nardo, G.; Del Pozzo, M.; Parisi, P.; Villa, M.P. Systemic corticosteroids could be used as bridge treatment in children with obstructive sleep apnea syndrome waiting for surgery. *Sleep Breath.* **2021**, *26*, 879–885. [CrossRef]
39. Don, D.M.; Goldstein, N.A.; Crockett, D.M.; Ward, S.D. Antimicrobial Therapy for Children With Adenotonsillar Hypertrophy and Obstructive Sleep Apnea: A Prospective Randomized Trial Comparing Azithromycin vs Placebo. *Otolaryngol. Neck Surg.* **2005**, *133*, 562–568. [CrossRef]
40. Zuliani, G.; Carron, M.; Gurrola, J.; Coleman, C.; Haupert, M.; Berk, R.; Coticchia, J. Identification of adenoid biofilms in chronic rhinosinusitis. *Int. J. Pediatr. Otorhinolaryngol.* **2006**, *70*, 1613–1617. [CrossRef]
41. Nath, A.; Emani, J.; Suskind, D.L.; Baroody, F.M. Predictors of Persistent Sleep Apnea After Surgery in Children Younger Than 3 Years. *JAMA Otolaryngol. Neck Surg.* **2013**, *139*, 1002–1008. [CrossRef] [PubMed]
42. Kearney, T.C.; Vazifedan, T.; Baldassari, C.M. Adenotonsillectomy outcomes in obese adolescents with obstructive sleep apnea. *J. Clin. Sleep Med.* **2022**, *18*, 2855–2860. [CrossRef] [PubMed]
43. Lee, S.Y.; Guilleminault, C.; Chiu, H.Y.; Sullivan, S.S. Mouth breathing, "nasal disuse", and pediatric sleep-disordered breathing. *Sleep Breath.* **2015**, *19*, 1257–1264. [CrossRef]
44. Huang, Y.-S.; Guilleminault, C. Pediatric Obstructive Sleep Apnea and the Critical Role of Oral-Facial Growth: Evidences. *Front. Neurol.* **2013**, *3*, 184. [CrossRef] [PubMed]
45. Guilleminault, C.; Huang, Y.S. From oral facial dysfunction to dysmorphism and the onset of pediatric OSA. *Sleep Med. Rev.* **2018**, *40*, 203–214. [CrossRef]
46. Amin, R.; Al-Saleh, S.; Narang, I. Domiciliary noninvasive positive airway pressure therapy in children. *Pediatr. Pulmonol.* **2015**, *51*, 335–348. [CrossRef]
47. Yui, M.S.; Tominaga, Q.; Lopes, B.C.P.; Eckeli, A.L.; Rabelo, F.A.W.; Küpper, D.S.; Valera, F.C.P. Nasal vs. oronasal mask during PAP treatment: A comparative DISE study. *Sleep Breath.* **2019**, *24*, 1129–1136. [CrossRef]
48. Castro-Codesal, M.L.; Olmstead, D.L.; MacLean, J.E. Mask interfaces for home non-invasive ventilation in infants and children. *Paediatr. Respir. Rev.* **2019**, *32*, 66–72. [CrossRef]
49. Ramirez, A.; Khirani, S.; Aloui, S.; Delord, V.; Borel, J.-C.; Pépin, J.-L.; Fauroux, B. Continuous positive airway pressure and noninvasive ventilation adherence in children. *Sleep Med.* **2013**, *14*, 1290–1294. [CrossRef]
50. Atag, E.; Krivec, U.; Ersu, R. Non-invasive Ventilation for Children With Chronic Lung Disease. *Front. Pediatr.* **2020**, *8*, 561639. [CrossRef]
51. Xanthopoulos, M.S.; Williamson, A.A.; Tapia, I.E. Positive airway pressure for the treatment of the childhood obstructive sleep apnea syndrome. *Pediatr. Pulmonol.* **2021**, *57*, 1897–1903. [CrossRef] [PubMed]

52. Parmar, A.; Baker, A.; Narang, I. Positive airway pressure in pediatric obstructive sleep apnea. *Paediatr. Respir. Rev.* **2019**, *31*, 43–51. [CrossRef] [PubMed]
53. Harsch, I.A.; Pour Schahin, S.; Radespiel-Tröger, M.; Weintz, O.; Jahreiß, H.; Fuchs, F.S.; Wiest, G.H.; Hahn, E.G.; Lohmann, T.; Konturek, P.C.; et al. Continuous Positive Airway Pressure Treatment Rapidly Improves Insulin Sensitivity in Patients with Obstructive Sleep Apnea Syndrome. *Am. J. Respir. Crit. Care Med.* **2004**, *169*, 156–162. [CrossRef] [PubMed]
54. Katz, S.L.; MacLean, J.; Hoey, L.; Horwood, L.; Barrowman, N.; Foster, B.; Hadjiyannakis, S.; Legault, L.; Bendiak, G.N.; Kirk, V.G.; et al. Insulin Resistance and Hypertension in Obese Youth With Sleep-Disordered Breathing Treated With Positive Airway Pressure: A Prospective Multicenter Study. *J. Clin. Sleep Med.* **2017**, *13*, 1039–1047. [CrossRef]
55. Johnstone, S.J.; Tardif, H.P.; Barry, R.J.; Sands, T. Nasal bilevel positive airway pressure therapy in children with a sleep-related breathing disorder and attention-deficit hyperactivity disorder: Effects on electrophysiological measures of brain function. *Sleep Med.* **2001**, *2*, 407–416. [CrossRef]
56. Hady, K.K.; Okorie, C.U.A. Positive Airway Pressure Therapy for Pediatric Obstructive Sleep Apnea. *Children* **2021**, *8*, 979. [CrossRef]
57. Oyegbile-Chidi, T. Continuous Positive Airway Pressure Use for Obstructive Sleep Apnea in Pediatric Patients. *Sleep Med. Clin.* **2022**, *17*, 629–638. [CrossRef]
58. Nixon, G.M.; Mihai, R.; Verginis, N.; Davey, M.J. Patterns of Continuous Positive Airway Pressure Adherence during the First 3 Months of Treatment in Children. *J. Pediatr.* **2011**, *159*, 802–807. [CrossRef]
59. Bhattacharjee, R.; Benjafield, A.V.; Armitstead, J.; Cistulli, P.A.; Nunez, C.M.; Pepin, J.-L.D.; Woehrle, H.; Yan, Y.; Malhotra, A. Adherence in children using positive airway pressure therapy: A big-data analysis. *Lancet Digit. Health* **2019**, *2*, e94–e101. [CrossRef]
60. Watach, A.J.; Xanthopoulos, M.S.; Afolabi-Brown, O.; Saconi, B.; Fox, K.A.; Qiu, M.; Sawyer, A.M. Positive airway pressure adherence in pediatric obstructive sleep apnea: A systematic scoping review. *Sleep Med. Rev.* **2020**, *51*, 101273. [CrossRef]
61. Mihai, R.; Vandeleur, M.; Pecoraro, S.; Davey, M.J.; Nixon, G.M. Autotitrating CPAP as a Tool for CPAP Initiation for Children. *J. Clin. Sleep Med.* **2017**, *13*, 713–719. [CrossRef] [PubMed]
62. Cielo, C.M.; Hernandez, P.; Ciampaglia, A.M.; Xanthopoulos, M.S.; Beck, S.E.; Tapia, I.E. Positive Airway Pressure for the Treatment of OSA in Infants. *Chest* **2020**, *159*, 810–817. [CrossRef] [PubMed]
63. Kang, E.K.; Xanthopoulos, M.S.; Kim, J.Y.; Arevalo, C.; Shults, J.; Beck, S.E.; Marcus, C.L.; Tapia, I.E. Adherence to Positive Airway Pressure for the Treatment of Obstructive Sleep Apnea in Children With Developmental Disabilities. *J. Clin. Sleep Med.* **2019**, *15*, 915–921. [CrossRef] [PubMed]
64. Marcus, C.L.; Rosen, G.; Ward, S.L.D.; Halbower, A.C.; Sterni, L.; Lutz, J.; Stading, P.J.; Bolduc, D.; Gordon, N. Adherence to and Effectiveness of Positive Airway Pressure Therapy in Children With Obstructive Sleep Apnea. *Pediatrics* **2006**, *117*, e442–e451. [CrossRef]
65. Bakker, J.P.; Weaver, T.E.; Parthasarathy, S.; Aloia, M.S. Adherence to CPAP: What should we be aiming for, and how can we get there? *Chest* **2019**, *155*, 1272–1287. [CrossRef]
66. Sawunyavisuth, B.; Ngamjarus, C.; Sawanyawisuth, K. Any Effective Intervention to Improve CPAP Adherence in Children with Obstructive Sleep Apnea: A Systematic Review. *Glob. Pediatr. Health* **2021**, *8*, 2333794X211019884. [CrossRef]
67. Mulholland, A.; Mihai, R.; Ellis, K.; Davey, M.J.; Nixon, G.M. Paediatric CPAP in the digital age. *Sleep Med.* **2021**, *84*, 352–355. [CrossRef]
68. Gozal, D.; Tan, H.-L.; Kheirandish-Gozal, L. Treatment of Obstructive Sleep Apnea in Children: Handling the Unknown with Precision. *J. Clin. Med.* **2020**, *9*, 888. [CrossRef]
69. Shoemaker, M.T.; Pierce, M.R.; Yoder, B.A.; DiGeronimo, R.J. High flow nasal cannula versus nasal CPAP for neonatal respiratory disease: A retrospective study. *J. Perinatol.* **2007**, *27*, 85–91. [CrossRef]
70. Dani, C.; Pratesi, S.; Migliori, C.; Bertini, G. High flow nasal cannula therapy as respiratory support in the preterm infant. *Pediatr. Pulmonol.* **2009**, *44*, 629–634. [CrossRef]
71. Joseph, L.; Goldberg, S.; Shitrit, M.; Picard, E. High-Flow Nasal Cannula Therapy for Obstructive Sleep Apnea in Children. *J. Clin. Sleep Med.* **2015**, *11*, 1007–1010. [CrossRef] [PubMed]
72. Nishimura, M. High-Flow Nasal Cannula Oxygen Therapy in Adults: Physiological Benefits, Indication, Clinical Benefits, and Adverse Effects. *Respir. Care* **2016**, *61*, 529–541. [CrossRef] [PubMed]
73. Narang, I.; Carberry, J.C.; Butler, J.E.; Gandevia, S.C.; Chiang, A.K.; Eckert, D.J. Physiological responses and perceived comfort to high-flow nasal cannula therapy in awake adults: Effects of flow magnitude and temperature. *J. Appl. Physiol.* **2021**, *131*, 1772–1782. [CrossRef] [PubMed]
74. Kushida, C.A.; Halbower, A.C.; Kryger, M.H.; Pelayo, R.; Assalone, V.; Cardell, C.-Y.; Huston, S.; Willes, L.; Wimms, A.J.; Mendoza, J. Evaluation of a New Pediatric Positive Airway Pressure Mask. *J. Clin. Sleep Med.* **2014**, *10*, 979–984. [CrossRef] [PubMed]
75. McGinley, B.M.; Patil, S.P.; Kirkness, J.P.; Smith, P.L.; Schwartz, A.R.; Schneider, H. A Nasal Cannula Can Be Used to Treat Obstructive Sleep Apnea. *Am. J. Respir. Crit. Care Med.* **2007**, *176*, 194–200. [CrossRef]
76. McGinley, B.; Halbower, A.; Schwartz, A.R.; Smith, P.L.; Patil, S.P.; Schneider, H. Effect of a High-Flow Open Nasal Cannula System on Obstructive Sleep Apnea in Children. *Pediatrics* **2009**, *124*, 179–188. [CrossRef]

77. Fishman, H.; Al-Shamli, N.; Sunkonkit, K.; Maguire, B.; Selvadurai, S.; Baker, A.; Amin, R.; Propst, E.J.; Wolter, N.E.; Eckert, D.J.; et al. Heated humidified high flow nasal cannula therapy in children with obstructive sleep apnea: A randomized cross-over trial. *Sleep Med.* **2023**, *107*, 81–88. [CrossRef]
78. Hawkins, S.; Huston, S.; Campbell, K.; Halbower, A. High-Flow, Heated, Humidified Air Via Nasal Cannula Treats CPAP-Intolerant Children With Obstructive Sleep Apnea. *J. Clin. Sleep Med.* **2017**, *13*, 981–989. [CrossRef]
79. Ignatiuk, D.; Schaer, B.; McGinley, B. High flow nasal cannula treatment for obstructive sleep apnea in infants and young children. *Pediatr. Pulmonol.* **2020**, *55*, 2791–2798. [CrossRef]
80. Verhelst, E.; Clinck, I.; Deboutte, I.; Vanderveken, O.; Verhulst, S.; Boudewyns, A. Positional obstructive sleep apnea in children: Prevalence and risk factors. *Sleep Breath.* **2019**, *23*, 1323–1330. [CrossRef]
81. Selvadurai, S.; Voutsas, G.; Massicotte, C.; Kassner, A.; Katz, S.L.; Propst, E.J.; Narang, I. Positional obstructive sleep apnea in an obese pediatric population. *J. Clin. Sleep Med.* **2020**, *16*, 1295–1301. [CrossRef]
82. Menon, A.; Kumar, M. Influence of body position on severity of obstructive sleep apnea: A systematic review. *ISRN Otolaryngol.* **2013**, *2013*, 670381. [CrossRef]
83. Saigusa, H.; Suzuki, M.; Higurashi, N.; Kodera, K. Three-dimensional Morphological Analyses of Positional Dependence in Patients with Obstructive Sleep Apnea Syndrome. *Anesthesiology* **2009**, *110*, 885–890. [CrossRef]
84. Squier, S.B.; Patil, S.P.; Schneider, H.; Kirkness, J.P.; Smith, P.L.; Schwartz, A.R.; Lambeth, C.; Kolevski, B.; Kairaitis, K.; Amatoury, J.; et al. Effect of end-expiratory lung volume on upper airway collapsibility in sleeping men and women. *J. Appl. Physiol.* **2010**, *109*, 977–985. [CrossRef]
85. Takahashi, S.; Ono, T.; Ishiwata, Y.; Kuroda, T. Effect of changes in the breathing mode and body position on tongue pressure with respiratory-related oscillations. *Am. J. Orthod. Dentofac. Orthop.* **1999**, *115*, 239–246. [CrossRef]
86. Xiao, L.; Baker, A.; Voutsas, G.; Massicotte, C.; Wolter, N.E.; Propst, E.J.; Narang, I. Positional device therapy for the treatment of positional obstructive sleep apnea in children: A pilot study. *Sleep Med.* **2021**, *85*, 313–316. [CrossRef] [PubMed]
87. Guimarães, K.C.; Drager, L.F.; Genta, P.R.; Marcondes, B.F.; Lorenzi-Filho, G. Effects of Oropharyngeal Exercises on Patients with Moderate Obstructive Sleep Apnea Syndrome. *Am. J. Respir. Crit. Care Med.* **2009**, *179*, 962–966. [CrossRef] [PubMed]
88. Villa, M.P.; Evangelisti, M.; Martella, S.; Barreto, M.; Del Pozzo, M. Can myofunctional therapy increase tongue tone and reduce symptoms in children with sleep-disordered breathing? *Sleep Breath.* **2017**, *21*, 1025–1032. [CrossRef]
89. Sutherland, K.; Weichard, A.J.; Davey, M.J.; Horne, R.S.; Cistulli, P.A.; Nixon, G.M. Craniofacial photography and association with sleep-disordered breathing severity in children. *Sleep Breath.* **2019**, *24*, 1173–1179. [CrossRef]
90. Fagundes, N.C.F.; Gianoni-Capenakas, S.; Heo, G.; Flores-Mir, C. Craniofacial features in children with obstructive sleep apnea: A systematic review and meta-analysis. *J. Clin. Sleep Med.* **2022**, *18*, 1865–1875. [CrossRef] [PubMed]
91. Camacho, M.; Chang, E.T.; Song, S.A.; Abdullatif, J.; Zaghi, S.; Pirelli, P.; Certal, V.; Guilleminault, C. Rapid maxillary expansion for pediatric obstructive sleep apnea: A systematic review and meta-analysis. *Laryngoscope* **2017**, *127*, 1712–1719. [CrossRef] [PubMed]
92. Hoxha, S.; Kaya-Sezginer, E.; Bakar-Ates, F.; Köktürk, O.; Toygar-Memikoğlu, U. Effect of semi-rapid maxillary expansion in children with obstructive sleep apnea syndrome: 5-month follow-up study. *Sleep Breath.* **2018**, *22*, 1053–1061. [CrossRef] [PubMed]
93. Fernández-Barriales, M.; de Mendoza, I.L.-I.; Pacheco, J.J.A.-F.; Aguirre-Urizar, J.M. Rapid maxillary expansion versus watchful waiting in pediatric OSA: A systematic review. *Sleep Med. Rev.* **2022**, *62*, 101609. [CrossRef]
94. Jacobs, S.; Mylemans, E.; Ysebaert, M.; Vermeiren, E.; De Guchtenaere, A.; Heuten, H.; Bruyndonckx, L.; De Winter, B.Y.; Van Hoorenbeeck, K.; Verhulst, S.L.; et al. The impact of obstructive sleep apnea on endothelial function during weight loss in an obese pediatric population. *Sleep Med.* **2021**, *86*, 48–55. [CrossRef] [PubMed]
95. Verhulst, S.L.; Van Gaal, L.; De Backer, W.; Desager, K. The prevalence, anatomical correlates and treatment of sleep-disordered breathing in obese children and adolescents. *Sleep Med. Rev.* **2008**, *12*, 339–346. [CrossRef] [PubMed]
96. Van de Perck, E.; Van Hoorenbeeck, K.; Verhulst, S.; Saldien, V.; Vanderveken, O.; Boudewyns, A. Effect of body weight on upper airway findings and treatment outcome in children with obstructive sleep apnea. *Sleep Med.* **2020**, *79*, 19–28. [CrossRef] [PubMed]
97. Van Eyck, A.; De Guchtenaere, A.; Van Gaal, L.; De Backer, W.; Verhulst, S.L.; Van Hoorenbeeck, K. Clinical Predictors of Residual Sleep Apnea after Weight Loss Therapy in Obese Adolescents. *J. Pediatr.* **2018**, *196*, 189–193.e1. [CrossRef]
98. Roche, J.; Isacco, L.; Masurier, J.; Pereira, B.; Mougin, F.; Chaput, J.-P.; Thivel, D. Are obstructive sleep apnea and sleep improved in response to multidisciplinary weight loss interventions in youth with obesity? A systematic review and meta-analysis. *Int. J. Obes.* **2020**, *44*, 753–770. [CrossRef]
99. Kelly, A.S.; Auerbach, P.; Barrientos-Perez, M.; Gies, I.; Hale, P.M.; Marcus, C.; Mastrandrea, L.D.; Prabhu, N.; Arslanian, S. A randomized, controlled trial of liraglutide for adolescents with obesity. *N. Engl. J. Med.* **2020**, *382*, 2117–2128. [CrossRef]
100. Dhillon, S. Phentermine/Topiramate: Pediatric First Approval. *Pediatr. Drugs* **2022**, *24*, 715–720. [CrossRef]
101. Furbetta, N.; Gragnani, F.; Cervelli, R.; Guidi, F.; Furbetta, F. Teenagers with obesity: Long-term results of laparoscopic adjustable gastric banding. *J. Pediatr. Surg.* **2020**, *55*, 732–736. [CrossRef] [PubMed]
102. Mashaqi, S.; Patel, S.I.; Combs, D.; Estep, L.; Helmick, S.; Machamer, J.; Parthasarathy, S. The Hypoglossal Nerve Stimulation as a Novel Therapy for Treating Obstructive Sleep Apnea—A Literature Review. *Int. J. Environ. Res. Public Health* **2021**, *18*, 1642. [CrossRef] [PubMed]

103. Skotko, B.G.; Macklin, E.A.; Muselli, M.; Voelz, L.; McDonough, M.E.; Davidson, E.; Allareddy, V.; Jayaratne, Y.S.N.; Bruun, R.; Ching, N.; et al. A predictive model for obstructive sleep apnea and Down syndrome. *Am. J. Med. Genet. Part A* **2017**, *173*, 889–896. [CrossRef]
104. Liu, P.; Kong, W.; Fang, C.; Zhu, K.; Dai, X.; Meng, X. Hypoglossal nerve stimulation in adolescents with down syndrome and obstructive sleep apnea: A systematic review and meta-analysis. *Front. Neurol.* **2022**, *25*, 1037926. [CrossRef] [PubMed]
105. Cielo, C.M.; Tapia, I.E. What's New in Pediatric Obstructive Sleep Apnea? *Sleep Med. Clin.* **2023**, *18*, 173–181. [CrossRef] [PubMed]
106. Stenerson, M.E.; Yu, P.K.; Kinane, T.B.; Skotko, B.G.; Hartnick, C.J. Long-term stability of hypoglossal nerve stimulation for the treatment of obstructive sleep apnea in children with Down syndrome. *Int. J. Pediatr. Otorhinolaryngol.* **2021**, *149*, 110868. [CrossRef]
107. Taranto-Montemurro, L.; Edwards, B.A.; Sands, S.A.; Marques, M.; Eckert, D.J.; White, D.P.; Wellman, A. Desipramine Increases Genioglossus Activity and Reduces Upper Airway Collapsibility during Non-REM Sleep in Healthy Subjects. *Am. J. Respir. Crit. Care Med.* **2016**, *194*, 878–885. [CrossRef]
108. Liu, X.; Sood, S.; Liu, H.; Horner, R.L. Opposing muscarinic and nicotinic modulation of hypoglossal motor output to genioglossus muscle in rats in vivo. *J. Physiol.* **2005**, *565*, 965–980. [CrossRef] [PubMed]

Disclaimer/Publisher's Note: The statements, opinions and data contained in all publications are solely those of the individual author(s) and contributor(s) and not of MDPI and/or the editor(s). MDPI and/or the editor(s) disclaim responsibility for any injury to people or property resulting from any ideas, methods, instructions or products referred to in the content.

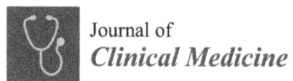

Article

Association of TNF-α (-308G/A) Gene Polymorphism with Changes in Circulating TNF-α Levels in Response to CPAP Treatment in Adults with Coronary Artery Disease and Obstructive Sleep Apnea

Yeliz Celik [1], Yüksel Peker [1,2,3,4,5,*], Tülay Yucel-Lindberg [6], Tilia Thelander [7] and Afrouz Behboudi [7]

1. Department of Pulmonary Medicine, Koc University School of Medicine, and Koc University Research Center for Translational Medicine (KUTTAM), Koc University, 34010 Istanbul, Turkey; yecelik@ku.edu.tr
2. Department of Molecular and Clinical Medicine, Sahlgrenska Academy, University of Gothenburg, 40530 Gothenburg, Sweden
3. Department of Clinical Sciences, Respiratory Medicine and Allergology, Faculty of Medicine, Lund University, 22185 Lund, Sweden
4. Division of Pulmonary, Allergy, and Critical Care Medicine, University of Pittsburgh School of Medicine, Pittsburgh, PA 15213, USA
5. Division of Sleep and Circadian Disorders, Brigham and Women's Hospital, and Harvard Medical School, Boston, MA 02115, USA
6. Department of Dental Medicine, Karolinska Institute, 17177 Stockholm, Sweden; tulay.lindberg@ki.se
7. Division of Biomedicine, School of Heath Sciences, University of Skövde, 54128 Skövde, Sweden; tilia.thelander@gmail.com (T.T.); afrouz.behboudi@his.se (A.B.)
* Correspondence: yuksel.peker@lungall.gu.se

Abstract: Rationale: We recently demonstrated that patients with coronary artery disease (CAD) and obstructive sleep apnea (OSA) carrying the tumor necrosis factor-alpha *(TNF-α) A* allele had increased circulating *TNF-α* levels compared with the ones carrying the *TNF-α G* allele. In the current study, we addressed the effect of *TNF-α* (-308G/A) gene polymorphism on circulating *TNF-α* levels following continuous positive airway pressure (CPAP) therapy. Methods: This study was a secondary analysis of the RICCADSA trial (NCT00519597) conducted in Sweden. CAD patients with OSA (apnea–hypopnea index) of ≥15 events/h and an Epworth Sleepiness Scale (ESS) score of <10 were randomized to CPAP or no-CPAP groups, and OSA patients with an ESS score of ≥10 were offered CPAP treatment. Blood samples were obtained at baseline and 12-month follow-up visits. *TNF-α* was measured by immunoassay (Luminex, R&D Systems). Genotyping of *TNF-α*-308G/A (single nucleotide polymorphism Rs1800629) was performed by polymerase chain reaction–restriction fragment length polymorphism. Results: In all, 239 participants (206 men and 33 women; mean age 64.9 (SD 7.7) years) with polymorphism data and circulating levels of *TNF-α* at baseline and 1-year follow-up visits were included. The median circulating *TNF-α* values fell in both groups between baseline and 12 months with no significant within- or between-group differences. In a multivariate linear regression model, a significant change in circulating *TNF-α* levels from baseline across the genotypes from GA to GA and GA to AA (standardized β-coefficient −0.129, 95% confidence interval (CI) −1.82; −0.12; $p = 0.025$) was observed in the entire cohort. The association was more pronounced among the individuals who were using the device for at least 4 h/night (n = 86; standardized β-coefficient −2.979 (95% CI −6.11; −1.21); $p = 0.004$)), whereas no significant association was found among the patients who were non-adherent or randomized to no-CPAP. The participants carrying the *TNF-α A* allele were less responsive to CPAP treatment regarding the decline in circulating *TNF-α* despite CPAP adherence (standardized β-coefficient −0.212, (95% CI −5.66; −1.01); $p = 0.005$). Conclusions: Our results suggest that *TNF-α* (-308G/A) gene polymorphism is associated with changes in circulating *TNF-α* levels in response to CPAP treatment in adults with CAD and OSA.

Citation: Celik, Y.; Peker, Y.; Yucel-Lindberg, T.; Thelander, T.; Behboudi, A. Association of TNF-α (-308G/A) Gene Polymorphism with Changes in Circulating TNF-α Levels in Response to CPAP Treatment in Adults with Coronary Artery Disease and Obstructive Sleep Apnea. *J. Clin. Med.* **2023**, *12*, 5325. https://doi.org/10.3390/jcm12165325

Academic Editor: Jari P. Ahlberg

Received: 14 July 2023
Revised: 10 August 2023
Accepted: 11 August 2023
Published: 16 August 2023

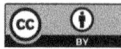

Copyright: © 2023 by the authors. Licensee MDPI, Basel, Switzerland. This article is an open access article distributed under the terms and conditions of the Creative Commons Attribution (CC BY) license (https://creativecommons.org/licenses/by/4.0/).

Keywords: coronary artery disease; obstructive sleep apnea; tumor necrosis factor

1. Introduction

Coronary artery disease (CAD) is associated with high mortality [1]. The traditionally recognized risk factors for CAD are age, male sex, hypertension, diabetes, and hyperlipidemia. It has also been proposed that the interaction between genetic and environmental factors influences the development of CAD [1–3].

Obstructive sleep apnea (OSA) is characterized by intermittent upper airway collapse during sleep, causing sleep fragmentation and intermittent hypoxia [4]. Almost 50% of CAD patients have OSA, and many of them do not report excessive daytime sleepiness (ESS), which is one of the cardinal symptoms of OSA [5]. Individuals with OSA have been reported to have an increased risk of incident CAD compared with adults without OSA [6].

Vascular inflammation plays a key role in the development of atherosclerotic plaques and CAD [7]. It has also been suggested that circulating levels of inflammatory markers can predict future cardiovascular events [8,9]. Elevated levels of high-sensitivity C-reactive protein (hs-CRP), interleukin (IL)-6, and tumor necrosis factor (TNF)-α have been reported in adults with OSA [10,11]. Treatment of OSA with continuous positive airway pressure (CPAP) has been suggested to normalize the levels of circulating inflammatory markers, supporting the link between systemic inflammation and OSA [12]. It has also been proposed that inflammation can be a predisposing factor for OSA [13–15], not just a consequence of OSA.

TNF-α is a pro-inflammatory cytokine that is important for the immune system and plays a notable role in the development of autoimmune and infectious diseases as well as atherosclerosis and CAD [16]. *TNF-α* also plays a crucial role in sleep regulation [17]. Many OSA patients have elevated levels of circulating *TNF-α* [18]. Existing data also suggest that genetic and environmental factors are involved in the development of OSA [19], and *TNF-α* has received special attention in this context [17,20]. There is an SNP (Rs1800629) in the promoter region of the *TNF-α* (position 308G/A); allele A at this position (*TNF-α*-308A) is suggested to be associated with a higher occurrence of OSA [21] as well as with the severity of this disorder [18,22–25]. There are also reports concerning the association of *TNF-α*-308G/A (rs1800629) polymorphism with the risk of many diseases, such as allograft rejection [26], asthma [27], chronic obstructive pulmonary disease [28], ischemic stroke [29], rheumatoid arthritis [30], and systemic lupus erythematosus [31]. An association between the *TNF-α*-308A allele and obesity has also been reported [17,21], whereas conflicting results have been reported regarding the relationship between *TNF-α*-308G/A polymorphism and CAD. One study suggested that *TNF-α*-308G/A polymorphism is associated with ST-elevation myocardial infarction and high plasma levels of biochemical ischemia markers [32], and a meta-analysis demonstrated a significant association between *TNF-α*-308G/A and the risk of acute myocardial infarction [33]. On the other hand, a recent meta-analysis showed no significant association [34].

We recently demonstrated that patients with CAD and OSA carrying the *TNF-α* A allele had increased circulating *TNF-α* levels compared with the ones carrying the *TNF-α* G allele [35] in the "Randomized Intervention with CPAP in CAD and OSA" (RICCADSA) cohort [36]. In the current study, we addressed the role of *TNF-α* (-308G/A) gene polymorphism on circulating *TNF-α* levels in response to 12 months of CPAP therapy.

2. Materials and Methods

2.1. Study Participants

The methodology of the main RICCADSA trial was described elsewhere [36]. In total, 511 CAD patients who underwent percutaneous coronary intervention (PCI) or coronary artery bypass grafting (CABG) in Skaraborg County of West Götaland, Sweden, were included in the RICCADSA trial between 2005 and 2010 (Figure 1). The participants with

OSA, defined as an apnea–hypopnea index (AHI) of ≥15/h, on the home sleep apnea test (HSAT) at screening and an Epworth Sleepiness Scale (ESS) score of <10 were randomized to CPAP or no-CPAP groups. Patients with ESS scores of ≥10 were categorized as having excessive daytime sleepiness (EDS) and were offered CPAP treatment. The CAD patients with AHI < 5/h were categorized as no-OSA in the main protocol. For the genetic analysis, blood samples were collected at the final visit in 2012/2013 from 384 eligible participants, and 239 patients with OSA were included as the final study population for the current $TNF\text{-}\alpha\text{-}308G/A$ polymorphism study to evaluate the changes in circulating $TNF\text{-}\alpha$ levels from baseline to 12 months after CPAP treatment (Figure 1).

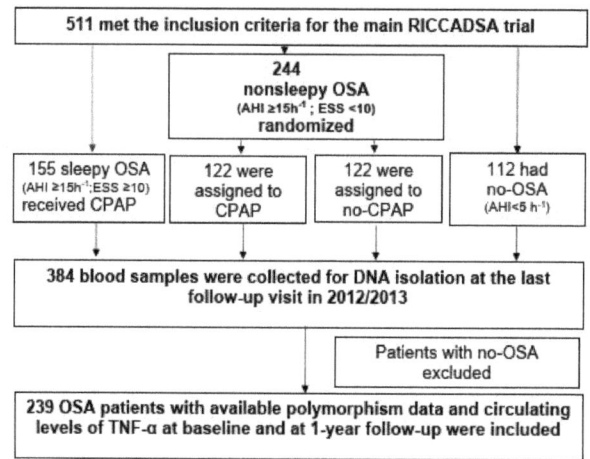

Figure 1. Analytic sample of the study population. Abbreviations: AHI, apneahypopnea index; CPAP, continuous positive airway pressure; ESS, Epworth Sleepiness Scale; OSA, obstructive sleep apnea; RICCADSA, Randomized Intervention with CPAP in Coronary Artery Disease and Sleep Apnea; TNF, tumor necrosis factor.

2.2. Study Oversight

The study protocol was approved by the Ethics Committee of the Medical Faculty of the University of Gothenburg (approval nr 207-05, 09.13.2005; amendment T744-10, 11.26.2010; amendment T512-11, 06.16.2011; additional approval for the molecular analysis, approval nr 814-17, 11.21.2017). Written informed consent was obtained from all participants. The main RICCADSA trial was registered with ClinicalTrials.gov (NCT 00519597).

2.3. Sleep Studies

The Embletta® Portable Digital System device (Embla, Broomfield, CO, USA) was used for the HSATs [36]. Apnea was defined as at least a 90% cessation of airflow, and hypopnea was defined as at least a 50% reduction in nasal pressure amplitude and/or thoracoabdominal movement for at least 10 s, following the Chicago criteria [37]. The total number of significant drops in SpO_2 exceeding 4% from the immediately preceding baseline was also recorded, and the oxygen desaturation index (ODI) was determined as the number of significant desaturations per hour.

2.4. Epworth Sleepiness Scale

The ESS [38] was assessed to measure subjective daytime sleepiness. The ESS has eight items asking about the risk of dozing off under 8 different situations, and a score of at least 10 out of 24 was defined as EDS.

2.5. Comorbidities

Demographics, smoking habits, and medical history of the study cohort were obtained from the medical records. Individuals with a body mass index (BMI) of ≥ 30 kg/m^2 were defined as obese, and abdominal obesity was defined as a waist-to-hip ratio (WHR) of ≥ 0.9 for men and a WHR of ≥ 0.8 for women [39].

2.6. TNF-α Circulating Concentration

All blood samples were collected in the morning (07:00–08.00 am) after overnight fasting using EDTA (ethylenediaminetetraacetic acid) tubes, as previously described [40]. The tubes underwent centrifugation, and the resulting plasma/serum samples were divided into aliquots and subsequently stored at $-70\ °C$ until analysis. Circulating *TNF-α* levels were measured in the plasma samples (undiluted) using commercially available MILLIPLEX MAP (based on Luminex technology) human adipokine assay kits according to the manufacturer's instructions (Merck Millipore, Burlington, MA, USA). The assay sensitivities (minimum detectable levels) for *TNF-α* were 0.14 pg/mL, and all samples exhibited levels within the standard curve, covering a spectrum of 0 to 10,000 pg/mL. The intra-assay variability ranged from 1.4% to 7.9%, while the inter-assay variability was below 21% for the assessment of *TNF-α* concentrations. These values were calculated from the mean of the percentage coefficient of variability from multiple reportable results across two different concentrations of the samples in one experiment or from two results each for two different concentrations of samples across several different experiments.

2.7. TNF-α Promotor -308G/A (Rs1800629) SNA Genotyping

As previously described in detail [35], genomic DNA was isolated from whole blood samples collected in EDTA-coated tubes using the PAXgene Blood DNA Kit (PreAnalytiX; Qiagen). The quality and concentration of DNA samples were determined using a nanodrop photometer (NanoDrop 2000; Thermo Scientific, Waltham, MA, USA), and DNA samples were stored at -80 degrees. *TNF-α* promoter -308A/G (Rs1800629) genotyping analysis was performed by polymerase chain reaction–restriction fragment length polymorphism (PCR–RFLP), as previously described [35].

2.8. Statistical Analysis

For descriptive statistics, variables were reported as medians with interquartile ranges (IQR) for continuous variables and as percentages for categorical variables. The Shapiro–Wilk test was used to test the normality assumption of the current data for all variables. Between-group differences stratified by CPAP allocation and CPAP usage in baseline characteristics, as well as changes from baseline in circulating *TNF-α* levels, were tested by the Mann–Whitney test for continuous variables and the Chi-square test for categorical data. Within-group differences in changes from baseline in circulating *TNF-α* levels were tested by the Wilcoxon signed-rank test. A univariate linear regression analysis was performed to test the association between the change from baseline to the 12-month follow-up in circulating *TNF-α* levels and age, sex, ESS, BMI, WHR, AHI, ODI, OSA, and comorbidities, as well as *TNF-α* genotypes (coded as GG = 0, GA = 1, and AA = 2) and *TNF-α* alleles (coded as G = 0, and A = 1), respectively. Multivariate models included the same significant covariates as the univariate analysis as well as the variables of age, BMI, and sex in order to align with the recent guidelines [41]. All statistical tests were two-sided, odds ratios (ORs) with 95% confidence interval (CI) were reported, and a *p*-value of <0.05 was considered significant. Statistical analyses were performed using SPSS® 28.0 for Windows® (SPSS Inc., Chicago, IL, USA).

3. Results

The study population consisted of 239 participants (mean age 64.9 $\pm$ 7.7 years; male, 86%). As presented in Table 1, patients allocated to the no-CPAP group were slightly older and less sleepy, and the proportion of individuals with diabetes at baseline was lower than that among the patients allocated to CPAP treatment. The circulating levels of *TNF-α* at baseline did not differ significantly between the groups.

Table 1. Baseline demographic and clinical characteristics of the OSA patients allocated to CPAP vs. no-CPAP groups.

	OSA on CPAP n = 169	OSA no-CPAP n = 70	*p*-Value
Age, yrs	64.1 (59.8–69.3)	67.4 (62.7–72.4)	0.019
Male sex, %	86.4	85.7	0.890
BMI, kg/m^2	28.3 (25.9–31.1)	(28.7 (26.2–30.0)	0.548
Obesity, %	32.0	24.3	0.238
WHR	0.96 (0.93–1.00)	0.96 (0.91–0.99)	0.153
Abdominal obesity, %	93.2	95.7	0.470
Current smoking, %	16.0	15.7	0.960
ESS score	10.0 (6.0–12.0)	6.0 (4.0–7.0)	<0.001
EDS (ESS score ≥ 10), %	56.8	0.0	<0.001
AHI, events/h	27.7 (18.7–39.2)	22.9 (17.8–35.7)	0.128
ODI, events/h	15.7 (9.4–24.8)	12.6 (7.2–22.9)	0.101
Hypertension	60.9	54.3	0.341
AMI at baseline	54.4	44.3	0.153
Lung disease, %	5.3	4.3	0.738
Diabetes, %	26.0	12.9	0.026
Stroke, %	4.8	10.1	0.121
Plasma *TNF-α* (pg/mL)	4.87 (3.43–6.99)	5.15 (3.92–6.54)	0.856

Continuous data are presented as median and 25–75% quartiles. Categorical data are presented as percentages. Abbreviations: AHI = Apnea–Hypopnea Index; BMI = Body Mass Index; EDS = Excessive Daytime Sleepiness (ESS score ≥ 10); ESS = Epworth Sleepiness Scale; *TNF-α* = tumor necrosis factor-alpha; ODI = Oxygen Desaturation Index; OSA = Obstructive Sleep Apnea; WHR = Waist–Hip Ratio.

As illustrated in Figure 2A, *TNF-α*-GG was the most prevalent genotype in both groups, whereas *TNF-α*-AA in the CPAP group and *TNF-α*-GA in the no-CPAP group were the least frequent ones, respectively.

The median circulating levels of *TNF-α* decreased from 4.87 (3.43–6.99) pg/mL to 4.62 (3.59–6.59) pg/mL in patients allocated to the CPAP group (*p* = 0.549) and from 5.15 (3.92–6.54) pg/mL to 4.50 (3.64–7.11) pg/mL in patients allocated to the no-CPAP group (*p* = 0.665), with no significant between-group differences in the magnitude of change from baseline.

When analyzing the study population after stratifying by CPAP usage, the baseline characteristics did not differ significantly, except for ESS scores and the proportion of individuals with baseline EDS, which were higher among patients who used the device for at least 4 h/night during the first 12 months (Table 2).

As illustrated in Figure 3A, *TNF-α*-GG was the most prevalent genotype and *TNF-α*-AA the least frequent one in both CPAP usage groups.

As illustrated in Figure 4, the median circulating levels of *TNF-α* decreased from 4.84 (3.48–7.53) pg/mL to 4.72 (3.63–7.20) pg/mL in patients who used the device for at least 4 h/night (*p* = 0.577) and from 5.24 (3.59–6.85) pg/mL to 4.51 (3.50–6.75) pg/mL in patients allocated to the no-CPAP group or who used the device for less than 4 h/night (*p* = 0.199), with no significant between-group differences in the magnitude of change from baseline.

In a multivariate linear regression model, a significant decline in the change from baseline in circulating *TNF-α* levels across the genotypes from GG to GA and GA to AA was observed in the entire cohort (Table 3). The association was more pronounced among individuals who were using the device for at least 4 h/night, whereas no significant association was found among the patients who were non-adherent or randomized to the no-CPAP group. ESS scores at baseline tended to be inversely correlated with the change in circulating *TNF-α* levels from baseline to 12 months in the entire cohort (Table 3).

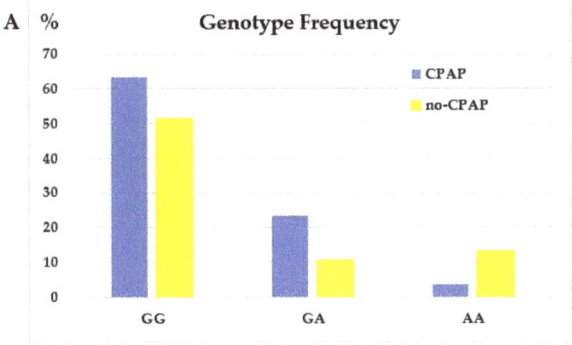

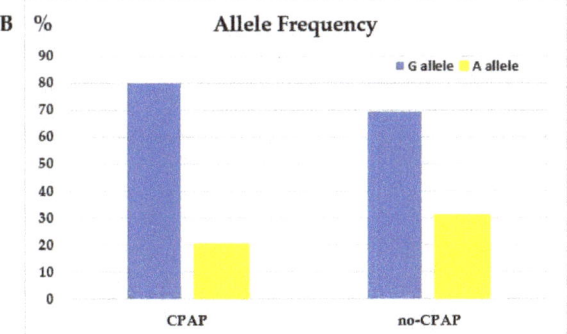

Figure 2. (**A**) Genotype frequency of *TNF-α*-308G/A promoter polymorphism and (**B**) allele frequency of *TNF-α*-308G/A promoter polymorphism in OSA patients allocated to CPAP vs. no-CPAP groups.

Table 2. Baseline demographic and clinical characteristics of the OSA patients stratified by CPAP usage.

	CPAP ≥ 4 h/Night (Adherent) n = 86	CPAP < 4 h/Night or no CPAP n = 153	*p*-Value
Age, yrs	64.4 (60.1–70.6)	65.2 (59.9–70.6)	0.602
Male sex, %	84.9	86.9	0.660
BMI, kg/m^2	28.2 (25.7–31.1)	28.7 (26.2–30.2)	0.875
Obesity, %	32.6	28.1	0.470
WHR	0.96 (0.92–1.02)	0.97 (0.93–1.01)	0.609
Abdominal obesity, %	92.8	94.6	0.586
Current smoking, %	12.8	17.6	0.324
ESS score	10.0 (6.0–11.0)	7.0 (4.0–10.0)	0.007
EDS (ESS score ≥ 10), %	53.5	32.7	0.002
AHI, events/h	28.2 (18.3–40.1)	25.3 (18.6–36.2)	0.293
ODI, events/h	17.2 (10.1–25.7)	14.2 (7.9–23.1)	0.052
Hypertension	60.5	58.2	0.729
AMI at baseline	54.7	49.7	0.460
Lung disease, %	5.3	4.3	0.738
Diabetes, %	27.9	19.0	0.110
Stroke, %	5.8	4.6	0.674
Plasma *TNF-α* (pg/mL)	4.87 (3.48–7.53)	5.24 (3.59–6.85)	0.631

Continuous data are presented as median and 25–75% quartiles. Categorical data are presented as percentages. Abbreviations: AHI = Apnea–Hypopnea Index; BMI = Body Mass Index; EDS= Excessive Daytime Sleepiness (ESS score ≥ 10); ESS = Epworth Sleepiness Scale; *TNF-α* = tumor necrosis factor-alpha; ODI = Oxygen Desaturation Index; OSA = Obstructive Sleep Apnea; WHR = Waist–Hip Ratio.

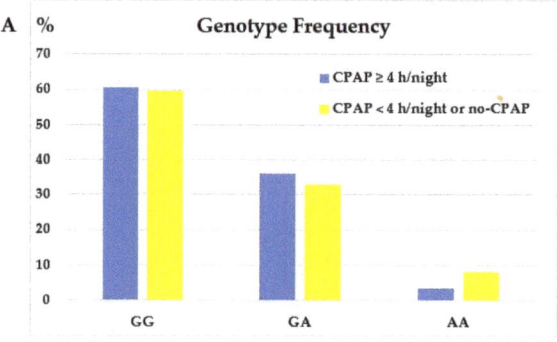

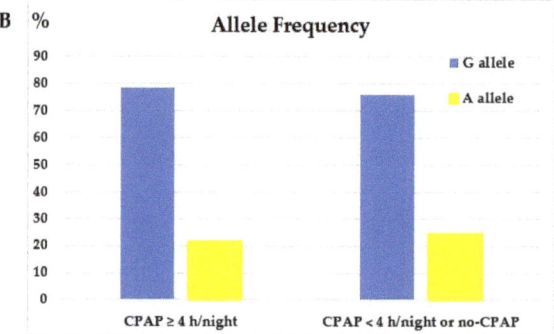

Figure 3. (**A**) Genotype frequency of *TNF-α*-308G/A promoter polymorphism and (**B**) allele frequency of *TNF-α*-308G/A promoter polymorphism in OSA patients stratified by CPAP usage.

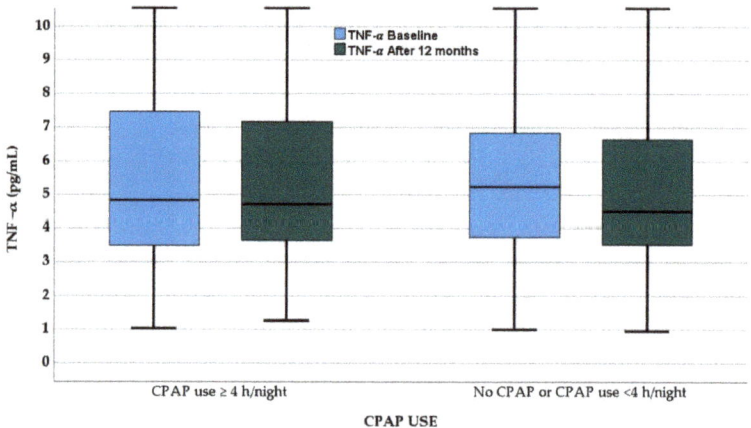

Figure 4. Circulating *TNF-α* levels at baseline and after 12 months of CPAP therapy in OSA patients stratified by CPAP usage categories.

As shown in Table 4, the participants carrying the *TNF-α* A allele were less responsive to CPAP treatment regarding the decline in circulating *TNF-α* levels despite CPAP adherence. Baseline AHI was also inversely correlated with a decline in the change from baseline in circulating *TNF-α* levels among patients who were adherent to CPAP. No significant changes were observed among patients who were randomized to the no-CPAP group or those who were using the device for less than 4 h/night, except for baseline AHI, which was associated with the change in circulating *TNF-α* levels (Table 4).

Table 3. Regression analyses of the association of the *TNF-α* genotypes with change in circulating *TNF-α* levels from baseline, adjusted for the confounding variables in CAD patients with OSA (entire cohort and subgroups based on the CPAP use).

		Standardized Coefficients β	95% Confidence Interval for Lower Bound	95% Confidence Interval for Upper Bound	*p*-Values
Entire Cohort	Genotypes *	−0.129	−1.82	−0.12	0.025
	Age	0.018	−0.05	0.07	0.762
	Male sex	−0.035	−1.91	1.00	0.540
	BMI	−0.005	−0.15	0.14	0.942
	AHI	−0.035	−0.04	0.02	0.573
	ESS	−0.115	−0.28	0.00	0.056
	Diabetes	0.017	−1.13	1.53	0.768
CPAP use ≥4 h/night	Genotypes *	−2.979	−6.11	−1.21	0.004
	Age	−0.057	−0.25	0.15	0.607
	Male sex	0.128	−1.61	6.21	0.246
	BMI	0.029	−0.29	0.38	0.803
	AHI	−0.183	−0.16	0.01	0.096
	ESS	−0.078	−0.46	0.22	0.481
	Diabetes	0.006	−3.03	3.21	0.955
CPAP use <4 h/night or no-CPAP	Genotypes *	−0.019	−0.93	0.73	0.816
	Age	0.026	−0.58	0.79	0.765
	Male sex	−0.079	−2.36	0.84	0.349
	BMI	−0.078	−0.23	0.09	0.368
	AHI	0.124	−0.01	0.07	0.149
	ESS	−0.055	−0.19	0.10	0.507
	Diabetes	−0.055	−1.82	0.91	0.509

Abbreviations: AHI = Apnea–Hypopnea Index; BMI = Body Mass Index; CAD = Coronary Artery Disease; CPAP = Continuous Positive Airway Pressure; ESS = Epworth Sleepiness Scale; OSA = Obstructive Sleep Apnea. * GG = 0, GA = 1, AA = 2.

Table 4. Regression analyses of the association of the *TNF-α* A allele with change in circulating *TNF-α* levels from baseline, adjusted for the confounding variables in CAD patients with concomitant OSA.

		Standardized Coefficients β	95% Confidence Interval for Lower Bound	95% Confidence Interval for Upper Bound	*p*-Values
Entire Cohort	*TNF-α* A Allele	−0.098	−2.08	−0.08	0.034
	Age	0.020	−0.04	0.07	0.676
	Male sex	0.027	−0.88	1.60	0.568
	BMI	−0.009	−0.13	0.11	0.858
	AHI	−0.060	−0.05	0.10	0.202
	CPAP h/night	0.011	−0.14	0.18	0.827
	ESS	−0.061	−0.19	0.41	0.208
	Diabetes	−0.017	−1.24	0.85	0.714
CPAP use ≥4 h/night	*TNF-α* A Allele	−0.212	−5.66	−1.01	0.005
	Age	−0.038	−0.18	0.11	0.627
	Male sex	0.102	−0.90	4.58	0.187
	BMI	0.018	−0.21	0.26	0.823
	AHI	−0.189	−0.14	−0.02	0.015
	ESS	−0.061	−0.34	0.15	0.434
	Diabetes	0.012	−2.03	2.38	0.876
CPAP use <4 h/night or no-CPAP	*TNF-α* A Allele	−0.014	−0.96	0.75	0.805
	Age	0.025	−0.04	0.06	0.670
	Male sex	−0.079	−1.87	0.35	0.180
	BMI	−0.078	−0.18	0.04	0.197
	AHI	0.123	−0.01	0.06	0.039
	ESS	−0.055	−0.15	0.05	0.347
	Diabetes	−0.055	−1.40	0.49	0.346

Abbreviations: AHI = Apnea–Hypopnea Index; BMI = Body Mass Index; CAD = Coronary Artery Disease; CPAP = Continuous Positive Airway Pressure; ESS = Epworth Sleepiness Scale; OSA = Obstructive Sleep Apnea.

4. Discussion

In the current revascularized CAD cohort with OSA, TNF-α-308G/A gene polymorphism was significantly correlated with the change in circulating TNF-α levels from baseline in response to 12 months of CPAP treatment, independent of age, sex, BMI, baseline AHI, ESS, and diabetes. The participants carrying the TNF-α A allele were less responsive to CPAP treatment in terms of the decline in circulating TNF-α levels despite adequate CPAP adherence levels.

To the best of our knowledge, this is the first study to address the association of TNF-α-308G/A polymorphism with change in circulating TNF-α levels in response to the alleviation of OSA with CPAP treatment in a Swedish cardiac population. Previous studies have suggested an association between the TNF-α -308A allele and OSA susceptibility in a British population [24] as well as in an obese Asian Indian population [22], whereas neutral results were reported in a Polish cohort [21] and a Turkish cohort [42]. Notwithstanding, two meta-analyses have supported the significant association between TNF-α -308G/A polymorphism and OSA [43,44].

In our entire cohort including adults without OSA as a control group, we found no significant difference between CAD patients with vs. without OSA in the frequency of TNF-α-308G/A polymorphism or TNF-α -308 alleles [35]. We found a similar -308A allele frequency in the no-OSA group, and, as interpreted in the previous report, this might be due to the confounding effect of other comorbidities, such as obesity, hypertension, and diabetes mellitus, given that individuals without OSA were not healthy controls [27]. Moreover, CAD *per se* is an inflammatory condition mediated by the activity of pro-inflammatory cytokines, including TNF-α [45]. The effect of TNF-α gene polymorphism on CAD pathogenesis has also been investigated previously, and TNF-α-308G/A polymorphism has been suggested to be involved in CAD development [45,46], whereas others reported no evidence for such an association [47]. Additionally, a recent meta-analysis suggested no significant relationship between TNF-α-308G/A polymorphism and the development of CAD [34].

Circulating levels of inflammatory markers predict future cardiovascular events in the general population [8] as well as in cardiac populations [9], and TNF-α levels are elevated in individuals with OSA compared with controls [25,48]. It has also been argued that inflammation can be a predisposing factor for OSA [13–15]; thus, this association could be bidirectional. In our first study on the effect of CPAP on inflammatory markers, including hs-CRP, IL-6, IL-8, and TNF-α, in the RICCADSA cohort, only IL-6 levels decreased after one year, both in the CPAP and no-CPAP arms [49]. This was probably indicative of a natural improvement in cardiac disease rather than the effect of CPAP treatment per se. We also demonstrated that patients with CAD and OSA carrying the TNF-α A allele had increased circulating TNF-α levels compared with the ones carrying the TNF-α G allele [35]. The TNF-α-308A allele is known to promote a two-fold increase in TNF transcription activity [50]. TNF-α is a mediator of the sleep regulatory system, and the fragmented sleep pattern associated with OSA is believed to increase circulatory levels of TNF-α [17]. Our current results clearly support a recent review of OSA heterogeneity regarding cardiovascular morbidities [1], suggesting that the response to CPAP treatment is modulated by genetic mechanisms, namely, in the current report, by TNF-α (-308G/A) gene polymorphism regarding the change in circulating levels of TNF-α from baseline. In other words, individuals with CAD and OSA carrying the TNF-α A allele seem to have an increased risk of elevated levels of circulating TNF-α, and the increased inflammatory activity is less likely to normalize despite CPAP use for at least 4 h/night. Whether or not those individuals should use the device even longer in order to reduce the levels of circulating TNF-α levels warrants further research. The clinical implications of our findings may also include that TNF-α-308G/A genotyping together with the analysis of TNF-α levels can be used for the prognostic evaluation of patients with CAD and concomitant OSA. For instance, patients carrying the A allele and higher levels of TNF-α could be included in a tighter follow-up scheme compared with those carrying the G allele.

We should acknowledge certain limitations. As also stated in the previous report [35], the power estimate for the entire RICCADSA cohort was conducted for the primary outcome and not for the secondary outcomes assessed in this study. Moreover, our results are limited to a Swedish CAD cohort and thus are not generalizable to adults with OSA in the general population or sleep clinic cohorts in other regions. Additionally, the follow-up period was relatively short in the context of the association of changes in circulating TNF-α levels at 12 months with long-term adverse outcomes. Finally, our results are limited to TNF-α (-308G/A) (rs1800629) polymorphism and not the TNF-α (-308G/A) (rs3611525) polymorphism. However, TNF-α-308G/A (rs1800629) and TNF-α-238G/A (rs361525) are located very close to each other and are hence tightly linked. In fact, in our sequencing results, we noticed that polymorphism in one 100% mirrored the other, and for the sake of simplicity, we chose to focus on and present only one of these SNPs. Accordingly, we propose that the TNF-α-308G/A (rs1800629) polymorphism analysis results can be extrapolated to TNF-α-238G/A (rs361525) SNP due to their tight linkage.

5. Conclusions

We conclude that TNF-α-308G/A gene polymorphism was significantly correlated with the change in the circulating TNF-α levels from baseline in response to 12 months of CPAP treatment in this revascularized Swedish CAD cohort, independent of age, sex, BMI, baseline AHI, ESS, and diabetes. The participants carrying the TNF-α A allele were less responsive to CPAP treatment in terms of the decline in circulating TNF-α levels despite adequate CPAP adherence levels. Further prospective studies in larger cohorts and different geographical locations are warranted in order to better clarify whether the combined gentrifying and protein level analysis can be used as a prognostic biomarker for improved clinical follow-up of patients with CAD and concomitant OSA.

Author Contributions: Conception and design: Y.P. and A.B. Analysis and interpretation: Y.P., Y.C., T.Y.-L., T.T. and A.B. Drafting the manuscript for important intellectual content: Y.C., Y.P. and A.B. All authors have read and agreed to the published version of the manuscript.

Funding: This study was supported by grants from the Swedish Research Council (521-2011-537 and 521-2013-3439); the Swedish Heart–Lung Foundation (20080592, 20090708, and 20100664); the "Agreement concerning research and education of doctors" of Västra Götalandsregionen (ALFGBG-11538 and ALFGBG-150801); the research fund at Skaraborg Hospital (VGSKAS-4731, VGSKAS-5908, VGSKAS-9134, VGSKAS-14781, VGSKAS-40271, and VGSKAS-116431); Skaraborg Research and Development Council (VGFOUSKB-46371); Lund University; the Heart Foundation of Kärnsjukhuset; the ResMed Foundation; and ResMed Ltd. None of the funders had any direct influence on the design of the study, the analysis of the data, data collection, the drafting of the manuscript, or the decision to publish.

Institutional Review Board Statement: The study protocol was approved by the Ethics Committee of the Medical Faculty of the University of Gothenburg (approval nr 207-05, 09.13.2005; amendment T744-10, 11.26.2010; amendment T512-11, 06.16.2011; additional approval for the molecular analysis, approval nr 814-17, 11.21.2017).

Informed Consent Statement: Written informed consent was obtained from all participants.

Data Availability Statement: Individual participant data that underlie the results reported in this article can be obtained by contacting the corresponding author, yuksel.peker@lungall.gu.se.

Conflicts of Interest: Y.C., T.Y.-L., T.T. and A.B. report no conflicts of interest. Y.P. received institutional grants from the ResMed Foundation.

References

1. Redline, S.; Azarbarzin, A.; Peker, Y. Obstructive sleep apnoea heterogeneity and cardiovascular disease. *Nat. Rev. Cardiol.* **2023**, *20*, 560–573. [CrossRef] [PubMed]
2. Musunuru, K.; Kathiresan, S. Genetics of Common, Complex Coronary Artery Disease. *Cell* **2019**, *177*, 132–145. [CrossRef]
3. Khera, A.V.; Kathiresan, S. Genetics of coronary artery disease: Discovery, biology and clinical translation. *Nat. Rev. Genet.* **2017**, *18*, 331–344. [CrossRef]

4. Young, T.; Palta, M.; Dempsey, J.; Peppard, P.E.; Nieto, F.J.; Hla, K.M. Burden of sleep apnea: Rationale, design, and major findings of the Wisconsin Sleep Cohort study. *WMJ Off. Publ. State Med. Soc. Wis.* **2009**, *108*, 246–249.
5. Peker, Y.; Franklin, K.; Hedner, J. Coronary artery disease and sleep apnea. In *Principles and Practice of Sleep Medicine*, 7th ed.; Roth, K., Goldstein, Dement, W.T., Eds.; Elsevier Inc.: Philadelphia, PA, USA, 2022; pp. 1453–1461, ISBN 978-0-323-66189-8.
6. Turgut Çelen, Y.; Peker, Y. Cardiovascular consequences of sleep apnea: II-Cardiovascular mechanisms. *Anatol. J. Cardiol.* **2010**, *10*, 168–175. [CrossRef] [PubMed]
7. Hansson, G.K. Inflammation, atherosclerosis, and coronary artery disease. *N. Engl. J. Med.* **2005**, *352*, 1685–1695. [CrossRef] [PubMed]
8. Cesari, M.; Penninx, B.W.; Newman, A.B.; Kritchevsky, S.B.; Nicklas, B.J.; Sutton-Tyrrell, K.; Pahor, M. Inflammatory markers and onset of cardiovascular events: Results from the Health ABC study. *Circulation* **2003**, *108*, 2317–2322. [CrossRef]
9. He, L.P.; Tang, X.Y.; Ling, W.H.; Chen, W.Q.; Chen, Y.M. Early C-reactive protein in the prediction of long-term outcomes after acute coronary syndromes: A meta-analysis of longitudinal studies. *Heart* **2010**, *96*, 339–346. [CrossRef]
10. Patt, B.T.; Jarjoura, D.; Haddad, D.N.; Sen, C.K.; Roy, S.; Flavahan, N.A.; Khayat, R.N. Endothelial dysfunction in the microcirculation of patients with obstructive sleep apnea. *Am. J. Respir. Crit. Care Med.* **2010**, *182*, 1540–1545. [CrossRef]
11. Arnardottir, E.S.; Mackiewicz, M.; Gislason, T.; Teff, K.L.; Pack, A.I. Molecular signatures of obstructive sleep apnea in adults: A review and perspective. *Sleep* **2009**, *32*, 447–470. [CrossRef]
12. Gabryelska, A.; Łukasik, Z.M.; Makowska, J.S.; Białasiewicz, P. Obstructive Sleep Apnea: From Intermittent Hypoxia to Cardiovascular Complications via Blood Platelets. *Front. Neurol.* **2018**, *9*, 635. [CrossRef]
13. Reid, M.B.; Lännergren, J.; Westerblad, H. Respiratory and limb muscle weakness induced by tumor necrosis factor-alpha: Involvement of muscle myofilaments. *Am. J. Respir. Crit. Care Med.* **2002**, *166*, 479–484. [CrossRef]
14. Boyd, J.H.; Petrof, B.J.; Hamid, Q.; Fraser, R.; Kimoff, R.J. Upper airway muscle inflammation and denervation changes in obstructive sleep apnea. *Am. J. Respir. Crit. Care Med.* **2004**, *170*, 541–546. [CrossRef] [PubMed]
15. Huang, T.; Goodman, M.; Li, X.; Sands, S.A.; Li, J.; Stampfer, M.J.; Saxena, R.; Tworoger, S.S.; Redline, S. C-reactive Protein and Risk of OSA in Four US Cohorts. *Chest* **2021**, *159*, 2439–2448. [CrossRef] [PubMed]
16. Nadeem, R.; Molnar, J.; Madbouly, E.M.; Nida, M.; Aggarwal, S.; Sajid, H.; Naseem, J.; Loomba, R. Serum inflammatory markers in obstructive sleep apnea: A meta-analysis. *J. Clin. Sleep Med.* **2013**, *9*, 1003–1012. [CrossRef]
17. Kheirandish-Gozal, L.; Gozal, D. Obstructive Sleep Apnea and Inflammation: Proof of Concept Based on Two Illustrative Cytokines. *Int. J. Mol. Sci.* **2019**, *20*, 459. [CrossRef]
18. Ming, H.; Tian, A.; Liu, B.; Hu, Y.; Liu, C.; Chen, R.; Cheng, L. Inflammatory cytokines tumor necrosis factor-α, interleukin-8 and sleep monitoring in patients with obstructive sleep apnea syndrome. *Exp. Ther. Med.* **2019**, *17*, 1766–1770. [CrossRef]
19. Mukherjee, S.; Saxena, R.; Palmer, L.J. The genetics of obstructive sleep apnoea. *Respirology* **2018**, *23*, 18–27. [CrossRef] [PubMed]
20. Kent, B.D.; Ryan, S.; McNicholas, W.T. The genetics of obstructive sleep apnoea. *Curr. Opin. Pulm. Med.* **2010**, *16*, 536–542. [CrossRef]
21. Popko, K.; Gorska, E.; Potapinska, O.; Wasik, M.; Stoklosa, A.; Plywaczewski, R.; Winiarska, M.; Gorecka, D.; Sliwinski, P.; Popko, M.; et al. Frequency of distribution of inflammatory cytokines IL-1, IL-6 and TNF-alpha gene polymorphism in patients with obstructive sleep apnea. *J. Physiol. Pharmacol.* **2008**, *59* (Suppl. S6), 607–614.
22. Bhushan, B.; Guleria, R.; Misra, A.; Luthra, K.; Vikram, N.K. TNF-alpha gene polymorphism and TNF-alpha levels in obese Asian Indians with obstructive sleep apnea. *Respir. Med.* **2009**, *103*, 386–392. [CrossRef]
23. Bhatt, S.P.; Guleria, R.; Vikram, N.K.; Vivekanandhan, S.; Singh, Y.; Gupta, A.K. Association of inflammatory genes in obstructive sleep apnea and non alcoholic fatty liver disease in Asian Indians residing in north India. *PLoS ONE* **2018**, *13*, e0199599. [CrossRef] [PubMed]
24. Riha, R.L.; Brander, P.; Vennelle, M.; McArdle, N.; Kerr, S.M.; Anderson, N.H.; Douglas, N.J. Tumour necrosis factor-α (−308) gene polymorphism in obstructive sleep apnoea–hypopnoea syndrome. *Eur. Respir. J.* **2005**, *26*, 673–678. [CrossRef] [PubMed]
25. Khalyfa, A.; Serpero, L.D.; Kheirandish-Gozal, L.; Capdevila, O.S.; Gozal, D. TNF-α gene polymorphisms and excessive daytime sleepiness in pediatric obstructive sleep apnea. *J. Pediatr.* **2011**, *158*, 77–82. [CrossRef] [PubMed]
26. Pawlik, A.; Domanski, L.; Rozanski, J.; Florczak, M.; Dabrowska-Zamojcin, E.; Dutkiewicz, G.; Gawronska-Szklarz, B. IL-2 and TNF-alpha promoter polymorphisms in patients with acute kidney graft rejection. *Transplant. Proc.* **2005**, *37*, 2041–2043. [CrossRef]
27. Aoki, T.; Hirota, T.; Tamari, M.; Ichikawa, K.; Takeda, K.; Arinami, T.; Shibasaki, M.; Noguchi, E. An association between asthma and TNF-308G/A polymorphism: Meta-analysis. *J. Hum. Genet.* **2006**, *51*, 677–685. [CrossRef]
28. Zang, S.; Wang, C.; Xi, B.; Li, X. Association between the tumour necrosis factor-α-308G/A polymorphism and chronic obstructive pulmonary disease: An update. *Respirology* **2011**, *16*, 107–115. [CrossRef]
29. Song, D.; Cheng, D. Associations of TNFα-308G/A and TNFα-238G/A Polymorphisms with Ischemic Stroke in East Asians and Non-East Asians: A Meta-Analysis. *Genet. Test Mol. Biomarkers* **2017**, *21*, 10–16. [CrossRef]
30. O'Rielly, D.D.; Roslin, N.M.; Beyene, J.; Pope, A. Rahman PTNF-alpha-308G/A polymorphism responsiveness to TNF-alpha blockade therapy in moderate to severe rheumatoid arthritis: A systematic review meta-analysis. *Pharmacogenom. J.* **2009**, *9*, 161–167. [CrossRef]
31. Guarnizo-Zuccardi, P.; Lopez, Y.; Giraldo, M.; Garcia, N.; Rodriguez, L.; Ramirez, L.; Uribe, O.; Garcia, L.; Vasquez, G. Cytokine gene polymorphisms in Colombian patients with systemic lupus erythematosus. *Tissue Antigens* **2007**, *70*, 376–382. [CrossRef]

32. Antonicelli, R.; Olivieri, F.; Cavallone, L.; Spazzafumo, L.; Bonaf, M.; Marchegiani, F.; Cardelli, M.; Galeazzi, R.; Giovagnetti, S.; Perna, G.P.; et al. Tumor necrosis factor-alpha gene-308G>A polymorphism is associated with ST-elevation myocardial infarction and with high plasma levels of biochemical ischemia markers. *Coron. Artery Dis.* **2005**, *16*, 489–493. [CrossRef] [PubMed]
33. Hua, X.P.; Qian, J.; Cao, C.B.; Xie, J.; Zeng, X.T.; Zhang, Z.J. Association between TNF-α rs1800629 polymorphism and the risk of myocardial infarction: A meta-analysis. *Genet. Mol. Res.* **2016**, *13*, gmr.15037292. [CrossRef]
34. Huang, R.; Zhao, S.R.; Li, Y.; Liu, F.; Gong, Y.; Xing, J.; Xu, Z.S. Association of tumor necrosis factor-α gene polymorphisms and coronary artery disease susceptibility: A systematic review and meta-analysis. *BMC Med. Genet.* **2020**, *21*, 29. [CrossRef]
35. Behboudi, A.; Thelander, T.; Yazici, D.; Celik, Y.; Yucel-Lindberg, T.; Thunström, E.; Peker, Y. Association of TNF-α (-308G/A) Gene Polymorphism with Circulating TNF-α Levels and Excessive Daytime Sleepiness in Adults with Coronary Artery Disease and Concomitant Obstructive Sleep Apnea. *J. Clin. Med.* **2021**, *10*, 3413. [CrossRef]
36. Peker, Y.; Glantz, H.; Eulenburg, C.; Wegscheider, K.; Herlitz, J.; Thunstrom, E. Effect of Positive Airway Pressure on Cardiovascular Outcomes in Coronary Artery Disease Patients with Nonsleepy Obstructive Sleep Apnea. The RICCADSA Randomized Controlled Trial. *Am. J. Respir. Crit. Care Med.* **2016**, *194*, 613–620. [CrossRef]
37. American Academy of Sleep Medicine Task Force. Sleep-related breathing disorders in adults: Recommendations for syndrome definition and measurement techniques in clinical research. The Report of an American Academy of Sleep Medicine Task Force. *Sleep* **1999**, *22*, 667–689. [CrossRef]
38. Johns, M.W. A new method for measuring daytime sleepiness: The Epworth sleepiness scale. *Sleep* **1991**, *14*, 540–545. [CrossRef] [PubMed]
39. World Health Organ. *Obesity: Preventing and Managing the Global Epidemic. Report of a WHO Consultation*; World Health Organ: Geneva, Switzerland, 2000; Volume 894, pp. i–xii.
40. Thunström, E.; Glantz, H.; Fu, M.; Yucel-Lindberg, T.; Petzold, M.; Lindberg, K.; Peker, Y. Increased inflammatory activity in nonobese patients with coronary artery disease and obstructive sleep apnea. *Sleep* **2015**, *38*, 463–471. [CrossRef] [PubMed]
41. Lederer, D.J.; Bell, S.C.; Branson, R.; Chalmers, J.D.; Marshall, R.; Maslove, D.M.; Ost, D.E.; Punjabi, N.M.; Schatz, M.; Smyth, A.R.; et al. Control of Confounding and Reporting of Results in Causal Inference Studies. Guidance for Authors from Editors of Respiratory, Sleep, and Critical Care Journals. *Ann. Am. Thorac. Soc.* **2019**, *16*, 22–28. [CrossRef]
42. Karkucak, M.; Ursavaş, A.; Ocakoğlu, G.; Görükmez, O.; Yakut, T.; Ercan, I.; Karadağ, M. Analysis of TNF-alpha G308A and C857T Gene Polymorphisms in Turkish Patients with Obstructive Sleep Apnea Syndrome. *Turk. Klin. J. Med. Sci.* **2012**, *32*, 1368–1373. [CrossRef]
43. Huang, J.; Liao, N.; Huang, Q.P.; Xie, Z.F. Association between tumor necrosis factor-α-308G/A polymorphism and obstructive sleep apnea: A meta-analysis. *Genet. Test Mol. Biomark.* **2012**, *16*, 246–251. [CrossRef]
44. Wu, Y.; Cao, C.; Wu, Y.; Zhang, C.; Zhu, C.; Ying, S.; Li, W. TNF-α-308G/A Polymorphism Contributes to Obstructive Sleep Apnea Syndrome Risk: Evidence Based on 10 Case-Control Studies. *PLoS ONE* **2014**, *9*, e106183. [CrossRef]
45. Kazemi, E.; Jamialahmadi, K.; Avan, A.; Mirhafez, S.R.; Mohiti, J.; Pirhoushiaran, M.; Hosseini, N.; Mohammadi, A.; Ferns, G.A.; Pasdar, A.; et al. Association of tumor necrosis factor-α-308G/A gene polymorphism with coronary artery diseases: An evidence-based study. *J. Clin. Lan. Anal.* **2018**, *32*, e22153. [CrossRef]
46. Nejati, P.; Naeimipour, S.; Salehi, A.; Shahbazi, M. Association of tumor necrosis factor-alpha gene promoter polymorphism and its mRNA expression level in coronary artery disease. *Meta Gene* **2018**, *18*, 122–126. [CrossRef]
47. Yuepeng, J.; Zhao, X.; Zhao, Y.; Li, L. Gene polymorphism associated with TNF-α (G308A) IL-6 (C174G) and susceptibility to coronary atherosclerotic heart disease: A meta-analysis. *Medicine* **2019**, *98*, e13813. [CrossRef] [PubMed]
48. Li, Q.; Zheng, X. Tumor necrosis factor alpha is a promising circulating biomarker for the development of obstructive sleep apnea syndrome: A meta-analysis. *Oncotarget* **2017**, *8*, 27616–27626. [CrossRef] [PubMed]
49. Thunström, E.; Glantz, H.; Yucel-Lindberg, T.; Lindberg, K.; Saygin, M.; Peker, Y. CPAP Does Not Reduce Inflammatory Biomarkers in Patients with Coronary Artery Disease and Nonsleepy Obstructive Sleep Apnea: A Randomized Controlled Trial. *Sleep* **2017**, *40*, zsx157. [CrossRef]
50. Kroeger, K.M.; Carville, K.S.; Abraham, L.J. The-308 tumor necrosis factor-alpha promoter polymorphism effects transcription. *Mol. Immunol.* **1997**, *34*, 391–399. [CrossRef]

Disclaimer/Publisher's Note: The statements, opinions and data contained in all publications are solely those of the individual author(s) and contributor(s) and not of MDPI and/or the editor(s). MDPI and/or the editor(s) disclaim responsibility for any injury to people or property resulting from any ideas, methods, instructions or products referred to in the content.

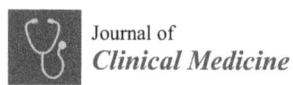

Article

The Correlation between the Severity of Obstructive Sleep Apnea and Insulin Resistance in a Japanese Population

Yukako Tomo [1], Ryo Naito [2,3,*], Yasuhiro Tomita [1], Satoshi Kasagi [1], Tatsuya Sato [4,5] and Takatoshi Kasai [1,2,3]

1. Sleep Center, Toranomon Hospital, Tokyo 105-0001, Japan; yukazou@gmail.com (Y.T.); ytomitatmy@gmail.com (Y.T.); skasagi@knd.biglobe.ne.jp (S.K.); kasai-t@mx6.nisiq.net (T.K.)
2. Department of Cardiovascular Biology and Medicine, Juntendo University Graduate School of Medicine, Tokyo 113-8421, Japan
3. Cardiovascular Respiratory Sleep Medicine, Juntendo University Graduate School of Medicine, Tokyo 113-8421, Japan
4. Department of Cellular Physiology and Signal Transduction, Sapporo Medical University School of Medicine, Sapporo 060-8556, Japan; sato.tatsuya@sapmed.ac.jp
5. Department of Cardiovascular, Renal and Metabolic Medicine, Sapporo Medical University School of Medicine, Sapporo 060-8556, Japan
* Correspondence: rnaitou@juntendo.ac.jp; Tel.: +81-3-3813-3111; Fax: +81-3-5689-0627

Abstract: Background: Repetitive episodes of apnea and hypopnea during sleep in patients with obstructive sleep apnea (OSA) are known to increase the risk of atherosclerosis. Underlying obesity and related disorders, such as insulin resistance, are indirectly related to the development of atherosclerosis. In addition, OSA is independently associated with insulin resistance; however, data regarding this relationship are scarce in Japanese populations. **Methods:** This study aimed to examine the relationship between the severity of OSA and insulin resistance in a Japanese population. We analyzed the data of consecutive patients who were referred for polysomnography under clinical suspicion of developing OSA and who did not have diabetes mellitus or any cardiovascular disease. Multiple regression analyses were performed to determine the relationship between the severity of OSA and insulin resistance. **Results:** The data from a total of 483 consecutive patients were analyzed. The median apnea-hypopnea index (AHI) was 40.9/h (interquartile range: 26.5, 59.1) and the median homeostasis model assessment for insulin resistance (HOMA-IR) was 2.00 (interquartile range: 1.25, 3.50). Multiple regression analyses revealed that the AHI, the lowest oxyhemoglobin saturation (SO_2), and the percentage of time spent on $SO_2 < 90\%$ were independently correlated with HOMA-IR (an adjusted R-squared value of 0.01278821, $p = 0.014$; an adjusted R-squared value of -0.01481952, $p = 0.009$; and an adjusted R-squared value of 0.018456581, $p = 0.003$, respectively). **Conclusions:** The severity of OSA is associated with insulin resistance assessed by HOMA-IR in a Japanese population.

Keywords: obstructive sleep apnea; insulin resistance; HOMA-IR

1. Introduction

Cardiovascular disease (CVD) is a leading cause of death worldwide. Knowing how to prevent CVD has been key for promoting health of the population and individuals around the world. The American Heart Association created a definition for the construct of cardiovascular health (CVH) in 2010 based on the idea that health is not regarded as merely the absence of disease [1]. It leveraged relevant existing evidence and emerging prevention concepts to formulate a definition that was intended to be accessible for all stakeholders, such as individuals, health practitioners, researchers for health, and policymakers, in order to focus efforts on improving CVH for all individuals. The initial definition of CVH was based on seven health behaviors, including indicators of dietary quality; participation in physical activity; exposure to cigarette smoking; and measures of body mass index, fasting blood glucose, total cholesterol, and blood pressure levels. Recently, the CVH has been updated with the inclusion of sleep as a novel CVH component [1]. Sleep is fundamental for human biology and essential for life. Epidemiological studies have identified inappropriate sleep hygiene as a risk factor for all-cause mortality, and subsequent research has explored potential mechanisms, including implications for cardiometabolic health. Much of the existing research has focused on sleep duration; however, sleep health is a multidimensional construct with overlapping components, such as duration, regularity, efficiency, self-satisfaction, impact on daytime alertness, as well as sleep-disordered breathing (SDB) [1].

Obstructive sleep apnea (OSA), which is a main type of SDB, is associated with the incidence and progression of metabolic and atherosclerotic diseases, including coronary artery disease, hypertension, and diabetes mellitus (DM) [2–5]. DM is mainly driven by insulin resistance and impaired secretion. Epidemiological studies have reported that OSA is associated with insulin resistance independent of confounders, such as obesity [6,7]. In a study of 150 overweight men, the apnea-hypopnea index (AHI) was associated with insulin resistance, independent of obesity [6]. Another case–control study of non-obese young men reported an association between OSA and insulin resistance, suggesting that OSA may provoke insulin resistance independent of obesity and age [7]. Japanese patients with OSA have different characteristics, such as comorbid obesity and anatomical abnormalities of the upper airway, from those in Europe and the United States. However, it remains unconclusive whether the severity of OSA in patients with OSA in Japan is associated with insulin resistance, even in the absence of diabetes mellitus and CVDs, which leads to insulin resistance with increased pro-inflammatory status. Therefore, we aimed to examine the relationship between the severity of OSA and insulin resistance in a Japanese population without diabetes mellitus and CVDs through exploratory data analyses.

2. Materials and Methods

2.1. Study Population

This is a retrospective observational study conducted at a single institution. Consecutive patients diagnosed with OSA using polysomnography at the sleep center of Toranomon Hospital, Tokyo, Japan, between 1 January 2006 and 1 October 2006, were enrolled in the study.

The exclusion criteria were as follows: (1) the presence of DM or undertreatment with any antidiabetic medication; (2) the presence of any CVD, including coronary artery disease, heart failure, or stroke; and (3) a history of renal failure undergoing dialysis treatment.

This study was conducted in accordance with the Declaration of Helsinki and was approved by the Ethics Board of Toranomon Hospital. In this study, sleep studies, anthropometric data collection, and blood sampling, which had already been performed as a routine clinical checkup, were analyzed. The requirement to obtain informed consent was waived by the Toranomon Hospital Ethics Board using opt-out methods.

2.2. Sleep Study

For sleep studies, overnight polysomnography was carried out, according to the standard protocols and criteria [8]. Electrocardiography, electroencephalography, electrooculography, and electromyography were performed, and thoracoabdominal motion was monitored with respiratory inductance plethysmography. Airflow was measured with an oronasal thermal airflow sensor and nasal pressure cannula, and oxyhemoglobin saturation (SO_2) was monitored with oximetry. Respiratory events (apneas or hypopneas) were counted according to the American Academy of Sleep Medicine scoring manual 2020 updates [9]. Apnea with and without rib cage and/or abdominal movement were defined as obstructive and central apnea, respectively. Hypopnea was defined as obstructive if any of the following conditions were present: (1) paradoxical chest or abdominal movements, (2) snoring, or (3) flow limitation during hypopnea events. Otherwise, hypopnea was classified as central.

2.3. Index of Insulin Resistance

The homeostasis model assessment for insulin resistance (HOMA-IR) was used as an index of insulin resistance, which was calculated as the fasting serum insulin level multiplied by the fasting glucose level multiplied by 405 [10]. Serum insulin and fasting glucose levels were measured using a commercially available assay at Toranomon Hospital before the polysomnography was performed.

2.4. Other Variables

The following variables were obtained from the clinical chart at the time of polysomnography: age; sex; body mass index (BMI); waist circumference; the presence of hypertension; and serum levels (total cholesterol, triglycerides, low-density lipoprotein cholesterol, high-density lipoprotein cholesterol, insulin, uric acid, and C-reactive protein). BMI was calculated as the body weight in kilograms divided by the square of body height in meters, and waist circumference was measured around the abdomen at the level between the top of the hip bone and the bottom of the ribs at the time of polysomnography. Hypertension is defined as systolic blood pressure $\geq$ 140 mm Hg, diastolic blood pressure $\geq$ 90 mm Hg, or under any antihypertensive medications.

2.5. Outcomes

Relationships between OSA severity, AHI, 3% oxygen desaturation index (ODI), lowest SO_2, the percentage of time spent on $SO_2 < 90\%$ (%TST $SO_2 < 90\%$), arousal index, and HOMA-IR were examined.

2.6. Statistical Analysis

The clinical data were presented as the mean $\pm$ standard deviation or median and interquartile range. Correlation analyses were performed to evaluate relationships between each index of OSA severity (AHI, 3% ODI, lowest SO_2, %TST $SO_2 < 90\%$, and arousal index) and HOMA-IR as the dependent variable adjusted for covariates (age, sex, and BMI), and the coefficient, standard error, t-test statistic (T), adjusted R-squared value, and the *p*-value were calculated. The indices of OSA severity were AHI, 3% ODI, lowest SO_2, %TST $SO_2 < 90\%$, and arousal index. As HOMA-IR was not normally distributed, log-transformed HOMA-IR (log HOMA-IR) was used in the analyses. Multiple regression analyses were performed to determine the association between OSA severity and HOMA-IR, with the other variables obtained at the time of polysomnography. Statistical significance was set at $p < 0.05$. All statistical analyses were performed using the SPSS statistical software (version 11.0; SPSS Inc., Chicago, IL, USA).

3. Results

A total of 483 patients were enrolled in this study. The participants' characteristics are presented in Table 1. The median age was 55.0 years (interquartile range (IQR): 44, 64) and 90.9% of the study population were men. The prevalence of hypertension was 54.0% and the median HOMA-IR was 2.00 (IQR: 1.25, 3.50). The polysomnographic data are presented in Table 2. The median AHI was 40.9 (IQR: 26.5, 59.1), the 3% ODI was 28.4 (IQR: 13.3, 50.5), the lowest SO_2 was 77 (IQR: 69, 82), the median arousal index was 39.1 (26.6, 56.3), and the median %TST $SO_2 < 90\%$ was 14.6 (IQR: 3.8, 44.3).

The relationships between the polysomnographic data and log HOMA-IR are shown in Table 3. The AHI, 3% ODI, %TST $SO_2 < 90\%$, and arousal index were positively correlated with log HOMA-IR (an adjusted R-squared value of 0.0038321, $p = 0.015$ for AHI; an adjusted R-squared value of 0.0030430, $p = 0.024$ for 3% ODI; an adjusted R-squared value of 0.003599, $p = 0.001$ for %TST $SO_2 < 90\%$; and an adjusted R-squared value of 0.00343508, $p = 0.028$ for the arousal index). The lowest SO_2 was inversely correlated with log HOMA-IR (an adjusted R-squared value of -0.0061958, $p = 0.004$). Multiple regression analyses revealed that AHI, 3% ODI, lowest SO_2, and %TST $SO_2 < 90\%$ were independently correlated with log HOMA-IR (an adjusted R-squared value of 0.01278821, $p = 0.014$ for

AHI; an adjusted R-squared value of −0.01481952, $p = 0.009$ for lowest SO$_2$; and an adjusted R-squared value of 0.018456581, $p = 0.003$ for %TST SO$_2$ < 90%) (Table 4).

Table 1. Baseline characteristics of the study participants.

	$n = 483$
Age, years	55.0 (44, 64)
Men, n (%)	439 (90.9)
BMI (kg/m^2)	26.6 (24.3, 29.4)
Waist circumference (cm)	95.3 ± 12.0
Hypertension, n (%)	261 (54.0)
Total cholesterol (mg/dL)	196 (174, 217)
Triglyceride (mg/dL)	139 (98, 197)
High-density lipoprotein cholesterol (mg/dL)	46 (40, 54)
Low-density lipoprotein cholesterol (mg/dL)	115.4 (97.2, 132.6)
Fasting blood glucose (mg/dL)	97 (91, 106)
Glycated hemoglobin (%)	5.4 (5.1, 5.8)
Insulin (μU/mL)	8 (5, 14)
Uric acid (mg/dL)	6.5 (5.5, 7.3)
C-reactive protein (mg/dL)	0.1 (0, 0.2)
HOMA-IR	2.00 (1.25, 3.50)

Continuous data are shown as mean ± standard deviation or median (interquartile range). Categorical data are shown as numbers (%). BMI, body mass index; HOMA-IR, homeostasis model assessment for insulin resistance.

Table 2. Polysomnographic findings.

	$n = 483$
AHI (/h)	40.9 (26.5, 59.1)
Awake SO$_2$ (%)	96 (94, 96)
Lowest SO$_2$ (%)	77 (69, 82)
%TST SO$_2$ < 90% (%)	14.6 (3.8, 44.3)
3% ODI (/h)	28.4 (13.3, 50.5)
Arousal index (/h)	39.1 (26.6, 56.3)
PLM arousal index (/h)	0.3 ± 1.3
Stage 1 (%)	31.4 (23.4, 44.5)
Stage 2 (%)	46.7 ± 12.6
Stage SWS (%)	2.8 (0.8, 6.5)
Stage REM (%)	10.3 (6.9, 14.2)

Data are shown as mean ± standard deviation or median (interquartile range). AHI, apnea-hypopnea index; SO$_2$, oxyhemoglobin saturation; TST, total sleep time; ODI, oxygen desaturation index; PLM, periodic eye movement; SWS, slow-wave sleep; REM, rapid eye movement.

Table 3. Relationships between the polysomnographic data and HOMA-IR.

	Coefficient	Standard Error	T	p	95% Confidence Interval	Adjusted R-Squared Value	Adjusted R-Squared Value for the Total Model	p-Value for the Total Model
AHI	0.0038	0.0016	2.45	0.015	0.0008, 0.0069	0.0675	0.313	<0.0001
3% ODI,	0.0030	0.0013	2.27	0.024	0.0004, 0.0057	0.0742	0.309	<0.0001
lowest SO$_2$,	−0.0062	0.0022	−2.88	0.004	−0.010, −0.0020	0.0612	0.312	<0.0001
%TST SO$_2$ < 90%,	0.0036	0.0010	3.46	0.001	0.0016, 0.0056	0.1092	0.318	<0.0001
arousal index	0.0034	0.0016	2.20	0.028	0.0004, 0.0065	0.0473	0.308	<0.0001

Age, sex, and BMI were included in each model. AHI, apnea-hypopnea index; ODI, oxygen desaturation index; SO$_2$, oxyhemoglobin saturation; TST, total sleep time; BMI, body mass index.

Table 4. Results of multiple regression analyses for the relationships between each index of OSA severity and HOMA-IR.

	Coefficient	Standard Error	T	p	95% Confidence Interval	Adjusted R-Squared Value	Adjusted R-Squared Value for the Total Model	p-Value for the Total Model
AHI	0.0015	0.000608	2.48	0.014	0.0003, 0.0027	0.0742	0.319	<0.0001
3% ODI,	0.0011	0.000566	1.91	0.057	−0.000037, 0.002189	0.0798	0.315	<0.0001
lowest SO_2,	−0.0026	0.000994	−2.61	0.009	−0.004550, −0.000643	0.0660	0.320	<0.0001
%TST SO_2 < 90%,	0.0014	0.000465	2.99	0.003	0.000475, 0.002304	0.1148	0.323	<0.0001
arousal index	0.0011	0.000632	1.79	0.074	−0.000110, 0.002375	0.0487	0.313	<0.0001

Age, sex, BMI, waist circumference, and presence of hypertension were included in each model. AHI, apnea-hypopnea index; ODI, oxygen desaturation index; SO_2, oxyhemoglobin saturation; TST, total sleep time; BMI, body mass index.

4. Discussion

Our study demonstrated that the indices of OSA severity (AHI, lowest SO_2, and %TST SO_2 < 90%) were correlated with insulin resistance, as assessed by HOMA-IR after adjusting for covariates in a Japanese population without diabetes mellitus and CVDs. The finding seems to be pathophysiologically valid because the high severity of OSA can be related to chronic sympathetic activity and systemic inflammation that can elicit insulin resistance. Although sleep disorders are often readily missed in routine medical care, they have been reported to be strongly associated with the development of CVDs. Therefore, the results of this study suggest that, at least in Japanese populations, even in the absence of known CVDs or diabetes mellitus, findings of insulin resistance may form the basis for suspecting the presence of OSA.

Epidemiological studies have reported an association between SDB and insulin resistance. A study reported that increased AHI was associated with worsening insulin resistance (odds ratio, 2.15; 95% confidence interval, 1.05 to 4.38), independent of obesity, in 150 obese men (mean BMI 30.5 ± 2.9 kg/m^2) without DM or cardiopulmonary disease [6]. Another case–control study of 52 young lean men (with a mean age of 23.4 ± 0.4 years and mean BMI of 22.6 ± 0.3 kg/m^2) without cardiometabolic disease reported that participants with OSA had 27% lower insulin sensitivity, estimated by the Matsuda index, and 37% higher insulin secretion after the ingestion of glucose load than those without OSA [7]. A longitudinal study assessing 141 non-diabetic men (with a mean age of 57.5 years and a mean BMI of 26.9 kg/m^2), with a mean follow-up of 11 years and 4 months, reported that an oxygen desaturation index >5/h was significantly associated with deteriorated insulin resistance assessed using the change in HOMA-IR from baseline to follow-up and a higher incidence of diabetes, partially supporting the findings of our study [11]. Nevertheless, the strong correlation between the severity of OSA observed in this study with insulin resistance reemphasizes that the presence of OSA can be a potent risk factor for atherosclerotic diseases via increased insulin resistance.

4.1. Mechanisms of the Association between OSA and Insulin Resistance

The presumed mechanisms underlying the association between OSA and insulin resistance include intermittent hypoxemia caused by OSA [12], inappropriate OSA-related sleep hygiene [13–15], increased sympathetic nerve activity, oxidative stress, and inflammation (Figure 1). In experimental animal models, intermittent hypoxia was shown to mediate hypoxia-inducible factor 1α expression in pancreatic beta cells, resulting in insulin resistance when the production of reactive oxygen species increases [16]. It has been speculated that initial hypoxia exposure may affect insulin clearance in the liver. From these findings, it is possible that the effects of hypoxia on insulin resistance may differ depending on the degree of hypoxia and the duration of exposure. Sleep fragmentation using auditory and mechanical stimulation in healthy subjects has been reported to reduce insulin sensitivity by 20–25% [15,17,18]. The mechanisms by which SDB induces insulin resistance is likely to be complex and cannot be explained by a single pathway, but the pathogenesis listed above may at least be involved in the sleep disturbances that can develop or exacerbate CVDs via the presence of insulin resistance.

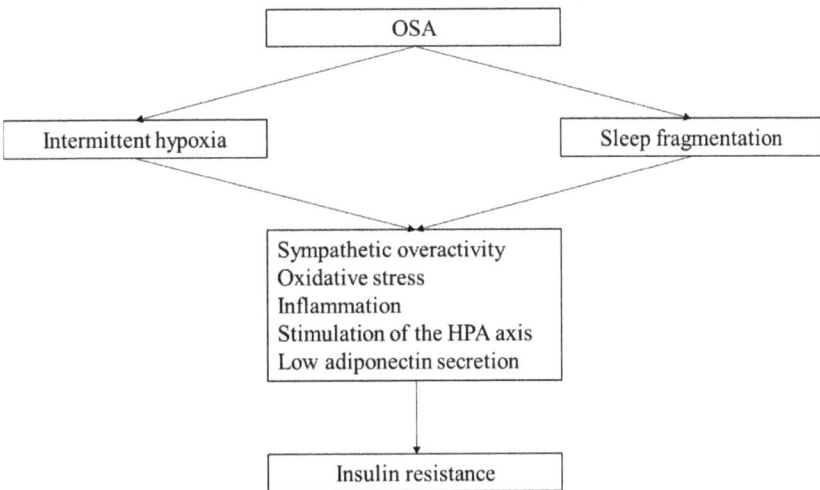

Figure 1. Mechanisms linking OSA and insulin resistance include sympathetic overactivity, oxidative stress, inflammation, the stimulation of the HPA axis and low adiponectin secretion induced by intermittent hypoxia and sleep fragmentation. HPA; hypothalamic–pituitary–adrenal.

4.2. Positive Airway Pressure Therapy for OSA and Insulin Resistance

Treatments for OSA include lifestyle modification mainly for obesity, postural therapy for patients with OSA whose severity of OSA fluctuate according to the body position, intraoral appliance, upper airway surgery, and CPAP therapy. Among the various treatment options for OSA, CPAP therapy has been an established choice to decrease AHI and improve symptoms due to OSA and quality of life, which has been covered by insurance since 1998 in Japan [2]. Variety of beneficial effects of CPAP for patients with OSA have been reported such as lowering blood pressure, suppression of sympathetic nerve activity, decrease in inflammatory markers, improvement of vascular endothelial function, left ventricular systolic and diastolic function, and nocturnal myocardial ischemia [2]. However, prognostic benefits of CPAP in patients with OSA concomitant with CVDs have been conflicting. An observational study examining prognostic effects of CPAP therapy in fifty-four patients with OSA and coronary artery disease reported that CPAP therapy was associated with reduction in a composite of cardiovascular events (cardiovascular death, acute coronary syndrome, hospitalization for heart failure, or coronary revascularization) with hazard ratio of 0.24 (95% confidence interval of 0.09–0.62) for CPAP as compared to the non-treatment group during a median follow-up of 86.5 months [19]. In contrast, large-scale randomized controlled trials investigating the effects of CPAP in patients with OSA and coronary artery disease did not agree with this finding, although low adherence to CPAP (with a mean usage time of CPAP < 4 h/night) was found to potentially affect the observed neutral finding [20–22]. The most recent trial of 1264 patients with acute coronary syndrome and OSA compared a range of cardiovascular events, including cardiovascular death, non-fatal myocardial infarction, non-fatal stroke, hospitalization for unstable angina pectoris, heart failure, and transient ischemic attack between CPAP and non-CPAP groups [22]. No significant reduction in the incident cardiovascular events was observed for the CPAP group (with a hazard ratio of 0.89 and a 95% confidence interval of 0.68–1.17) during a median follow-up of 3.35 years. Similarly, the prognostic benefits of CPAP therapy on reducing the number of cardiovascular events in patients with CVDs, including heart failure, ventricular arrhythmias, stroke, aortic disease, and other vascular diseases, have not yet been demonstrated in randomized controlled trials.

Although our study demonstrated the relationship between the severity of OSA and insulin resistance, evidence on whether positive airway pressure therapy for OSA improves insulin resistance has not yet been established. A small randomized controlled trial that assessed the effect of CPAP therapy on glycated hemoglobin in 50 patients with OSA and type 2 DM (with a mean age of 61 ± 9 years and a mean BMI of 32.5 ± 4.5 kg/m^2) reported that CPAP therapy for 6 months decreased glycated hemoglobin compared to the no-CPAP group (with an intergroup adjusted difference of −0.4 (95% confidence interval of −0.7 to −0.04), p = 0.029) [23]. HOMA-IR was also significantly reduced in the CPAP group (with an intergroup adjusted difference of −2.58 and a 95% confidence interval of −4.75 to −0.41, p = 0.023). Furthermore, serum biomarker levels of IL-1β, IL-6, and adiponectin also improved in the CPAP group compared with the control group, suggesting the effects of CPAP therapy on improving glucose metabolism and reversing proinflammatory status [23]. Another randomized trial assessed the incremental effect of combined intervention, including a weight loss intervention and CPAP, in which 146 patients with obesity, moderate-to-severe OSA, and serum levels of C-reactive protein (CRP) greater than 1.0 mg/L were allocated to three groups (CPAP alone, weight loss intervention alone, or CPAP with a weight loss intervention) [24]. In the 24th week of the interventions, CRP levels, insulin resistance levels, and serum triglyceride levels were reduced in the patients assigned to weight loss only and those assigned to the combined interventions, while none of these changes were observed in the group treated using CPAP alone. Reductions in insulin resistance and serum triglyceride levels were greater in the combination treatment group than in the group treated using CPAP therapy alone. In per-protocol analyses, which included 90 participants who met prespecified criteria for adherence to CPAP therapy (used for an average of at least 4 h per night on at least 70% of the total number of nights) [24]. On the other hand, a study in which the effects of CPAP on glycemic variability were assessed in 203 patients of SDB with or without diabetes mellitus (mean age 67.5 ± 14.1 years) was also conducted. Glycemic variability assessed by continuous glucose monitoring showed that CPAP reduced the mean amplitude of glycemic excursion from 75.3 to 53.0 mg/dl in the non-DM group, but a similar finding was not observed in the DM group, suggesting the difficulty of improving glucose metabolism using CPAP therapy in patients with advanced glucose metabolism disorders [25]. A meta-analysis of nine randomized controlled trials (443 patients) comparing CPAP treatment with sham CPAP groups, placebo groups, or no-treatment groups, with the goal of improving insulin resistance and glucose metabolism in non-diabetic adults with OSA, reported that CPAP therapy significantly improved HOMA-IR (with a mean difference = −0.39 Ui (CI: −0.69 to −0.08), p < 0.05, and I^2 = 57%) as compared to the non-CPAP group, while no significant differences in fasting glucose was observed [26]. The other meta-analysis, in which 23 studies (19 prospective studies and 4 randomized controlled trials with a total of 965 patients) were included, assessed the effect of CPAP therapy on HOMA-IR, fasting blood glucose, and fasting insulin in non-diabetic and pre-diabetic patients with OSA. CPAP therapy showed significant reductions in the pooled standard difference regarding the means of HOMA-IR (−0.442, p = 0.001) from baseline levels compared with the control group, while no significant differences were observed for fasting blood glucose and fasting insulin from baseline levels between the CPAP and the control groups [27]. Despite the findings of these meta-analyses, we cannot conclude the generalizability of these findings due to the small sample size of each study included in the meta-analyses and the difference in study populations and designs. Further large-scale studies are needed to determine the effects of CPAP on insulin resistance. Given that diets play an important role in the development of obesity which can cause OSA and cardiovascular disease through metabolic disorders and inflammation, and given that specific diets such as Washoku (Japanese diet) and the Mediterranean diet have been regarded as healthy diets [28], research on dietary patterns in relation to the prevention of cardio-metabolic diseases is warranted in order to reduce the burden of CVDs. Furthermore, the development of artificial intelligence may enable the implementation of personalized medicine in various medical fields, such as sleep medicine, whereby treatment effects, adverse effects, and net benefits are communicated to medical practitioners in advance, leading them to choose the best possible treatment for each patient. While the advent of such technology-based prediction models and the potential benefits of utilizing the models for patients with OSA and concomitant cardiovascular risks and diseases are acceptable, we must bear in mind that physicians and other medical practitioners are essential players in preventing cardiovascular events in these patients by encouraging them to adhere to a healthy diet, including salt restriction and a reduction in calory intake, physical activity, the maintenance of healthy body weight, smoking cessation, sobriety, and other self-management, all of which are recommended to improve CVH.

4.3. Limitations

We acknowledge that this study has several limitations. First, this was a retrospective analysis of a single-center observational study in an urban area with a relatively small sample size. Since sleep disorders can be influenced by occupational and residential settings, we cannot rule out the possibility that a multicenter study that includes rural areas may lead to different results. Second, unknown confounders, such as diet, physical activity, and other lifestyle factors may have affected the results, even after the multivariate analysis. Therefore, our data should be interpreted carefully, and further studies with larger sample sizes are required to confirm our findings. Although the reliability of HOMA-IR depends on the precision of the insulin radioimmunoassay, we lack detailed information on the assay used to measure insulin in this study. Since the majority of the study participants are men, our findings may not be applicable for women. Finally, although this study included subjects without DM or known CVDs, the possibility of asymptomatic or latent CVDs being present cannot be completely excluded.

5. Conclusions

Our study demonstrated that the severity of OSA was independently correlated with insulin resistance, as assessed using HOMA-IR in a Japanese population with OSA who do not have DM and CVDs.

Author Contributions: T.K.—methodology, investigation, review and editing, and supervision; Y.T. (Yukako Tomo) and R.N.—original draft preparation; Y.T. (Yasuhiro Tomita), T.S. and S.K.—supervision. All the authors have read and approved the final draft. All authors have read and agreed to the published version of the manuscript.

Funding: This study was partly supported by JSPS KAKENHI (grant numbers: JP21K08116 and JP21K16034); a Grant-in-Aid for Scientific Research (grant numbers: 20FC1027 and 23FC1031) from the Ministry of Health, Labor, and Welfare of Japan; and a research grant from the Japanese Center for Research on Women in Sport, Juntendo University. These funding sources did not play any other role in this study.

Institutional Review Board Statement: This study was conducted in accordance with the Declaration of Helsinki and approved by the Ethics Board of Toranomon Hospital (code: 1864, approved on 13 September 2016).

Informed Consent Statement: The requirement to obtain informed consent was waived by the Toranomon Hospital Ethics Board using opt-out methods.

Data Availability Statement: The deidentified participant data will be shared by the corresponding author upon reasonable request.

Conflicts of Interest: Ryo Naito and Takatoshi Kasai are affiliated with a department funded by Philips Respironics, ResMed, and Fukuda Denshi. The remaining authors have no conflicts of interest to declare.

References

1. Lloyd-Jones, D.M.; Allen, N.B.; Anderson, C.A.; Black, T.; Brewer, L.C.; Foraker, R.E.; Grandner, M.A.; Lavretsky, H.; Perak, A.M.; Sharma, G.; et al. Life's Essential 8: Updating and Enhancing the American Heart Association's Construct of Cardiovascular Health: A Presidential Advisory from the American Heart Association. *Circulation* **2022**, *146*, E18–E43. [CrossRef]
2. Kasai, T.; Floras, J.S.; Bradley, T.D. Sleep apnea and cardiovascular disease: A bidirectional relationship. *Circulation* **2012**, *126*, 1495–1510. [CrossRef] [PubMed]
3. Kent, B.D.; McNicholas, W.T.; Ryan, S. Insulin resistance, glucose intolerance and diabetes mellitus in obstructive sleep apnoea. *J. Thorac. Dis.* **2015**, *7*, 1343–1357. [CrossRef] [PubMed]
4. Pamidi, S.; Aronsohn, R.S.; Tasali, E. Obstructive sleep apnea: Role in the risk and severity of diabetes. *Best Pract. Res. Clin. Endocrinol. Metab.* **2010**, *24*, 703–715. [CrossRef] [PubMed]
5. Rajan, P.; Greenberg, H. Obstructive sleep apnea as a risk factor for type 2 diabetes mellitus. *Nat. Sci. Sleep.* **2015**, *7*, 113–125. [CrossRef] [PubMed]
6. Punjabi, N.M.; Sorkin, J.D.; Katzel, L.I.; Goldberg, A.P.; Schwartz, A.R.; Smith, P.L. Sleep-disordered Breathing and Insulin Resistance in Middle-aged and Overweight Men. *Am. J. Respir. Crit. Care Med.* **2002**, *165*, 677–682. [CrossRef] [PubMed]
7. Pamidi, S.; Wroblewski, K.; Broussard, J.; Day, A.; Hanlon, E.C.; Abraham, V.; Tasali, E. Obstructive Sleep Apnea in Young Lean Men. *Diabetes Care* **2012**, *35*, 2384–2389. [CrossRef] [PubMed]
8. American Academy of Sleep Medicine (Ed.) *Sleep Technicians and Technologists*; AASM Facility Standards for Accreditation: Darien, IL, USA, 2020.
9. American Academy of Sleep Medicine. *The AASM Manual for the Scoring of Sleep and Associated Events: Rules, Terminology and Technical Specifications*; Version 2.6; American Academy of Sleep Medicine: Westchester, IL, USA, 2020.
10. Matthews, D.R.; Hosker, J.P.; Rudenski, A.S.; Naylor, B.A.; Treacher, D.F.; Turner, R.C. Homeostasis model assessment: Insulin resistance and ?-cell function from fasting plasma glucose and insulin concentrations in man. *Diabetologia* **1985**, *28*, 412–419. [CrossRef] [PubMed]
11. Lindberg, E.; Theorell-Haglöw, J.; Svensson, M.; Gislason, T.; Berne, C.; Janson, C. Sleep Apnea and Glucose Metabolism. *Chest* **2012**, *142*, 935–942. [CrossRef]
12. Louis, M.; Punjabi, N.M. Effects of acute intermittent hypoxia on glucose metabolism in awake healthy volunteers. *Appl. Physiol.* **2009**, *106*, 1538–1544. [CrossRef]
13. Spiegel, K.; Leproult, R.; Van Cauter, E. Impact of sleep debt on metabolic and endocrine function. *Lancet* **1999**, *354*, 1435–1439. [CrossRef] [PubMed]
14. Broussard, J.L.; Ehrmann, D.A.; Van Cauter, E.; Tasali, E.; Brady, M.J. Impaired Insulin Signaling in Human Adipocytes After Experimental Sleep Restriction: A Randomized, Crossover Study. *Ann. Intern. Med.* **2012**, *157*, 549. [CrossRef] [PubMed]
15. Stamatakis, K.A.; Punjabi, N.M. Effects of Sleep Fragmentation on Glucose Metabolism in Normal Subjects. *Chest* **2010**, *137*, 95–101. [CrossRef] [PubMed]
16. Prabhakar, N.R.; Peng, Y.J.; Nanduri, J. Hypoxia-inducible factors and obstructive sleep apnea. *J. Clin. Investig.* **2020**, *130*, 5042–5051. [CrossRef] [PubMed]
17. Tasali, E.; Leproult, R.; Ehrmann, D.A.; Van Cauter, E. Slow-wave sleep and the risk of type 2 diabetes in humans. *Proc. Natl. Acad. Sci. USA* **2008**, *105*, 1044–1049. [CrossRef] [PubMed]
18. Herzog, N.; Jauch-Chara, K.; Hyzy, F.; Richter, A.; Friedrich, A.; Benedict, C.; Oltmanns, K.M. Selective slow wave sleep but not rapid eye movement sleep suppression impairs morning glucose tolerance in healthy men. *Psychoneuroendocrinology* **2013**, *38*, 2075–2082. [CrossRef] [PubMed]
19. Milleron, O.; Pillière, R.; Foucher, A.; de Roquefeuil, F.; Aegerter, P.; Jondeau, G.; Raffestin, B.G.; Dubourg, O. Benefits of obstructive sleep apnoea treatment in coronary artery disease: A long-term follow-up study. *Eur. Hear J.* **2004**, *25*, 728–734. [CrossRef] [PubMed]
20. McEvoy, R.D.; Antic, N.A.; Heeley, E.; Luo, Y.; Ou, Q.; Zhang, X.; Mediano, O.; Chen, R.; Drager, L.F.; Liu, Z.; et al. CPAP for Prevention of Cardiovascular Events in Obstructive Sleep Apnea. *N. Engl. J. Med.* **2016**, *375*, 919–931. [CrossRef] [PubMed]
21. Peker, Y.; Glantz, H.; Eulenburg, C.; Wegscheider, K.; Herlitz, J.; Thunström, E. Effect of Positive Airway Pressure on Cardiovascular Outcomes in Coronary Artery Disease Patients with Nonsleepy Obstructive Sleep Apnea. The RICCADSA Randomized Controlled Trial. *Am. J. Respir. Crit. Care Med.* **2016**, *194*, 613–620. [CrossRef]
22. Sánchez-De-La-Torre, M.; Sánchez-De-La-Torre, A.; Bertran, S.; Abad, J.; Duran-Cantolla, J.; Cabriada, V.; Mediano, O.; Masdeu, M.J.; Alonso, M.L.; Masa, J.F.; et al. Effect of obstructive sleep apnoea and its treatment with continuous positive airway pressure on the prevalence of cardiovascular events in patients with acute coronary syndrome (ISAACC study): A randomised controlled trial. *Lancet Respir. Med.* **2020**, *8*, 359–367. [CrossRef]
23. Martínez-Cerón, E.; Barquiel, B.; Bezos, A.-M.; Casitas, R.; Galera, R.; García-Benito, C.; Hernanz, A.; Alonso-Fernández, A.; Garcia-Rio, F. Effect of Continuous Positive Airway Pressure on Glycemic Control in Patients with Obstructive Sleep Apnea and Type 2 Diabetes. A Randomized Clinical Trial. *Am. J. Respir. Crit. Care Med.* **2016**, *194*, 476–485. [CrossRef] [PubMed]

24. Chirinos, J.A.; Gurubhagavatula, I.; Teff, K.; Rader, D.J.; Wadden, T.A.; Townsend, R.; Foster, G.D.; Maislin, G.; Saif, H.; Broderick, P.; et al. CPAP, Weight Loss, or Both for Obstructive Sleep Apnea. *N. Engl. J. Med.* **2014**, *370*, 2265–2275. [CrossRef] [PubMed]
25. Nakata, K.; Miki, T.; Tanno, M.; Ohnishi, H.; Yano, T.; Muranaka, A.; Sato, T.; Oshima, H.; Tatekoshi, Y.; Mizuno, M.; et al. Distinct impacts of sleep-disordered breathing on glycemic variability in patients with and without diabetes mellitus. *PLoS ONE* **2017**, *12*, e0188689. [CrossRef] [PubMed]
26. Abud, R.; Salgueiro, M.; Drake, L.; Reyes, T.; Jorquera, J.; Labarca, G. Efficacy of continuous positive airway pressure (CPAP) preventing type 2 diabetes mellitus in patients with obstructive sleep apnea hypopnea syndrome (OSAHS) and insulin resistance: A systematic review and meta-analysis. *Sleep Med.* **2019**, *62*, 14–21. [CrossRef] [PubMed]
27. Chen, L.; Kuang, J.; Pei, J.-H.; Chen, H.-M.; Chen, Z.; Li, Z.-W.; Yang, H.-Z.; Fu, X.-Y.; Wang, L.; Chen, Z.-J.; et al. Continuous positive airway pressure and diabetes risk in sleep apnea patients: A systemic review and meta-analysis. *Eur. J. Intern. Med.* **2017**, *39*, 39–50. [CrossRef]
28. Singh, R.B.; Fedacko, J.; Fatima, G.; Magomedova, A.; Watanabe, S.; Elkilany, G. Why and How the Indo-Mediterranean Diet May Be Superior to Other Diets: The Role of Antioxidants in the Diet. *Nutrients* **2022**, *14*, 898. [CrossRef]

Disclaimer/Publisher's Note: The statements, opinions and data contained in all publications are solely those of the individual author(s) and contributor(s) and not of MDPI and/or the editor(s). MDPI and/or the editor(s) disclaim responsibility for any injury to people or property resulting from any ideas, methods, instructions or products referred to in the content.

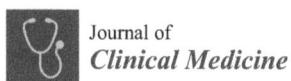

Review

The Future of Telemedicine for Obstructive Sleep Apnea Treatment: A Narrative Review

Sébastien Bailly [1,†], Monique Mendelson [1,†], Sébastien Baillieul [1], Renaud Tamisier [1] and Jean-Louis Pépin [1,2,*]

1. HP2 Laboratory, Inserm U1300, Grenoble Alps University, 38000 Grenoble, France; sbailly@chu-grenoble.fr (S.B.); mmendelson@chu-grenoble.fr (M.M.); sbaillieul@chu-grenoble.fr (S.B.); rtamisier@chu-grenoble.fr (R.T.)
2. Laboratoire EFCR, CHU de Grenoble, CS10217, 38043 Grenoble, France
* Correspondence: jpepin@chu-grenoble.fr
† These authors contributed equally to this work.

Abstract: Obstructive sleep apnea is a common type of sleep-disordered breathing associated with multiple comorbidities. Nearly a billion people are estimated to have obstructive sleep apnea, which carries a substantial economic burden, but under-diagnosis is still a problem. Continuous positive airway pressure (CPAP) is the first-line treatment for OSAS. Telemedicine-based interventions (TM) have been evaluated to improve access to diagnosis, increase CPAP adherence, and contribute to easing the follow-up process, allowing healthcare facilities to provide patient-centered care. This narrative review summarizes the evidence available regarding the potential future of telemedicine in the management pathway of OSA. The potential of home sleep studies to improve OSA diagnosis and the importance of remote monitoring for tracking treatment adherence and failure and to contribute to developing patient engagement tools will be presented. Further studies are needed to explore the impact of shifting from teleconsultations to collaborative care models where patients are placed at the center of their care.

Keywords: telemedicine; obstructive sleep apnea; diagnosis; continuous positive airway pressure; adherence; artificial intelligence; collaborative care; virtual sleep laboratory

1. Introduction

Obstructive sleep apnea (OSA) is one of the most common chronic diseases and affects nearly one billion people worldwide [1,2]. The prevalence of OSA is expected to continue to rise due to the epidemic of obesity, physical inactivity, and diabetes, all of which are risk factors for OSA [3]. Patients with OSA present significant heterogeneity and diversity in clinical presentation and responses to treatment [4–6]. Moreover, OSA, in its heterogenous presentation, is related to comorbidities' occurrence, and co-evolution and aggregation can emerge over time [7–9]. The first-line treatment for OSA is continuous positive airway pressure (CPAP), which opens and stabilizes the upper airways during sleep. Currently, millions of patients are treated by CPAP worldwide and CPAP treatment relies essentially on ambulatory care. CPAP is highly effective in improving patient-reported outcome measures (PROMs) and cardiovascular risk only in adherent patients. Several studies show that all-cause mortality is associated with CPAP adherence or CPAP continuation [10–12].

Traditionally, the diagnosis of OSA relies on overnight polysomnography conducted in a sleep clinic, a process often characterized by lengthy waiting lists and high demand for human resources, as well as carrying the potential for misdiagnosis and severity misclassification (i.e., due to night-to-night variability in the apnea–hypopnea index (AHI) [13–20]). Thus, among the current requirements for an accurate diagnostic workup of OSA, it is recommended that at-home multi-night testing becomes mainstream practice [21]. This

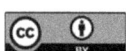

situation requires the development and validation of new end-to-end digital medicine solutions supported by artificial intelligence [22].

Moreover, despite the benefits of CPAP treatment, CPAP adherence remains low. A study based on half a million patients showed that up to 50% of patients stop CPAP therapy in the first 3 years after initiation [23]. Thus, a new organization of the follow-up management pathway will be necessary in the future. Reinventing the diagnostic tools alone is a first step; however, there is a need to transform the entire patient journey from the suspicion of OSA to ongoing treatment management follow-up.

Telemedicine is defined as the remote delivery of healthcare services, leveraging telecommunications technology to facilitate the exchange of medical information between patients and healthcare providers. Telemedicine has the potential to offer patients convenient access to healthcare [24] and offers remarkable potential to lower healthcare costs and enhance access to various care services for underserved populations [25]. Telemedicine is already used in various pathologies and it has been shown that it is an acceptable alternative to in-person care as evidenced in a recent study examining the feasibility, effectiveness, and acceptance of virtual visits as compared to in-person visits among clinical electrophysiology patients during the COVID-19 pandemic [26].

OSA treatment is well designed for telemedicine with remote telemonitoring, which is already deployed in pediatric (for review: [27]) and adult populations. In France, a new national CPAP telemonitoring and pay-for-performance scheme for homecare providers was implemented in 2018 and now involves 98% of CPAP-treated patients in France. This enables healthcare professionals to track sleep patterns and treatment adherence without the need for frequent in-person visits. The COVID-19 pandemic has led to the development of remote medical consultation systems, which have helped to advance telemedicine approaches in the context of OSA. Conversely, the COVID-19 pandemic also exacerbated existing challenges in accessing sleep laboratories, leading to significant variability in the duration of accessing diagnostic exams for OSA [28,29]. This delay in diagnosis and subsequent treatment poses limitations, particularly given the reliance on one-night sleep measures that fail to capture the full variability of the condition. However, amongst these challenges, telemedicine has emerged as a promising solution, offering out-of-lab exams that demonstrate comparable performance to traditional polysomnography (PSG) for diagnosing sleep apnea [30–32]. Few studies to date have investigated the cost-effectiveness of telemedicine in the management of OSA. Nevertheless, a randomized controlled trial comparing a telemedicine-based CPAP follow-up strategy compared with standard face-to-face management showed that telemedicine is cost-effective mostly due to savings on transport and less lost productivity (indirect costs) [33].

In this narrative review, we aim to investigate what could be the future of telemedicine in the treatment of OSA by exposing how home sleep studies driven by technological innovations and artificial intelligence can improve the diagnosis of OSA by decreasing delays in diagnosis and increasing access to evaluations. We will also present the importance of remote monitoring for tracking treatment adherence as well as treatment failure and the potential of remote monitoring to contribute to the development of patient engagement tools and telerehabilitation programs. Lastly, we will present the shift from teleconsultations to collaborative care models that place the patient at the center of his/her care. Lastly, we will present the pitfalls of telemedicine and the challenges remaining in the development of remote management pathways.

2. Home Sleep Studies Driven by Technology Innovations and Artificial Intelligence Analysis

Traditionally, the diagnosis of OSA relies on overnight polysomnography conducted in sleep clinics, often leading to lengthy waiting periods due to high demand and the intensive need for human resources. Polysomnography is complex to implement and also requires specific expertise for analysis. Furthermore, it is widely acknowledged that a single night of polysomnography can result in the misclassification of disease severity for approximately one third of patients with mild-to-moderate sleep apnea [17]. This discrepancy stems from significant night-to-night fluctuations in the apnea–hypopnea index (AHI) and inconsistencies in sleep quality [13–15]. These factors include wake/sleep habits, alcohol or drug consumption, social jetlag, rostral fluid shift, natural night-to-night changes in sleep architecture (i.e., respective proportions of time spent in non-rapid eye movement [NREM] and rapid eye movement [REM] sleep), and changes in body and head positions during sleep [34–37].

The American Academy of Sleep Medicine has endorsed clinical practice guidelines supporting home sleep apnea testing (HSAT) using technically appropriate devices for diagnosing OSA in "uncomplicated adult patients presenting with signs and symptoms that indicate an increased risk of moderate to severe OSA" (strong recommendation) [38]. The impact of the "first night effect" is notably significant within sleep laboratories, as the unfamiliar setting can result in shifts in sleep architecture, alterations in sleeping positions, and consequent variations in respiratory event measures [15]. Thus, among the current necessities for a precise diagnosis of OSA, it is imperative that multi-night testing at home becomes standard practice [21]. Although implementing such a strategy has faced challenges, including potential increases in healthcare expenses and inconvenience for patients, the advent of new digital medical solutions promises to streamline the process of multi-night testing at home, enabling the establishment of efficient and cost-effective diagnostic pathways [17,39–41].

Home sleep studies (home sleep apnea testing or HSAT) offer a more accessible and convenient alternative to traditional in-lab sleep studies. Patients can conduct sleep studies in the comfort of their homes, which may increase overall participation in diagnostic assessments, especially among those who might find attending a sleep clinic challenging and expensive [42]. This advancement signifies a new potential avenue for expanding access to both diagnosis and treatment for OSA, addressing critical gaps in care exacerbated by the pandemic. A major step forward in the seamless integration of new diagnostics would be the validation and availability of a select set of innovative sensors and metrics capable of consolidating comprehensive information necessary to understand the pathophysiology of sleep disorders and assess disease severity [31,43]. Numerous technologies have emerged for the diagnosis of sleep apnea in the home environment, with promising techniques such as mandibular jaw movements (MJMs), photoplethysmography (PPG), and peripheral arterial tone demonstrating high performance in various research and clinical contexts [44]. Developing access to a telemedicine solution for OSA diagnosis could involve a virtual sleep laboratory, as proposed previously [22], with a view to improving (and increasing) access to adequate treatment for OSA, which remains an under-diagnosed chronic sleep disorder. Such a virtual sleep laboratory would propose preliminary screening with a recommendation for a home sleep test, if appropriate, (ideally, over several nights), data collection, and interpretation in a digital pipeline, strictly adhering to data protection rules [22,45,46].

3. Remote Monitoring, Treatment Adherence, and Treatment Failures

Once OSA is diagnosed, the first-line treatment for OSA is CPAP. Machine or web-based tracking systems that generate information for both the healthcare provider and the patient are a new aspect of CPAP devices. Over the last 20 years, telemedicine technology has been applied in the field of CPAP. This has facilitated the follow-up process and allowed healthcare providers to provide more consistent care. Despite advancements in device technology over the past two decades, CPAP termination rates remain persistently high [23], highlighting a significant adherence challenge. Interestingly, factors such as OSA severity, measured by the apnea–hypopnea index, and technical features of CPAP devices appear to have minimal impact on adherence rates. Instead, attention must be directed towards recognizing and addressing other influential factors such as comorbidities, psychological factors, relationship dynamics, socioeconomic status, access to care, and cultural diversity [47–49]. Tailored interventions should be developed to address these multifaceted determinants of CPAP adherence, focusing not only on enhancing device usage but also on promoting overall lifestyle changes, encompassing physical activity and dietary habits. Access to these personalized strategies can be facilitated through improved visualization tools on CPAP remote monitoring platforms and the widespread adoption of telemedicine services, incorporating innovative analytics like artificial intelligence to enhance efficacy and accessibility.

Remote monitoring platforms also offer a valuable means of detecting potential failures in positive airway pressure (PAP) treatment and facilitating timely interventions. Initially, these platforms can help pinpoint instances of elevated or fluctuating residual apnea–hypopnea index (AHI) levels under PAP therapy, as highlighted in a study by Midelet et al. [50,51]. Additionally, through telemedicine, healthcare providers can effectively identify cases of high residual AHI attributed to specific issues with PAP equipment. Treatment failure induced by mask change can be directly monitored from PAP remote monitoring data using automated algorithms which are able to automatically assess the change in rAHI level related to a mask change and produce a significant alert which can be used as a telemedicine tool [51]. Another possibility is to identify the point in time in the remote monitoring data at which an elevated residual AHI may be indicative of an exacerbation of cardiovascular comorbidities, leading to a clinical alert for the patient's healthcare provider [52–54]. This implies the integration of some machine learning algorithms directly in the remote process, such as some machine learning algorithms to consider rAHI variability [55].

This integration of remote monitoring and telemedicine not only enhances the early detection of treatment inefficiencies but also enables targeted interventions to optimize patient outcomes and improve overall therapy adherence. The French health system has demonstrated for the first time that a national deployment is feasible and financial performance incentives encourage homecare providers to redirect resources and interactions towards individuals who have the lowest adherence to CPAP.

4. Patient Education and Engagement and Telerehabilitation Programs

In line with the widespread use of remote monitoring platforms, over the past few years there has been an increase in the access to online medical information, a proliferation of health apps on mobile phones and wearable devices, and a rising utilization of patient portals within electronic medical records [56–58]. Taken together, this clearly demonstrates that patients increasingly want to be engaged in their own health management. As mentioned previously, the ability of CPAP devices to record data on usage, efficacy, leak, and other parameters has transformed the management of patients on CPAP. Telemedicine provides a unique opportunity to collect objective data regarding adherence, efficacy, and leak data, along with patient reported outcome measures (PROMs). A recent study evaluating the impact of PROMs on CPAP usage in a real-world setting demonstrated a relationship between PROMs and CPAP use, in particular self-reported sleepiness and its response to therapy [59]. The authors of this study highlighted the potential of capturing PROMs using digital solutions during the course of treatment in order to enhance patient outcomes by providing actionable insights.

Patient engagement can be achieved through web-based access to CPAP therapy data and other asynchronous telemedicine approaches. A recent Cochrane review examined the effects of supportive, educational, and behavioral interventions on CPAP adherence. These different intervention types increase CPAP usage with varying degrees of effectiveness, which may be related to the heterogeneous nature of the factors affecting CPAP use [60]. Behavioral therapy was shown to increase machine usage by 79 min per night, and ongoing supportive interventions increase machine use by about 42 min per night. This is significantly greater than the MCID of 30 min [61].

The use of telemonitoring platforms at CPAP initiation provide an opportunity to combine lifestyle interventions and patient engagement, supported by telemedicine for integrated care in OSA. An example of holistic telerehabilitation lifestyle intervention at

CPAP initiation has recently been described using the intervention mapping framework [62] and the results of this multi-center randomized controlled trial can be used to inform the design of future interventions [63].

Telemedicine can provide application tools to collect PROMs which can be considered as a predictor of patient's outcome. The development of such tools allows us to collect PROMs over time and to be able to assess, with a dynamic process, the association between PROMs' changes and patient outcomes, such as CPAP adherence or sleepiness [59,64]. Causal inference approaches can be used to analyze retrospective databases and provide real-world based evidence of the impact of advanced management tools based on telemedicine approaches on PROMs, such as CPAP adherence [65].

5. From Teleconsultations to Collaborative Care Models

To move towards personalized care in OSA [66], management pathways should be designed to provide a comprehensive solution that takes into account the heterogeneity of clinical phenotypes and the dynamics of lifespan trajectories of individuals with OSA. The implementation of remote management that relies on the participation of homecare providers and sleep physicians [67] offers the unique opportunity to provide holistic treatment plans that place the patient at the center of his/her care. Remote management pathways rely on virtual consultation and follow-up visits that are delivered either by telephone or videoconferencing [68]. Virtual care was shown to be as effective as in-person consultations for improving sleepiness in CPAP-treated OSA patients [69]. The authors of this meta-analysis suggest that, on the basis of the patient's preference, remote management of patients with OSA using CPAP should be available as an alternative care strategy to in-person follow-up [69].

The telemonitoring of CPAP treatment is another important component of remote management pathways. Telemonitoring has been shown to be as effective as in-person care for improving PAP adherence [65,70] and does not imply increased costs [69]. Telemonitoring is transforming patient follow-up by being implanted in dedicated virtual platforms [50]. Enhancing patients' participation in care through remote management pathways could facilitate the advancement of shared decision-making in the realm of OSA management [71].

Multimodal telemonitoring proves effective among OSA patients with increased cardiovascular risk, enhancing adherence to CPAP therapy and improving patient-centered outcomes including daytime sleepiness and quality of life [72]. However, its efficacy was not evident among patients with lower cardiovascular risk [73].

A recent randomized controlled trial in patients with OSA and obesity (168 patients recruited at 16 centers in Japan) examined the effects of the implementation of CPAP telemonitoring enhanced with body weight management tools (scales), BP measures, and a pedometer that could transmit data from devices wirelessly [74]. The group that benefited from multimodal telemonitoring exhibited a higher percentage of weight reduction ($\geq 3\%$) compared to the standard PAP telemonitoring group.

Recent studies have shed light on the potential of wearable digital health technologies to transform healthcare by making behavioral and physiological patterns in daily life, outside the clinic, visible to healthcare professionals. A recent series in the New England Journal of Medicine has highlighted the value of these technologies in diabetes [75], two types of cardiovascular disease [57], and in the management of depression [56].

6. Pitfalls of Telemedicine

While showing promising potential for enhancing CPAP adherence and overall management of OSA, several challenges remain for the development of remote management pathways. A primary obstacle lies in the disparity experienced by certain populations [i.e., "The digital divide" [76]], such as the elderly, who could gain significant advantages from telemedicine services, but encounter challenges stemming from technical, cultural, and financial barriers [68]. However, in certain countries like France, adherence to CPAP therapy monitored remotely serves as a prerequisite for health insurance coverage of CPAP devices, and reimbursement rates are proportionate to adherence levels. Another area for improvement involves the absence of standardized calculation methods for CPAP indices across manufacturers [51], along with the necessity for thorough validation of devices utilized in multimodal telemonitoring of various health-related parameters [45]. Finally, numerous regulatory matters concerning data safety and healthcare regulation remain unresolved, and additional enhancements should concentrate on delineating the pertinent data for medical diagnosis and follow-up purposes [77].

7. Conclusions

Sleep apnea syndrome affects many people around the world, and is undoubtedly under-diagnosed. Given the heterogeneity of diagnosis and treatment, it is essential to develop personalized approaches. Telemedicine is one of the promising solutions for the years to come which could enable the development of individualized, digitized care pathways, as summarized in Figure 1. However, it will be important to ensure that digital development does not work to the detriment of patients, particularly those who are far removed from these systems. Telemedicine is a tool of the future, but it must be seen as one possible approach among others.

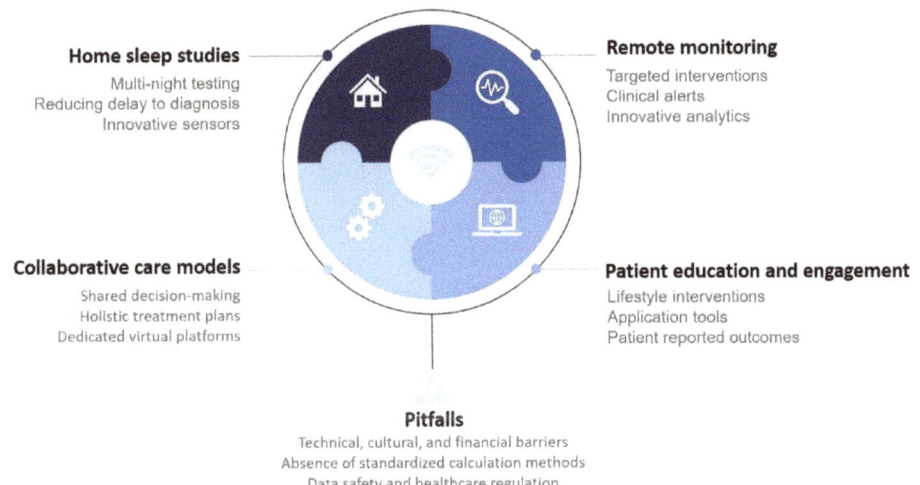

Figure 1. Overview of the future of telemedicine in obstructive sleep apnea.

Author Contributions: Conceptualization, S.B. (Sébastien Bailly), M.M., S.B. (Sébastien Baillieul), R.T. and J.-L.P.; methodology, S.B. (Sébastien Bailly), M.M., S.B. (Sébastien Baillieul), R.T. and J.-L.P.; validation, S.B. (Sébastien Bailly), M.M., S.B. (Sébastien Baillieul), R.T. and J.-L.P.; writing—original draft preparation, S.B. (Sébastien Bailly), M.M., S.B. (Sébastien Baillieul), R.T. and J.-L.P.; writing—review and editing, S.B. (Sébastien Bailly), M.M., S.B. (Sébastien Baillieul), R.T. and J.-L.P. All authors have read and agreed to the published version of the manuscript.

Funding: J.-L.P., R.T. and S.B. (Sébastien Bailly). are supported by the French National Research Agency in the framework of the "Investissements d'avenir" program (ANR-15-IDEX-02) and the "e-health and integrated care and trajectories medicine and MIAI artificial intelligence (ANR-19-P3IA-0003)" Chairs of excellence from the Grenoble Alpes University Foundation.

Institutional Review Board Statement: Not applicable.

Informed Consent Statement: Not applicable.

Data Availability Statement: Not applicable.

Conflicts of Interest: The authors declare no conflicts of interest.

References

1. Benjafield, A.V.; Ayas, N.T.; Eastwood, P.R.; Heinzer, R.; Ip, M.S.M.; Morrell, M.J.; Nunez, C.M.; Patel, S.R.; Penzel, T.; Pepin, J.L.; et al. Estimation of the global prevalence and burden of obstructive sleep apnoea: A literature-based analysis. *Lancet Respir. Med.* **2019**, *7*, 687–698. [CrossRef]
2. Levy, P.; Kohler, M.; McNicholas, W.T.; Barbe, F.; McEvoy, R.D.; Somers, V.K.; Lavie, L.; Pepin, J.L. Obstructive sleep apnoea syndrome. *Nat. Rev. Dis. Primers* **2015**, *1*, 15015. [CrossRef]
3. Hudgel, D.W.; Patel, S.R.; Ahasic, A.M.; Bartlett, S.J.; Bessesen, D.H.; Coaker, M.A.; Fiander, P.M.; Grunstein, R.R.; Gurubhagavatula, I.; Kapur, V.K.; et al. The Role of Weight Management in the Treatment of Adult Obstructive Sleep Apnea. An Official American Thoracic Society Clinical Practice Guideline. *Am. J. Respir. Crit. Care Med.* **2018**, *198*, e70–e87. [CrossRef]
4. Bailly, S.; Grote, L.; Hedner, J.; Schiza, S.; McNicholas, W.T.; Basoglu, O.K.; Lombardi, C.; Dogas, Z.; Roisman, G.; Pataka, A.; et al. Clusters of sleep apnoea phenotypes: A large pan-European study from the European Sleep Apnoea Database (ESADA). *Respirology* **2021**, *26*, 378–387. [CrossRef] [PubMed]
5. Keenan, B.T.; Kim, J.; Singh, B.; Bittencourt, L.; Chen, N.H.; Cistulli, P.A.; Magalang, U.J.; McArdle, N.; Mindel, J.W.; Benediktsdottir, B.; et al. Recognizable clinical subtypes of obstructive sleep apnea across international sleep centers: A cluster analysis. *Sleep* **2018**, *41*, zsx214. [CrossRef] [PubMed]
6. Mazzotti, D.R.; Keenan, B.T.; Lim, D.C.; Gottlieb, D.J.; Kim, J.; Pack, A.I. Symptom Subtypes of Obstructive Sleep Apnea Predict Incidence of Cardiovascular Outcomes. *Am. J. Respir. Crit. Care Med.* **2019**, *200*, 493–506. [CrossRef]
7. Javaheri, S.; Barbe, F.; Campos-Rodriguez, F.; Dempsey, J.A.; Khayat, R.; Javaheri, S.; Malhotra, A.; Martinez-Garcia, M.A.; Mehra, R.; Pack, A.I.; et al. Sleep Apnea: Types, Mechanisms, and Clinical Cardiovascular Consequences. *J. Am. Coll. Cardiol.* **2017**, *69*, 841–858. [CrossRef] [PubMed]
8. Torres, G.; Sanchez de la Torre, M.; Pinilla, L.; Barbe, F. Obstructive sleep apnea and cardiovascular risk. *Clin. Investig. Arterioscler.* **2024**, *26*. [CrossRef] [PubMed]
9. Zhang, Y.; Yu, B.; Qi, Q.; Azarbarzin, A.; Chen, H.; Shah, N.A.; Ramos, A.R.; Zee, P.C.; Cai, J.; Daviglus, M.L.; et al. Metabolomic profiles of sleep-disordered breathing are associated with hypertension and diabetes mellitus development. *Nat. Commun.* **2024**, *15*, 1845. [CrossRef]
10. Gerves-Pinquie, C.; Bailly, S.; Goupil, F.; Pigeanne, T.; Launois, S.; Leclair-Visonneau, L.; Masson, P.; Bizieux-Thaminy, A.; Blanchard, M.; Sabil, A.; et al. Positive Airway Pressure Adherence, Mortality, and Cardiovascular Events in Patients with Sleep Apnea. *Am. J. Respir. Crit. Care Med.* **2022**, *206*, 1393–1404. [CrossRef]
11. Pepin, J.L.; Bailly, S.; Rinder, P.; Adler, D.; Benjafield, A.V.; Lavergne, F.; Josseran, A.; Sinel-Boucher, P.; Tamisier, R.; Cistulli, P.A.; et al. Relationship Between CPAP Termination and All-Cause Mortality: A French Nationwide Database Analysis. *Chest* **2022**, *161*, 1657–1665. [CrossRef] [PubMed]
12. Sanchez-de-la-Torre, M.; Gracia-Lavedan, E.; Benitez, I.D.; Sanchez-de-la-Torre, A.; Moncusi-Moix, A.; Torres, G.; Loffler, K.; Woodman, R.; Adams, R.; Labarca, G.; et al. Adherence to CPAP Treatment and the Risk of Recurrent Cardiovascular Events: A Meta-Analysis. *JAMA* **2023**, *330*, 1255–1265. [CrossRef]
13. Punjabi, N.M.; Patil, S.; Crainiceanu, C.; Aurora, R.N. Variability and Misclassification of Sleep Apnea Severity Based on Multi-Night Testing. *Chest* **2020**, *158*, 365–373. [CrossRef] [PubMed]
14. Roeder, M.; Bradicich, M.; Schwarz, E.I.; Thiel, S.; Gaisl, T.; Held, U.; Kohler, M. Night-to-night variability of respiratory events in obstructive sleep apnoea: A systematic review and meta-analysis. *Thorax* **2020**, *75*, 1095–1102. [CrossRef] [PubMed]
15. Roeder, M.; Kohler, M. It's Time for Multiple Sleep Night Testing in OSA. *Chest* **2020**, *158*, 33–34. [CrossRef]
16. Lechat, B.; Loffler, K.A.; Reynolds, A.C.; Naik, G.; Vakulin, A.; Jennings, G.; Escourrou, P.; McEvoy, R.D.; Adams, R.J.; Catcheside, P.G.; et al. High night-to-night variability in sleep apnea severity is associated with uncontrolled hypertension. *NPJ Digit. Med.* **2023**, *6*, 57. [CrossRef]
17. Lechat, B.; Naik, G.; Reynolds, A.; Aishah, A.; Scott, H.; Loffler, K.A.; Vakulin, A.; Escourrou, P.; McEvoy, R.D.; Adams, R.J.; et al. Multinight Prevalence, Variability, and Diagnostic Misclassification of Obstructive Sleep Apnea. *Am. J. Respir. Crit. Care Med.* **2022**, *205*, 563–569. [CrossRef] [PubMed]
18. Lechat, B.; Nguyen, D.P.; Reynolds, A.; Loffler, K.; Escourrou, P.; McEvoy, R.D.; Adams, R.; Catcheside, P.G.; Eckert, D.J. Single-Night Diagnosis of Sleep Apnea Contributes to Inconsistent Cardiovascular Outcome Findings. *Chest* **2023**, *164*, 231–240. [CrossRef]
19. Lechat, B.; Scott, H.; Manners, J.; Adams, R.; Proctor, S.; Mukherjee, S.; Catcheside, P.; Eckert, D.J.; Vakulin, A.; Reynolds, A.C. Multi-night measurement for diagnosis and simplified monitoring of obstructive sleep apnoea. *Sleep. Med. Rev.* **2023**, *72*, 101843. [CrossRef]
20. Martinot, J.B.; Le-Dong, N.N.; Tamisier, R.; Bailly, S.; Pepin, J.L. Determinants of apnea-hypopnea index variability during home sleep testing. *Sleep. Med.* **2023**, *111*, 86–93. [CrossRef]
21. Abreu, A.; Punjabi, N.M. How Many Nights Are Really Needed to Diagnose Obstructive Sleep Apnea? *Am. J. Respir. Crit. Care Med.* **2022**, *206*, 125–126. [CrossRef] [PubMed]
22. Pepin, J.L.; Tamisier, R.; Baillieul, S.; Ben Messaoud, R.; Foote, A.; Bailly, S.; Martinot, J.B. Creating an Optimal Approach for Diagnosing Sleep Apnea. *Sleep. Med. Clin.* **2023**, *18*, 301–309. [CrossRef] [PubMed]

23. Pepin, J.L.; Bailly, S.; Rinder, P.; Adler, D.; Szeftel, D.; Malhotra, A.; Cistulli, P.A.; Benjafield, A.; Lavergne, F.; Josseran, A.; et al. CPAP Therapy Termination Rates by OSA Phenotype: A French Nationwide Database Analysis. *J. Clin. Med.* **2021**, *10*, 936. [CrossRef] [PubMed]
24. Dorsey, E.R.; Topol, E.J. State of Telehealth. *N. Engl. J. Med.* **2016**, *375*, 154–161. [CrossRef] [PubMed]
25. Norden, J.G.; Wang, J.X.; Desai, S.A.; Cheung, L. Utilizing a novel unified healthcare model to compare practice patterns between telemedicine and in-person visits. *Digit. Health* **2020**, *6*, 2055207620958528. [CrossRef] [PubMed]
26. Mariani, M.V.; Pierucci, N.; Forleo, G.B.; Schiavone, M.; Bernardini, A.; Gasperetti, A.; Mitacchione, G.; Mei, M.; Giunta, G.; Piro, A.; et al. The Feasibility, Effectiveness and Acceptance of Virtual Visits as Compared to In-Person Visits among Clinical Electrophysiology Patients during the COVID-19 Pandemic. *J. Clin. Med.* **2023**, *12*, 620. [CrossRef] [PubMed]
27. Rizzo, L.; Barbetta, E.; Ruberti, F.; Petz, M.; Tornesello, M.; Deolmi, M.; Fainardi, V.; Esposito, S. The Role of Telemedicine in Children with Obstructive Sleep Apnea Syndrome (OSAS): A Review of the Literature. *J. Clin. Med.* **2024**, *13*, 2108. [CrossRef] [PubMed]
28. Grote, L.; McNicholas, W.T.; Hedner, J. on behalf of the ESADA collaborators. Sleep apnoea management in Europe during the COVID-19 pandemic: Data from the European Sleep Apnoea Database (ESADA). *Eur. Respir. J.* **2020**, *55*, 2001323. [CrossRef]
29. Schobel, C.; Werther, S.; Teschler, H.; Taube, C. Telemedicine in respiratory sleep medicine: COVID-19 pandemic unmasks the need for a process-oriented, replicable approach for implementation in clinical routine. *J. Thorac. Dis.* **2020**, *12*, S261–S263. [CrossRef]
30. Arnal, P.J.; Thorey, V.; Debellemaniere, E.; Ballard, M.E.; Bou Hernandez, A.; Guillot, A.; Jourde, H.; Harris, M.; Guillard, M.; Van Beers, P.; et al. The Dreem Headband compared to polysomnography for electroencephalographic signal acquisition and sleep staging. *Sleep* **2020**, *43*, zsaa097. [CrossRef]
31. Lee, T.; Cho, Y.; Cha, K.S.; Jung, J.; Cho, J.; Kim, H.; Kim, D.; Hong, J.; Lee, D.; Keum, M.; et al. Accuracy of 11 Wearable, Nearable, and Airable Consumer Sleep Trackers: Prospective Multicenter Validation Study. *JMIR Mhealth Uhealth* **2023**, *11*, e50983. [CrossRef] [PubMed]
32. Tauman, R.; Berall, M.; Berry, R.; Etzioni, T.; Shrater, N.; Hwang, D.; Marai, I.; Manthena, P.; Rama, A.; Spiegel, R.; et al. Watch-PAT is Useful in the Diagnosis of Sleep Apnea in Patients with Atrial Fibrillation. *Nat. Sci. Sleep.* **2020**, *12*, 1115–1121. [CrossRef] [PubMed]
33. Isetta, V.; Negrin, M.A.; Monasterio, C.; Masa, J.F.; Feu, N.; Alvarez, A.; Campos-Rodriguez, F.; Ruiz, C.; Abad, J.; Vazquez-Polo, F.J.; et al. A Bayesian cost-effectiveness analysis of a telemedicine-based strategy for the management of sleep apnoea: A multicentre randomised controlled trial. *Thorax* **2015**, *70*, 1054–1061. [CrossRef] [PubMed]
34. Lorenzo, J.L.; Barbanoj, M.J. Variability of sleep parameters across multiple laboratory sessions in healthy young subjects: The "very first night effect". *Psychophysiology* **2002**, *39*, 409–413. [CrossRef] [PubMed]
35. Stoberl, A.S.; Schwarz, E.I.; Haile, S.R.; Turnbull, C.D.; Rossi, V.A.; Stradling, J.R.; Kohler, M. Night-to-night variability of obstructive sleep apnea. *J. Sleep. Res.* **2017**, *26*, 782–788. [CrossRef] [PubMed]
36. Tamaki, M.; Nittono, H.; Hayashi, M.; Hori, T. Examination of the first-night effect during the sleep-onset period. *Sleep* **2005**, *28*, 195–202. [CrossRef] [PubMed]
37. White, L.H.; Lyons, O.D.; Yadollahi, A.; Ryan, C.M.; Bradley, T.D. Night-to-night variability in obstructive sleep apnea severity: Relationship to overnight rostral fluid shift. *J. Clin. Sleep. Med.* **2015**, *11*, 149–156. [CrossRef] [PubMed]
38. Kapur, V.K.; Auckley, D.H.; Chowdhuri, S.; Kuhlmann, D.C.; Mehra, R.; Ramar, K.; Harrod, C.G. Clinical Practice Guideline for Diagnostic Testing for Adult Obstructive Sleep Apnea: An American Academy of Sleep Medicine Clinical Practice Guideline. *J. Clin. Sleep. Med.* **2017**, *13*, 479–504. [CrossRef] [PubMed]
39. Kelly, J.L.; Ben Messaoud, R.; Joyeux-Faure, M.; Terrail, R.; Tamisier, R.; Martinot, J.B.; Le-Dong, N.N.; Morrell, M.J.; Pepin, J.L. Diagnosis of Sleep Apnoea Using a Mandibular Monitor and Machine Learning Analysis: One-Night Agreement Compared to in-Home Polysomnography. *Front. Neurosci.* **2022**, *16*, 726880. [CrossRef]
40. Le-Dong, N.N.; Martinot, J.B.; Coumans, N.; Cuthbert, V.; Tamisier, R.; Bailly, S.; Pepin, J.L. Machine Learning-based Sleep Staging in Patients with Sleep Apnea Using a Single Mandibular Movement Signal. *Am. J. Respir. Crit. Care Med.* **2021**, *204*, 1227–1231. [CrossRef]
41. Pepin, J.L.; Sauvaget, O.; Borel, J.C.; Rolland, C.; Sapene, M.; Amroussia, I.; Bailly, S.; Tamisier, R. Continuous positive airway pressure-treated patients' behaviours during the COVID-19 crisis. *ERJ Open Res.* **2020**, *6*, 00508–2020. [CrossRef] [PubMed]
42. Di Pumpo, M.; Nurchis, M.C.; Moffa, A.; Giorgi, L.; Sabatino, L.; Baptista, P.; Sommella, L.; Casale, M.; Damiani, G. Multiple-access versus telemedicine home-based sleep apnea testing for obstructive sleep apnea (OSA) diagnosis: A cost-minimization study. *Sleep. Breath.* **2022**, *26*, 1641–1647. [CrossRef] [PubMed]
43. Masoumian Hosseini, M.; Masoumian Hosseini, S.T.; Qayumi, K.; Hosseinzadeh, S.; Sajadi Tabar, S.S. Smartwatches in healthcare medicine: Assistance and monitoring; a scoping review. *BMC Med. Inform. Decis. Mak.* **2023**, *23*, 248. [CrossRef] [PubMed]
44. de Zambotti, M.; Goldstein, C.; Cook, J.; Menghini, L.; Altini, M.; Cheng, P.; Robillard, R. State of the Science and Recommendations for Using Wearable Technology in Sleep and Circadian Research. *Sleep* **2023**, *47*, zsad325. [CrossRef] [PubMed]
45. Baumert, M.; Cowie, M.R.; Redline, S.; Mehra, R.; Arzt, M.; Pepin, J.L.; Linz, D. Sleep characterization with smart wearable devices: A call for standardization and consensus recommendations. *Sleep* **2022**, *45*, zsac183. [CrossRef] [PubMed]

46. Verhaert, D.V.M.; Betz, K.; Gawalko, M.; Hermans, A.N.L.; Pluymaekers, N.; van der Velden, R.M.J.; Philippens, S.; Vorstermans, B.; Simons, S.O.; den Uijl, D.W.; et al. A VIRTUAL Sleep Apnoea management pathway For the work-up of Atrial fibrillation patients in a digital Remote Infrastructure: VIRTUAL-SAFARI. *Europace* **2022**, *24*, 565–575. [CrossRef] [PubMed]
47. Duval, J.; Mouroux, C.; Foury, S.; Pepin, J.L.; Bailly, S. Patient motivation ranked by caregivers at continuous positive airway pressure initiation is predictive of adherence and 1-year therapy termination rate. *Sleep. Breath* **2023**, *epub ahead of print*. [CrossRef]
48. Gentina, T.; Gentina, E.; Douay, B.; Micoulaud-Franchi, J.A.; Pepin, J.L.; Bailly, S. Investigating associations between social determinants, self-efficacy measurement of sleep apnea and CPAP adherence: The SEMSA study. *Front. Neurol.* **2023**, *14*, 1148700. [CrossRef] [PubMed]
49. Mendelson, M.; Duval, J.; Bettega, F.; Tamisier, R.; Baillieul, S.; Bailly, S.; Pepin, J.L. The individual and societal prices of non-adherence to continuous positive airway pressure, contributors, and strategies for improvement. *Expert. Rev. Respir. Med.* **2023**, *17*, 305–317. [CrossRef] [PubMed]
50. Bottaz-Bosson, G.; Midelet, A.; Mendelson, M.; Borel, J.C.; Martinot, J.B.; Le Hy, R.; Schaeffer, M.C.; Samson, A.; Hamon, A.; Tamisier, R.; et al. Remote Monitoring of Positive Airway Pressure Data: Challenges, Pitfalls, and Strategies to Consider for Optimal Data Science Applications. *Chest* **2023**, *163*, 1279–1291. [CrossRef]
51. Midelet, A.; Borel, J.C.; Tamisier, R.; Le Hy, R.; Schaeffer, M.C.; Daabek, N.; Pepin, J.L.; Bailly, S. Apnea-hypopnea index supplied by CPAP devices: Time for standardization? *Sleep. Med.* **2021**, *81*, 120–122. [CrossRef]
52. Prigent, A.; Pellen, C.; Texereau, J.; Bailly, S.; Coquerel, N.; Gervais, R.; Liegaux, J.M.; Luraine, R.; Renaud, J.C.; Serandour, A.L.; et al. CPAP telemonitoring can track Cheyne-Stokes respiration and detect serious cardiac events: The AlertApnee Study. *Respirology* **2022**, *27*, 161–169. [CrossRef] [PubMed]
53. Prigent, A.; Serandour, A.L.; Luraine, R.; Poineuf, J.S.; Bosseau, C.; Pepin, J.L. Interrelated atrial fibrillation and leaks triggering and maintaining central sleep apnoea and periodic breathing in a CPAP-treated patient. *Respirol. Case Rep.* **2020**, *8*, e00666. [CrossRef] [PubMed]
54. Rossetto, A.; Midelet, A.; Baillieul, S.; Tamisier, R.; Borel, J.C.; Prigent, A.; Bailly, S.; Pepin, J.L. Factors Associated With Residual Apnea-Hypopnea Index Variability During CPAP Treatment. *Chest* **2023**, *163*, 1258–1265. [CrossRef]
55. Midelet, A.; Bailly, S.; Tamisier, R.; Borel, J.C.; Baillieul, S.; Le Hy, R.; Schaeffer, M.C.; Pepin, J.L. Hidden Markov model segmentation to demarcate trajectories of residual apnoea-hypopnoea index in CPAP-treated sleep apnoea patients to personalize follow-up and prevent treatment failure. *EPMA J.* **2021**, *12*, 535–544. [CrossRef]
56. Fedor, S.; Lewis, R.; Pedrelli, P.; Mischoulon, D.; Curtiss, J.; Picard, R.W. Wearable Technology in Clinical Practice for Depressive Disorder. *N. Engl. J. Med.* **2023**, *389*, 2457–2466. [CrossRef]
57. Spatz, E.S.; Ginsburg, G.S.; Rumsfeld, J.S.; Turakhia, M.P. Wearable Digital Health Technologies for Monitoring in Cardiovascular Medicine. *N. Engl. J. Med.* **2024**, *390*, 346–356. [CrossRef] [PubMed]
58. Varma, N.; Han, J.K.; Passman, R.; Rosman, L.A.; Ghanbari, H.; Noseworthy, P.; Avari Silva, J.N.; Deshmukh, A.; Sanders, P.; Hindricks, G.; et al. Promises and Perils of Consumer Mobile Technologies in Cardiovascular Care: JACC Scientific Statement. *J. Am. Coll. Cardiol.* **2024**, *83*, 611–631. [CrossRef] [PubMed]
59. Cistulli, P.A.; Armitstead, J.P.; Malhotra, A.; Yan, Y.; Vuong, V.; Sterling, K.L.; Barrett, M.A.; Nunez, C.M.; Pepin, J.L.; Benjafield, A.V. Relationship between Self-reported Sleepiness and Positive Airway Pressure Treatment Adherence in Obstructive Sleep Apnea. *Ann. Am. Thorac. Soc.* **2023**, *20*, 1201–1209. [CrossRef] [PubMed]
60. Askland, K.; Wright, L.; Wozniak, D.R.; Emmanuel, T.; Caston, J.; Smith, I. Educational, supportive and behavioural interventions to improve usage of continuous positive airway pressure machines in adults with obstructive sleep apnoea. *Cochrane Database Syst. Rev.* **2020**, *4*, CD007736. [CrossRef]
61. Patil, S.P.; Ayappa, I.A.; Caples, S.M.; Kimoff, R.J.; Patel, S.R.; Harrod, C.G. Treatment of Adult Obstructive Sleep Apnea With Positive Airway Pressure: An American Academy of Sleep Medicine Systematic Review, Meta-Analysis, and GRADE Assessment. *J. Clin. Sleep. Med.* **2019**, *15*, 301–334. [CrossRef]
62. Latrille, C.; Chapel, B.; Heraud, N.; Bughin, F.; Hayot, M.; Boiche, J. An individualized mobile health intervention to promote physical activity in adults with obstructive sleep apnea: An intervention mapping approach. *Digit. Health* **2023**, *9*, 20552076221150744. [CrossRef]
63. Bughin, F.; Mendelson, M.; Jaffuel, D.; Pepin, J.L.; Gagnadoux, F.; Goutorbe, F.; Abril, B.; Ayoub, B.; Aranda, A.; Alagha, K.; et al. Impact of a telerehabilitation programme combined with continuous positive airway pressure on symptoms and cardiometabolic risk factors in obstructive sleep apnea patients. *Digit. Health* **2023**, *9*, 20552076231167009. [CrossRef] [PubMed]
64. Bhattacharjee, R.; Benjafield, A.V.; Armitstead, J.; Cistulli, P.A.; Nunez, C.M.; Pepin, J.D.; Woehrle, H.; Yan, Y.; Malhotra, A.; medXcloud, g. Adherence in children using positive airway pressure therapy: A big-data analysis. *Lancet Digit. Health* **2020**, *2*, e94–e101. [CrossRef]
65. Malhotra, A.; Crocker, M.E.; Willes, L.; Kelly, C.; Lynch, S.; Benjafield, A.V. Patient Engagement Using New Technology to Improve Adherence to Positive Airway Pressure Therapy: A Retrospective Analysis. *Chest* **2018**, *153*, 843–850. [CrossRef]
66. Martinez-Garcia, M.A.; Campos-Rodriguez, F.; Barbe, F.; Gozal, D.; Agusti, A. Precision medicine in obstructive sleep apnoea. *Lancet Respir. Med.* **2019**, *7*, 456–464. [CrossRef]
67. Pepin, J.L.; Baillieul, S.; Tamisier, R. Reshaping Sleep Apnea Care: Time for Value-based Strategies. *Ann. Am. Thorac. Soc.* **2019**, *16*, 1501–1503. [CrossRef]
68. Verbraecken, J. Telemedicine in Sleep-Disordered Breathing. *Sleep. Med. Clin.* **2021**, *16*, 417–445. [CrossRef] [PubMed]

69. Alsaif, S.S.; Kelly, J.L.; Little, S.; Pinnock, H.; Morrell, M.J.; Polkey, M.I.; Murphie, P. Virtual consultations for patients with obstructive sleep apnoea: A systematic review and meta-analysis. *Eur. Respir. Rev.* **2022**, *31*, 220180. [CrossRef] [PubMed]
70. Fox, N.; Hirsch-Allen, A.J.; Goodfellow, E.; Wenner, J.; Fleetham, J.; Ryan, C.F.; Kwiatkowska, M.; Ayas, N.T. The impact of a telemedicine monitoring system on positive airway pressure adherence in patients with obstructive sleep apnea: A randomized controlled trial. *Sleep* **2012**, *35*, 477–481. [CrossRef]
71. Overby, C.T.; Sutharshan, P.; Gulbrandsen, P.; Dammen, T.; Hrubos-Strom, H. Shared decision making: A novel approach to personalized treatment in obstructive sleep apnea. *Sleep. Med. X* **2022**, *4*, 100052. [CrossRef]
72. Pepin, J.L.; Jullian-Desayes, I.; Sapene, M.; Treptow, E.; Joyeux-Faure, M.; Benmerad, M.; Bailly, S.; Grillet, Y.; Stach, B.; Richard, P.; et al. Multimodal Remote Monitoring of High Cardiovascular Risk Patients With OSA Initiating CPAP: A Randomized Trial. *Chest* **2019**, *155*, 730–739. [CrossRef] [PubMed]
73. Tamisier, R.; Treptow, E.; Joyeux-Faure, M.; Levy, P.; Sapene, M.; Benmerad, M.; Bailly, S.; Grillet, Y.; Stach, B.; Muir, J.F.; et al. Impact of a Multimodal Telemonitoring Intervention on CPAP Adherence in Symptomatic OSA and Low Cardiovascular Risk: A Randomized Controlled Trial. *Chest* **2020**, *158*, 2136–2145. [CrossRef] [PubMed]
74. Murase, K.; Minami, T.; Hamada, S.; Gozal, D.; Takahashi, N.; Nakatsuka, Y.; Takeyama, H.; Tanizawa, K.; Endo, D.; Akahoshi, T.; et al. Multimodal Telemonitoring for Weight Reduction in Patients With Sleep Apnea: A Randomized Controlled Trial. *Chest* **2022**, *162*, 1373–1383. [CrossRef] [PubMed]
75. Hughes, M.S.; Addala, A.; Buckingham, B. Digital Technology for Diabetes. *N. Engl. J. Med.* **2023**, *389*, 2076–2086. [CrossRef] [PubMed]
76. Greenhalgh, T.; Rosen, R.; Shaw, S.E.; Byng, R.; Faulkner, S.; Finlay, T.; Grundy, E.; Husain, L.; Hughes, G.; Leone, C.; et al. Planning and Evaluating Remote Consultation Services: A New Conceptual Framework Incorporating Complexity and Practical Ethics. *Front. Digit. Health* **2021**, *3*, 726095. [CrossRef]
77. Verbraecken, J. More than sleepiness: Prevalence and relevance of nonclassical symptoms of obstructive sleep apnea. *Curr. Opin. Pulm. Med.* **2022**, *28*, 552–558. [CrossRef]

Disclaimer/Publisher's Note: The statements, opinions and data contained in all publications are solely those of the individual author(s) and contributor(s) and not of MDPI and/or the editor(s). MDPI and/or the editor(s) disclaim responsibility for any injury to people or property resulting from any ideas, methods, instructions or products referred to in the content.

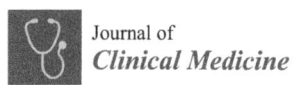

Review

Potential Therapeutic Targets in Obesity, Sleep Apnea, Diabetes, and Fatty Liver Disease

Christina Gu [1,*], Nicole Bernstein [1], Nikita Mittal [1], Soumya Kurnool [1], Hannah Schwartz [2], Rohit Loomba [1] and Atul Malhotra [1,*]

[1] Department of Medicine, University of California San Diego, 9500 Gilman Drive, La Jolla, CA 92037, USA; nbernstein@health.ucsd.edu (N.B.); nmittal@health.ucsd.edu (N.M.); skurnool@health.ucsd.edu (S.K.); roloomba@health.ucsd.edu (R.L.)

[2] Weill Cornell Medicine, 1300 York Ave, New York, NY 10285, USA; has4021@med.cornell.edu

* Correspondence: cxgu@health.ucsd.edu (C.G.); amalhotra@health.ucsd.edu (A.M.)

Abstract: Obesity and metabolic syndrome affect the majority of the US population. Patients with obesity are at increased risk of developing type 2 diabetes (T2DM), obstructive sleep apnea (OSA), and metabolic dysfunction-associated steatotic liver disease (MASLD), each of which carry the risk of further complications if left untreated and lead to adverse outcomes. The rising prevalence of obesity and its comorbidities has led to increased mortality, decreased quality of life, and rising healthcare expenditures. This phenomenon has resulted in the intensive investigation of exciting therapies for obesity over the past decade, including more treatments that are still in the pipeline. In our present report, we aim to solidify the relationships among obesity, T2DM, OSA, and MASLD through a comprehensive review of current research. We also provide an overview of the surgical and pharmacologic treatment classes that target these relationships, namely bariatric surgery, the glucagon-like peptide-1 (GLP-1), glucose-dependent insulinotropic polypeptide (GIP), and glucagon receptor agonists.

Keywords: obesity; metabolic syndrome; MASLD; NAFLD; hepatic steatosis; OSA; CPAP; diabetes; GLP-1; GIP; glucagon; bariatric surgery

Citation: Gu, C.; Bernstein, N.; Mittal, N.; Kurnool, S.; Schwartz, H.; Loomba, R.; Malhotra, A. Potential Therapeutic Targets in Obesity, Sleep Apnea, Diabetes, and Fatty Liver Disease. *J. Clin. Med.* **2024**, *13*, 2231. https://doi.org/10.3390/jcm13082231

Academic Editor: Silvano Dragonieri

Received: 9 March 2024
Revised: 7 April 2024
Accepted: 10 April 2024
Published: 12 April 2024

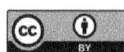

Copyright: © 2024 by the authors. Licensee MDPI, Basel, Switzerland. This article is an open access article distributed under the terms and conditions of the Creative Commons Attribution (CC BY) license (https://creativecommons.org/licenses/by/4.0/).

1. Introduction

Obesity has been increasingly pervasive over the past several decades, although the mechanism of the rising prevalence remains unclear [1]. Current estimates suggest that just over one-third of the US population is considered to have a healthy weight (defined by BMI 18.5–24.9 kg/m^2), one-third fall in the overweight category (BMI 25–29.9 kg/m^2), and one-third is obese (BMI $\geq$ 30 kg/m^2) [2]. Current projections suggest one in two Americans will meet criteria for obesity by 2030. The mechanisms underlying obesity and the metabolic syndrome are intricate and complex. Obstructive sleep apnea (OSA), type 2 diabetes (T2DM), and metabolic dysfunction-associated steatotic liver disease (MASLD) are common comorbidities of obesity. While T2DM affects roughly 10% of the US population (www.cdc.gov/diabetes, accessed on 22 January 2024), it is estimated that OSA affects nearly 1 billion people worldwide [3]. It is estimated that about 25% of the U.S. population has non-alcoholic-associated fatty liver disease (NAFLD), recently renamed to MASLD, and about 20% of those with NAFLD have non-alcoholic steatohepatitis (NASH). As early as 2018, the leading cause of liver transplantation in U.S. women was shown to be NASH [4]. The rising prevalence of obesity and the resultant pervasiveness of its comorbidities, namely T2DM, OSA, and MASLD, hold critical adverse implications in healthcare, including rising mortality risk, impaired quality of life, and increased healthcare spending [2]. The complications from these disease states themselves also give rise to further problems, including cardiovascular, microvascular, skeletal, gastrointestinal, and neurocognitive diseases. The close association among these disease states begs the questions: What are the shared mechanisms underlying obesity and its comorbidities? What current US Food and Drug Administration-approved therapies might be beneficial for comorbid conditions? Looking ahead, what future therapies on the horizon might also target these mechanisms? Current literature has established connections between various permutations of the metabolic syndrome comorbidities (obesity, T2DM, OSA, and MASLD); however, the complex nature of the physiological axes connecting these diseases is still under investigation (Figure S1). Thus far, the current literature has yet to include a comprehensive review of T2DM, OSA, and MASLD in the context of obesity. Notably, OSA is also an underrecognized independent risk factor for the development of both T2DM and MASLD.

In this report, we first aim to discuss the current understanding of the interplay among obesity, T2DM, OSA, and MASLD. Next, we describe current therapeutic approaches to the metabolic syndrome axis and discuss how various treatment classes, including GLP-1 receptor agonists and triple G triagonists (combined glucagon, glucagon-like peptide-1, and glucose-dependent insulinotropic polypeptide receptor agonists), may transform our understanding of the physiological interconnectedness of these diseases. Finally, we draw attention to the potential therapeutic benefit of continuous positive airway pressure (CPAP) on disease states beyond OSA. The overarching aim of our review is to highlight the interconnectedness of T2DM, OSA, and MASLD and to provide an overview for the direct and indirect effects of obesity treatment on all of these diseases.

2. Relationship between OSA and T2DM

Sleep disturbances have commonly been associated with the development of obesity in epidemiological studies [5,6]. This finding could be explained by physiological studies that have shown suppression of leptin and increases in ghrelin with sleep deprivation, both of which are changes predicted to stimulate appetite and promote obesity [7]. It is unsurprising then, that short sleep has also been associated with incident diabetes mellitus, as well as the worsening of markers of insulin regulation [6,8–10]. OSA itself has been established as an independent risk factor for several metabolic and cardiovascular disease states, including hypertension, insulin resistance, fatty liver disease, atherosclerosis, and dyslipidemia. Treatment for sleep apnea can lead to improvements in blood pressure, although the impact of OSA treatment on glycemic control is less clear [11,12].

Multiple pathways are theorized to explain a causative effect of intermittent hypoxemia and sleep fragmentation on the development of insulin resistance and glucose dysregulation. One such pathway is via increased sympathetic neural activity. Laboratory assessments of patients with untreated OSA have demonstrated both increased sympathetic hormonal levels and activity that persists in the daytime and is reduced by consistent CPAP therapy [13,14]. Most processes involved in glucose control, including pancreatic insulin secretion and hepatic glucose production, are inhibited by elevated sympathetic tone [15]. In addition, cholinergic activity is directly linked to the secretion of incretin hormones, such as glucagon-like peptide-1 and glucose-dependent insulinotropic polypeptide. These incretin hormones act to augment insulin release. These findings suggest that patients with OSA are more predisposed to developing sympathetic hyperactivity and parasympathetic withdrawal, which collectively mediate glucose intolerance and thus T2DM [16]. Chronic intermittent hypoxia has been proposed to cause glucose intolerance through other proposed pathways, including the development of oxidative stress, systemic inflammation, activation of the hypothalamic–pituitary–adrenal (HPA) axis, pancreatic beta-cell apoptosis, and the alteration of adipokines, each of which leads to downstream effects on beta cell dysfunction and insulin resistance.

T2DM is also proposed to contribute to worsening OSA. Some observational evidences suggest that patients with diabetes and autonomic neuropathy demonstrate altered control of respiration and upper airway reflexes that promote airway patency, as seen in sleep-disordered breathing patterns among patients with diabetes [17,18]. This reverse causative relationship is also supported by a high prevalence of OSA among patients who are younger and non-obese with type 1 diabetes [19].

Unfortunately, a major subgroup of patients with T2DM are undertreated for OSA [20–22]. The Sleep-Ahead study showed that 87% of patients with T2DM and obesity also had clinically important OSA. After these patients and their providers received the diagnosis of OSA, over 95% of these patients with OSA remained untreated a year later [21–23]. Despite mixed results in studies assessing the impact of CPAP on glycemic control [11,24], the importance of addressing OSA in T2DM patients to reduce cardiometabolic risk is emphasized. Amongst patients with T2DM, there is a need for increased awareness to promote OSA as a valuable therapeutic target with implications on cardiometabolic health.

3. Relationship between OSA and MASLD

Hypoxia has been shown to accelerate the development of MASLD. One study using mouse models [25] demonstrated that hypoxia contributed to liver abnormalities only in the presence of obesity. Mice with diet-induced obesity were subject to chronic intermittent hypoxia; compared to lean mice that received the same hypoxic conditions, the obese mice exhibited markedly increased serum AST, ALT, and alkaline phosphatase levels and fasting glucose from baseline. In addition, the obese mice exhibited significantly higher levels of hepatic steatosis and inflammation on histology. Similar findings were reproduced in human studies. A study by Polotsky et al. [26] focused on patients presenting for bariatric surgery found that those with severe nocturnal hypoxemia tended to exhibit histologic signs of worse hepatic inflammation, including hepatocyte ballooning and perivesicular fibrosis, when compared to patients with mild sleep apnea. These findings are supported by other studies that observed nocturnal hypoxic episodes as a contributor to hyperlipidemia and steatohepatitis and as a possible risk factor for MASLD [27,28].

Considerable data from rodent studies have suggested that hypoxic effects on lipid metabolism may be responsible for the development of MASLD. In gene expression analysis studies, chronic intermittent hypoxia has been demonstrated to cause the upregulation of multiple genes responsible for the biosynthesis of cholesterol, triglycerides, fatty acid, and phospholipids [29]. It is not surprising then that increased enzymatic activity in hepatocytes would lead to increased lipid accumulation and hepatic steatosis. Other proposed indirect mechanisms include pancreatic beta-cell apoptosis and overactivation of the sympathetic nervous system, both of which lead to insulin resistance and thus predispose individuals to MASLD.

To date, most studies that have investigated the link between MASLD and OSA have focused on the increased risk of developing liver injury and inflammation among individuals with OSA. However, few have examined whether the inverse is true. One such study [30] reported that among patients with biopsy-proven MASLD, those with concurrent hepatic fibrosis had higher overall rates of OSA, compared to those without fibrosis. Another study demonstrated that the apnea–hypopnea index was significantly higher among those with moderate to severe MASLD, compared to those without MASLD [31–33]. The study by Chung et al. [34], which used a surrogate fatty liver index (FLI) score to identify MASLD, found that the risk for receiving an OSA diagnosis increased in a dose-dependent manner as FLI increased. This relationship remained consistent regardless of BMI and the presence of abdominal obesity and offers FLI as a potential tool used to identify individuals at high risk of OSA. These studies, although not necessarily suggestive of a causative effect by MASLD upon the development of OSA, do again underscore a close association between the two.

4. Relationship between T2DM and MASLD

Insulin resistance is believed to play a pivotal role in the development of fatty liver disease. On a cellular level, insulin signaling is initiated through the binding and activation of its cell-surface receptor, which triggers a cascade of phosphorylation and dephosphorylation events that ultimately lead to the translocation of glucose transporters into the cell membrane. The transporters then facilitate glucose influx down a concentration gradient from the extracellular space into the cytoplasm. Defects at any step of this cascade will result in issues with glucose uptake into cells and abnormalities with insulin sensitivity. Features seen in patients with obesity and diabetes, such as hyperglycemia, hyperinsulinemia, and the presence of free fatty acids, have been implicated in altering insulin signaling. Once peripheral insulin resistance has been established, hyperinsulinemia subsequently leads to increased fatty acid delivery into the liver, leading to increased hepatic triglyceride production and hepatic steatosis. Hepatic steatosis itself has been shown to lead to hepatic insulin resistance, which may contribute to the overall worsening of peripheral insulin resistance. Additionally, high levels of free fatty acids and hyperinsulinemia in the body have also been shown to lead to the production of free radicals, resulting in oxidative stress and an inflammatory response, including cytokine production, which are believed to further promote both insulin resistance and steatohepatitis. These latter mechanisms underlying the development of insulin resistance that have been reproduced in multiple molecular studies do suggest that the relationship between T2DM and MASLD may be bidirectional, or perhaps cyclic, in nature [35].

In clinical studies, the close association of T2DM and MASLD has been clearly illustrated. In a national survey of middle-aged patients with and without T2DM, it was found that the rate of steatosis was significantly higher in those with overweightness and obesity with T2DM versus without T2DM. T2DM was also found to significantly increase the proportion of those at moderate-to-high risk of fibrosis by two-fold [36], suggesting that T2DM may be predictive of the development of fibrosis in MASLD. Another study by Sung et al. compared the effect of ultrasound-diagnosed MASLD on the risk of developing incident T2DM among 12,000 South Korean adults over the span of 5 years [37]. After adjusting for confounding factors, MASLD doubled the risk of developing T2DM. Other cohort studies have consistently shown that MASLD is predictive of T2DM, whether the diagnosis of MASLD is made by imaging or biopsy [38]. In addition, MASLD has also been shown to increase microvascular complications of T2DM, including chronic kidney disease and retinopathy.

The recognition of this shared elevated risk underscores the importance of vigilant monitoring in individuals with the dual burden of MASLD and T2DM. Due to the impact of insulin resistance on the pathophysiology of MASLD, potential pharmacologic treatments for MASLD have focused on hypoglycemic agents, including metformin, SGLT2-I, PPAR agonists, GLP-1 receptor agonists, and multi-agonists [39]. These diabetes drug classes have shown varying levels of benefit in reducing liver enzyme levels, liver fat content, and histologic features of inflammation and fibrosis.

5. Treatment Approaches

In the above review, we discussed current literature that inform our current understanding of how obesity, diabetes, sleep apnea, and fatty liver disease are inter-related. Here, we discuss the surgical and pharmacologic treatments that act upon these relationships to benefit patients with metabolic syndrome. We also expand on the potential efficacy of CPAP for patients with OSA and other concomitant metabolic diseases.

6. Overview of Bariatric Surgery

Bariatric surgery has been established as a highly effective option for patients with obesity to achieve sustained weight loss. Common, established procedures include sleeve gastrectomy (SG), Roux-en-Y gastric bypass (RYGB), gastric banding, and biliopancreatic diversion with duodenal switch [40]. A review of the literature suggests that among the different types of bariatric surgery, SG and RYGB have the highest efficacy for major weight reduction, with similar long-term results. A randomized controlled trial comparing the two methods, the SM-BOSS trial by Peterli et al. [41], evaluated adults with morbid obesity undergoing sleeve gastrectomy compared with gastric bypass over the course of 5 years. At the end of the study, the SG group lost 61% BMI, compared to the RYGB group, which lost 68%, a difference that was not statistically significant. Overall complications within the first 30 days occurred more often in the RYGB group than the SG group. However, the rates of developing severe complications in this study, such as severe GERD after SG and severe dumping syndrome after RYGB, which required further surgeries, were not statistically significant. Similar effects of bariatric surgery on weight loss were seen in other studies, which also noted improved comorbidities, including diabetes and hypertension [42,43].

There is clear evidence that bariatric surgery achieves meaningful remission rates of T2DM. Two meta-analyses reviewed the long-term effects of surgery on glycemic control over more than 2–5 years. These found that bariatric procedures were likely to achieve sustained weight loss, A1c lowering, overall blood glucose reduction, and, in many cases, diabetes remission. In addition, it was also shown that bariatric surgery had a significant reduction on the incidence of complications, as well as overall mortality, among patients who received at least 5 years of follow-up [44,45]. Another longer-term study was the Swedish Obese Subjects (SOS) trial, a 15-year prospective matched cohort study which observed a diabetes remission rate of 30% among those who had received bariatric surgery, with fewer incidences of micro- and macrovascular complications [46]. In fact, a recent study found that participants had higher rates of diabetes remission after bariatric surgery, compared to medical/lifestyle management, at up to 12 years of follow-up [47].

With regards to its effects on liver disease, several studies have also shown improvement in MASLD both after SG and RYGB. In a meta-analysis [48], patients undergoing RYGB achieved significant reductions in steatohepatitis and fibrosis, while patients undergoing LSG had a significant reduction in steatohepatitis only. Studies have shown mixed data regarding the superiority of one bariatric method in reversal of MASLD. Interestingly, there is a cohort of patients that appear to develop new or progressively worsening MASLD after bariatric surgery. In 2019, Lee et al. [49] showed that 12% of patients (95% CI, 5–20%) developed new or worsening MASLD after bariatric surgery. Further examination of those with worsening disease after surgery suggests that those who lose weight more rapidly may be more susceptible, which is possibly related to malnutrition or malabsorption. Of note, this meta-analysis included variations in bariatric surgery beyond SG and RYGB, such as gastric banding and gastroplasty. Although studies show an overall benefit of bariatric surgery on the amelioration of MASLD, there is a significant portion of patients that may develop new or worsening disease; this is an important clinical consideration prior to surgical intervention.

The prevalence of patients with OSA among patients undergoing bariatric surgery should not be understated; some screening studies estimate that as many as 72% of the bariatric surgery population has OSA [50,51]. Dramatic and sustainable weight loss, as seen in these surgeries, does see remarkable improvement and, in some cases, even the resolution of OSA. There is substantial evidence that weight reduction alleviates upper airway collapsibility and reduces upper airway resistance, thereby promoting increased oxygenation and the reduction of apneic episodes [52]. A large-scale UK national registry cohort study by Currie et al. [53] followed over four-thousand bariatric surgery cases over the span of nine years, including SG, RYGB, and gastric banding. SG and RYGB were associated with a 50% increased likelihood of OSA remission, compared with gastric banding, consistent with the greater degree of weight loss seen in both SG and RYGB surgeries. It is important to recognize, however, that even with weight reduction, the presence of obstructive sleep apnea is not always totally reversible, and its degree of resolution is highly variable [54]. In the UK registry cohort study, about half of the remaining cases at follow-up by the end of the study duration saw a complete resolution of OSA. Other studies have also illustrated that some patients may redevelop OSA, despite maintaining weight loss [54,55].

7. Overview of GLP-1 and GIP–GLP-1 Agonists

Incretins are peptide hormones that are released from the intestine and brainstem in response to nutrient consumption and act primarily to lower serum glucose and increase satiety. The backbone of medical therapies used to treat metabolic syndrome utilizes analogs of the main incretin hormones: glucagon-like peptide-1 (GLP-1) and glucose-dependent insulinotropic polypeptide (GIP). GLP-1 is a 30-amino-acid-long peptide chain produced by enteroendocrine L cells in the distal ileum and colon and by neurons in the nucleus of the solitary tract of the brainstem. It acts to stimulate insulin production in pancreatic beta cells in a glucose-dependent manner and decreases glucagon secretion from pancreatic alpha cells. GLP-1 additionally has extra-pancreatic effects through the direct suppression of the appetite center and the slowing of gastric emptying, thus increasing satiety and reducing food-seeking behavior. GIP is a 4-amino-acid peptide secreted by K cells in the duodenum and jejunum. This short peptide hormone is stimulated by glucose hyperosmolarity in the intestine to induce insulin secretion. Given these properties, GLP-1 and GIP agonists have been subjected to intensive pharmacologic investigation for the treatment of obesity and T2DM (Figure S2).

The current FDA-approved GLP-1 receptor agonists for treating both T2DM and obesity include once-daily liraglutide, weekly semaglutide, and weekly tirzepatide injections. Tirzepatide, a dual GIP–GLP-1 agonist, is the latest to be approved and has demonstrated significant results in weight reduction and glucose control when compared with its predecessors. The phase 3 SURMOUNT-1 trial examined the efficacy of tirzepatide on weight loss against a placebo over the span of 72 weeks [56]. All three doses of tirzepatide being studied (5, 10, and 15 mg) found a significantly greater weight reduction than with the placebo after as soon as 20 weeks. These results were greater than the mean placebo-adjusted weight reduction with liraglutide and semaglutide but with a similar safety profile. Weight reduction with tirzepatide was also accompanied by other cardiometabolic benefits, including reductions in blood pressure, waist circumference, fasting glucose, fasting cholesterol levels, and aspartate aminotransferase levels, when compared with the placebo. Similarly, the SURPASS-3 MRI study was another phase 3 trial that examined tirzepatide but with a specific focus on its effects on liver changes as measured by MRI; this demonstrated meaningful reductions in liver fat content, volume of visceral adipose tissue, and abdominal subcutaneous adipose tissue among patients with T2DM receiving 52 weeks of 10 mg or 15 mg tirzepatide when compared with those taking insulin degludec [57]. The impact of these medications on OSA is yet to be established and is a topic of ongoing investigation, particularly the efficacy of tirzepatide on OSA reversal [58].

8. Overview of Triple G Triagonists

Currently in the pharmacologic pipeline is a class of medications called triple G receptor agonists, or triagonists. These act via three receptors; the mechanisms of GIP and GLP-1 receptor agonists have been described above. The third "G" is glucagon, which is a 29-amino-acid peptide hormone produced by pancreatic alpha cells. Glucagon is known for its hyperglycemic effects via the liver and works in a feedback loop with GIP and GLP-1 to achieve glucose homeostasis. Additionally, glucagon is also a catabolic peptide, acting to increase lipolysis and thermogenesis. Some biochemical studies have shown that glucagon exerts its effects in the CNS by promoting satiety as well. Through the fine-tuning of the combined triple peptide analog, preclinical studies have demonstrated that the resultant triple G receptor agonist can promote glucagon's catabolic effects without exacerbating hyperglycemia [59].

One such triple G triagonist, retatrutide, has shown promising results in the treatment of obesity, T2DM, and MASLD. Initial data from three studies were revealed at the 2023 ADA conference. The Triple-Hormone-Receptor Agonist Retatrutide for Obesity was a phase 2 trial which examined retatrutide at various doses and dose-escalation regimens in patients with obesity [60]. Jastreboff et al. found that over the course of 48 weeks, all participants on the two highest doses of 8mg and 12mg lost at least 5% of weight, and those who were on 12 mg lost 24% of body weight on average. Those on 12 mg had a mean reduction of 19.6 cm waist circumference. The overall safety profile was similar to other GLP-1 agonists previously approved for obesity treatment, with the most common side effect being adverse GI events. A sub-study from the trial recruited participants with obesity and MASLD and utilized MRI and liver injury biomarkers to track changes in hepatic steatosis. Findings at the ADA press release [61] revealed that those with MASLD had a normalization of fat levels in the liver after 48 weeks of treatment on the highest dose of retatrutide, suggesting that MASLD can be treatable and reversible. A third study by Rosenstock et al. examined the efficacy and safety profile of retatrutide for the treatment of T2DM [62]. Participants lowered their A1c by 1.3–2% after taking 4–12 mg for about six months, compared to no change with the placebo and a 1.4% reduction with dulaglutide.

Data regarding the effect of triple G agonists on OSA specifically are still sparse, although phase 3 trials for retatrutide are projected to enroll patients with OSA. Given the impacts of these drugs on weight loss, glycemic control, and fatty liver disease, it is reasoned that patients with OSA may still see benefit.

9. Implications of CPAP Therapy on T2DM and MASLD

As evidenced above, OSA has high prevalence and tightly co-exists with other metabolic diseases, including central obesity, dyslipidemia, diabetes, and fatty liver disease. The direct effects of CPAP therapy on these metabolic disease states, however, is still under investigation. Short-term, randomized control trials evaluating CPAP efficacy on glycemic control for patients with concurrent OSA and prediabetes have demonstrated overall improved insulin sensitivity. One such study by Pamidi et al. [63] randomized participants to receiving either 8 h of nightly CPAP or a placebo over 2 weeks. Although the study did not find a difference in fasting glucose between the two groups, it did demonstrate improvement in response to glucose tolerance tests and in measured fasting insulin levels. Norepinephrine levels were also markedly lower in those receiving CPAP, which again supports the theory that a reduction in sympathetic activity could mediate improved glycemic control. However, a meta-analysis of RCTs examining CPAP effects on T2DM over a longer period concluded that CPAP does not significantly improve A1c or fasting glucose [64]. CPAP effects on MASLD are also under investigation. As described above, there are robust literature that demonstrate chronic intermittent hypoxic episodes as a contributor to oxidative stress on the liver, accelerated progression to steatohepatitis, and increased inflammation and fibrosis [28–31]. Reversal of hypoxic insults to the liver with CPAP alone, however, has yielded mixed results to date. One study examined the effects of 6 months of CPAP treatment for patients with both MASLD and OSA [65]. When controlling for weight changes over the duration of the study, the authors found no significant difference between the placebo and CPAP use on intrahepatic triglyceride content as measured by MRI, on FibroScan results, or serum liver function tests. A few other studies have shown that liver enzymes may be elevated in those with OSA and may also be lowered with CPAP [66]; however, these studies provide only indirect data with regards to specific liver tissue effects from CPAP use. Given the previous research findings that have supported chronic intermittent hypoxia as an important risk factor for glucose intolerance and hepatic steatosis, it is unclear why the results of CPAP trials on patients with T2DM and MASLD have been largely negative. Considerations for future studies include changes in trial design to promote better CPAP adherence and more direct methods to measure T2DM and MASLD outcomes. Alternative treatments for OSA should also be considered in these trials to better reflect real-world clinical practice, such as the use of oral appliances or surgical treatments.

10. Future Directions

For both clinicians and researchers, a number of practical questions remain for our understanding of and management of OSA. First, the specific mechanisms underlying obesity-related sleep apnea are still not entirely clear. Abnormalities in pharyngeal anatomy and the tongue have been reported, as well as the impact of abdominal obesity on end-expiratory lung volume [67–70]. However, other abnormalities in control of breathing and upper airway dilator muscle function have been suggested as potential issues [71].

Second, the optimal therapy for OSA for patients with obesity has not yet been found. Ongoing studies will likely inform this discussion. However, it seems highly likely that treatments of both obesity and OSA will be necessary to optimize clinical outcomes in afflicted patients [72]. Third, it is not yet clear whether there are predictors of cardiometabolic outcomes in obese people with OSA that could be used to stratify risk. Robust biomarkers and predictive markers could be used to identify high-risk patients and potentially stratify interventional approaches for those patients most likely to benefit. Approaches including mass spectroscopy could be used to discover new biomarkers, which predict the risk of OSA and associated complications [73,74].

Additional questions remain for the management of patients with T2DM and MASLD as well. There are few U.S. Food and Drug Administration-approved drugs that exist to treat MASLD [75], and the mainstay of therapy continues to focus on lifestyle interventions targeting dietary changes and weight loss. Given what we know now, more work needs to be performed to establish standardized screening criteria that help recognize those at risk of developing MASLD who require more aggressive therapy, whether this is in the form of the early initiation of tirzepatide or referral to bariatric surgery. Similarly, given the role that insulin resistance and autonomic neuropathy might play on the development of MASLD and OSA, respectively, more defined screening tools for the recognition of liver and sleep abnormalities may be necessary for patients with diabetes. It is also unclear whether patients with mild OSA but concomitant T2DM or MASLD require a more aggressive push toward starting CPAP therapy. More prospective studies are needed to better inform these questions.

Finally, although not directly addressed in this review article, diet is a foundational pillar underlying metabolism that is still not fully understood. Changes in how and what we eat have been suggested to play a role in the development of metabolic syndrome. Many specific food components and nutrients, as well as various dietary patterns, are undergoing studies to test their therapeutic potential. Polyphenolic compounds, for example, which are naturally occurring in fruits, vegetables, and cereals, may be one group of metabolites utilized for treatment, given their antidiabetic and cardioprotective properties [54]. Dietary formulations, including the Mediterranean diet, which is rich in polyphenols, may also hold promise in reducing oxidative stress in sleep apnea.

11. Conclusions

Understanding the intricate connections between obesity, OSA, T2DM, and MASLD is paramount for developing effective therapeutic strategies. Sleep, often overlooked, plays a crucial role in the progression of these conditions. The ongoing research, as exemplified by the SURPASS-3 MRI study and triple G medication studies, offers promising avenues for addressing NAFLD and improving overall health outcomes. By integrating sleep health considerations into treatment approaches, there exists the potential for preventing and managing obesity, OSA, and T2DM, thereby enhancing the quality of life for individuals affected by these conditions.

Supplementary Materials: The following supporting information can be downloaded at: https://www.mdpi.com/article/10.3390/jcm13082231/s1, Figure S1: An overview of the proposed mechanisms underlying MASLD, OSA, and T2DM and some of the current therapies that target these associations. Figure S2: An overview of GIP–GLP-1 effects on glucose and satiety.

Funding: This research received no external funding.

Data Availability Statement: No new data were created or analyzed in this study. Data sharing is not applicable to this article.

Conflicts of Interest: The authors declare no conflict of interest.

References

1. McTigue, K.; Kuller, L. Cardiovascular risk factors, mortality, and overweight. *JAMA* **2008**, *299*, 1260–1261. [CrossRef] [PubMed]
2. McTigue, K.; Larson, J.C.; Valoski, A.; Burke, G.; Kotchen, J.; Lewis, C.E.; Stefanick, M.L.; Van Horn, L.; Kuller, L. Mortality and cardiac and vascular outcomes in extremely obese women. *JAMA* **2006**, *296*, 79–86. [CrossRef] [PubMed]
3. Benjafield, A.V.; Ayas, N.T.; Eastwood, P.R.; Heinzer, R.; Ip, M.S.M.; Morrell, M.J.; Nunez, C.M.; Patel, S.R.; Penzel, T.; Pepin, J.L.; et al. Estimation of the global prevalence and burden of obstructive sleep apnoea: A literature-based analysis. *Lancet Respir. Med.* **2019**, *7*, 687–698. [CrossRef] [PubMed]
4. Noureddin, M.; Vipani, A.; Bresee, C.; Todo, T.; Kim, I.K.; Alkhouri, N.; Setiawan, V.W.; Tran, T.; Ayoub, W.S.; Lu, S.C.; et al. NASH Leading Cause of Liver Transplant in Women: Updated Analysis of Indications For Liver Transplant and Ethnic and Gender Variances. *Am. J. Gastroenterol.* **2018**, *113*, 1649–1659. [CrossRef] [PubMed]
5. Patel, S.R.; Ayas, N.T.; Malhotra, M.R.; White, D.P.; Schernhammer, E.S.; Speizer, F.E.; Stampfer, M.J.; Hu, F.B. A prospective study of sleep duration and mortality risk in women. *Sleep* **2004**, *27*, 440–444. [CrossRef] [PubMed]
6. Patel, S.R.; Malhotra, A.; White, D.P.; Gottlieb, D.J.; Hu, F.B. Association between reduced sleep and weight gain in women. *Am. J. Epidemiol.* **2006**, *164*, 947–954. [CrossRef] [PubMed]
7. Spiegel, K.; Tasali, E.; Penev, P.; Van Cauter, E. Brief communication: Sleep curtailment in healthy young men is associated with decreased leptin levels, elevated ghrelin levels, and increased hunger and appetite. *Ann. Intern. Med.* **2004**, *141*, 846–850. [CrossRef] [PubMed]
8. Spiegel, K.; Leproult, R.; Van Cauter, E. Impact of Sleep Debt on metabolic and endocrine function. *Lancet* **1999**, *23*, 1435–1439. [CrossRef] [PubMed]
9. Tasali, E.; Leproult, R.; Ehrmann, D.A.; Van Cauter, E. Slow-wave sleep and the risk of type 2 diabetes in humans. *Proc. Natl. Acad. Sci. USA* **2008**, *105*, 1044–1049. [CrossRef]
10. Tasali, E.; Wroblewski, K.; Kahn, E.; Kilkus, J.; Schoeller, D.A. Effect of Sleep Extension on Objectively Assessed Energy Intake Among Adults With Overweight in Real-life Settings: A Randomized Clinical Trial. *JAMA Intern. Med.* **2022**, *182*, 365–374. [CrossRef]
11. Weinstock, T.G.; Wang, X.; Rueschman, M.; Ismail-Beigi, F.; Aylor, J.; Babineau, D.C.; Mehra, R.; Redline, S. A controlled trial of CPAP therapy on metabolic control in individuals with impaired glucose tolerance and sleep apnea. *Sleep* **2012**, *35*, 617B–625B. [CrossRef] [PubMed]
12. Bakker, J.P.; Edwards, B.A.; Gautam, S.P.; Montesi, S.B.; Duran-Cantolla, J.; Aizpuru, F.; Barbe, F.; Sanchez-de-la-Torre, M.; Malhotra, A. Blood pressure improvement with continuous positive airway pressure is independent of obstructive sleep apnea severity. *J. Clin. Sleep Med.* **2014**, *10*, 365–369. [CrossRef] [PubMed]
13. Somers, V.K.; Dyken, M.E.; Clary, M.P.; Abboud, F.M. Sympathetic neural mechanisms in obstructive sleep apnea. *J. Clin. Investig.* **1995**, *96*, 1897–1904. [CrossRef] [PubMed]
14. Narkiewicz, K.; Kato, M.; Phillips, B.G.; Pesek, C.A.; Davison, D.E.; Somers, V.K. Nocturnal continuous positive airway pressure decreases daytime sympathetic traffic in obstructive sleep apnea. *Circulation* **1999**, *100*, 2332–2335. [CrossRef] [PubMed]
15. Bloom, S.R.; Edwards, A.V.; Hardy, R.N. The role of the autonomic nervous system in the control of glucagon, insulin and pancreatic polypeptide release from the pancreas. *J. Physiol.* **1978**, *280*, 9–23. [CrossRef] [PubMed]
16. Hilton, M.F.; Chappell, M.J.; Bartlett, W.A.; Malhotra, A.; Beattie, J.M.; Cayton, R.M. The sleep apnoea/hypopnoea syndrome depresses waking vagal tone independent of sympathetic activation. *Eur. Respir. J.* **2001**, *17*, 1258–1266. [CrossRef]
17. Bottini, P.; Redolfi, S.; Dottorini, M.L.; Tantucci, C. Autonomic neuropathy increases the risk of obstructive sleep apnea in obese diabetics. *Respiration* **2008**, *75*, 265–271. [CrossRef]
18. Lecube, A.; Sampol, G.; Hernandez, C.; Romero, O.; Ciudin, A.; Simo, R. Characterization of sleep breathing pattern in patients with type 2 diabetes: Sweet sleep study. *PLoS ONE* **2015**, *10*, e0119073. [CrossRef] [PubMed]
19. Banghoej, A.M.; Nerild, H.H.; Kristensen, P.L.; Pedersen-Bjergaard, U.; Fleischer, J.; Jensen, A.E.; Laub, M.; Thorsteinsson, B.; Tarnow, L. Obstructive sleep apnoea is frequent in patients with type 1 diabetes. *J. Diabetes Complicat.* **2017**, *31*, 156–161. [CrossRef]
20. Punjabi, N.M.; Polotsky, V.Y. Disorders of glucose metabolism in sleep apnea. *J. Appl. Physiol.* **2005**, *99*, 1998–2007. [CrossRef]
21. Foster, G.D.; Borradaile, K.E.; Sanders, M.H.; Millman, R.; Zammit, G.; Newman, A.B.; Wadden, T.A.; Kelley, D.; Wing, R.R.; Pi-Sunyer, F.X.; et al. A randomized study on the effect of weight loss on obstructive sleep apnea among obese patients with type 2 diabetes: The Sleep AHEAD study. *Arch. Intern. Med.* **2009**, *169*, 1619–1626. [CrossRef] [PubMed]
22. Foster, G.D.; Sanders, M.H.; Millman, R.; Zammit, G.; Borradaile, K.E.; Newman, A.B.; Wadden, T.A.; Kelley, D.; Wing, R.R.; Sunyer, F.X.; et al. Obstructive sleep apnea among obese patients with type 2 diabetes. *Diabetes Care* **2009**, *32*, 1017–1019. [CrossRef] [PubMed]
23. Kuna, S.T.; Reboussin, D.M.; Strotmeyer, E.S.; Millman, R.P.; Zammit, G.; Walkup, M.P.; Wadden, T.A.; Wing, R.R.; Pi-Sunyer, F.X.; Spira, A.P.; et al. Effects of Weight Loss on Obstructive Sleep Apnea Severity. Ten-Year Results of the Sleep AHEAD Study. *Am. J. Respir. Crit. Care Med.* **2021**, *203*, 221–229. [CrossRef] [PubMed]
24. Brooks, B.; Cistulli, P.A.; Borkman, M.; Ross, G.; McGhee, S.; Grunstein, R.R.; Sullivan, C.E.; Yue, D.K. Obstructive sleep apnea in obese noninsulin-dependent diabetic patients: Effect of continuous positive airway pressure treatment on insulin responsiveness. *J. Clin. Endocrinol. Metab.* **1994**, *79*, 1681–1685. [PubMed]
25. Drager, L.F.; Li, J.; Reinke, C.; Bevans-Fonti, S.; Jun, J.C.; Polotsky, V.Y. Intermittent hypoxia exacerbates metabolic effects of diet-induced obesity. *Obesity* **2011**, *19*, 2167–2174. [CrossRef] [PubMed]

26. Polotsky, V.Y.; Patil, S.P.; Savransky, V.; Laffan, A.; Fonti, S.; Frame, L.A.; Steele, K.E.; Schweizter, M.A.; Clark, J.M.; Torbenson, M.S.; et al. Obstructive sleep apnea, insulin resistance, and steatohepatitis in severe obesity. *Am. J. Respir. Crit. Care Med.* **2009**, *179*, 228–234. [CrossRef] [PubMed]
27. Kallwitz, E.R.; Herdegen, J.; Madura, J.; Jakate, S.; Cotler, S.J. Liver enzymes and histology in obese patients with obstructive sleep apnea. *J. Clin. Gastroenterol.* **2007**, *41*, 918–921. [CrossRef] [PubMed]
28. Mishra, P.; Nugent, C.; Afendy, A.; Bai, C.; Bhatia, P.; Afendy, M.; Fang, Y.; Elariny, H.; Goodman, Z.; Younossi, Z.M. Apnoeic-hypopnoeic episodes during obstructive sleep apnoea are associated with histological nonalcoholic steatohepatitis. *Liver Int.* **2008**, *28*, 1080–1086. [CrossRef] [PubMed]
29. Li, J.; Grigoryev, D.N.; Ye, S.Q.; Thorne, L.; Schwartz, A.R.; Smith, P.L.; O'Donnell, C.P.; Polotsky, V.Y. Chronic intermittent hypoxia upregulates genes of lipid biosynthesis in obese mice. *J. Appl. Physiol.* **2005**, *99*, 1643–1648. [CrossRef]
30. Petta, S.; Marrone, O.; Torres, D.; Buttacavoli, M.; Camma, C.; Di Marco, V.; Licata, A.; Lo Bue, A.; Parrinello, G.; Pinto, A.; et al. Obstructive Sleep Apnea Is Associated with Liver Damage and Atherosclerosis in Patients with Non-Alcoholic Fatty Liver Disease. *PLoS ONE* **2015**, *10*, e0142210. [CrossRef]
31. Mesarwi, O.A.; Shin, M.K.; Drager, L.F.; Bevans-Fonti, S.; Jun, J.C.; Putcha, N.; Torbenson, M.S.; Pedrosa, R.P.; Lorenzi-Filho, G.; Steele, K.E.; et al. Lysyl Oxidase as a Serum Biomarker of Liver Fibrosis in Patients with Severe Obesity and Obstructive Sleep Apnea. *Sleep* **2015**, *38*, 1583–1591. [CrossRef] [PubMed]
32. Mesarwi, O.A.; Loomba, R.; Malhotra, A. Obstructive Sleep Apnea, Hypoxia, and Nonalcoholic Fatty Liver Disease. *Am. J. Respir. Crit. Care Med.* **2019**, *199*, 830–841. [CrossRef] [PubMed]
33. Corey, K.E.; Misdraji, J.; Gelrud, L.; King, L.Y.; Zheng, H.; Malhotra, A.; Chung, R.T. Obstructive Sleep Apnea Is Associated with Nonalcoholic Steatohepatitis and Advanced Liver Histology. *Dig. Dis. Sci.* **2015**, *60*, 2523–2528. [CrossRef]
34. Chung, G.E.; Cho, E.J.; Yoo, J.J.; Chang, Y.; Cho, Y.; Park, S.H.; Shin, D.W.; Han, K.; Yu, S.J. Nonalcoholic fatty liver disease is associated with the development of obstructive sleep apnea. *Sci. Rep.* **2021**, *11*, 13473. [CrossRef]
35. Marusic, M.; Paic, M.; Knobloch, M.; Prso, A.M.L. NAFLD, Insulin Resistance, and Diabetes Mellitus Type 2. *Can. J. Gastroenterol. Hepatol.* **2021**, *2021*, 6613827. [CrossRef]
36. Barb, D.; Repetto, E.M.; Stokes, M.E.; Shankar, S.S.; Cusi, K. Type 2 diabetes mellitus increases the risk of hepatic fibrosis in individuals with obesity and nonalcoholic fatty liver disease. *Obesity* **2021**, *29*, 1950–1960. [CrossRef]
37. Sung, K.C.; Jeong, W.S.; Wild, S.H.; Byrne, C.D. Combined influence of insulin resistance, overweight/obesity, and fatty liver as risk factors for type 2 diabetes. *Diabetes Care* **2012**, *35*, 717–722. [CrossRef] [PubMed]
38. Mantovani, A.; Petracca, G.; Beatrice, G.; Tilg, H.; Byrne, C.D.; Targher, G. Non-alcoholic fatty liver disease and risk of incident diabetes mellitus: An updated meta-analysis of 501 022 adult individuals. *Gut* **2021**, *70*, 962–969. [CrossRef]
39. Targher, G.; Corey, K.E.; Byrne, C.D.; Roden, M. The complex link between NAFLD and type 2 diabetes mellitus—Mechanisms and treatments. *Nat. Rev. Gastroenterol. Hepatol.* **2021**, *18*, 599–612. [CrossRef]
40. Aderinto, N.; Olatunji, G.; Kokori, E.; Olaniyi, P.; Isarinade, T.; Yusuf, I.A. Recent advances in bariatric surgery: A narrative review of weight loss procedures. *Ann. Med. Surg.* **2023**, *85*, 6091–6104. [CrossRef]
41. Peterli, R.; Wolnerhanssen, B.K.; Peters, T.; Vetter, D.; Kroll, D.; Borbely, Y.; Schultes, B.; Beglinger, C.; Drewe, J.; Schiesser, M.; et al. Effect of Laparoscopic Sleeve Gastrectomy vs Laparoscopic Roux-en-Y Gastric Bypass on Weight Loss in Patients With Morbid Obesity: The SM-BOSS Randomized Clinical Trial. *JAMA* **2018**, *319*, 255–265. [CrossRef] [PubMed]
42. Durmush, E.K.; Ermerak, G.; Durmush, D. Short-term outcomes of sleeve gastrectomy for morbid obesity: Does staple line reinforcement matter? *Obes. Surg.* **2014**, *24*, 1109–1116. [CrossRef] [PubMed]
43. Neagoe, R.; Muresan, M.; Timofte, D.; Darie, R.; Razvan, I.; Voidazan, S.; Muresan, S.; Sala, D. Long-term outcomes of laparoscopic sleeve gastrectomy—A single-center prospective observational study. *Videosurgery Miniinv.* **2019**, *14*, 242–248. [CrossRef] [PubMed]
44. Sheng, B.; Truong, K.; Spitler, H.; Zhang, L.; Tong, X.; Chen, L. The Long-Term Effects of Bariatric Surgery on Type 2 Diabetes Remission, Microvascular and Macrovascular Complications, and Mortality: A Systematic Review and Meta-Analysis. *Obes. Surg.* **2017**, *27*, 2724–2732. [CrossRef] [PubMed]
45. Yu, J.; Zhou, X.; Li, L.; Li, S.; Tan, J.; Li, Y.; Sun, X. The long-term effects of bariatric surgery for type 2 diabetes: Systematic review and meta-analysis of randomized and non-randomized evidence. *Obes. Surg.* **2015**, *25*, 143–158. [CrossRef] [PubMed]
46. Sjostrom, L.; Peltonen, M.; Jacobson, P.; Ahlin, S.; Andersson-Assarsson, J.; Anveden, A.; Bouchard, C.; Carlsson, B.; Karason, K.; Lonroth, H.; et al. Association of bariatric surgery with long-term remission of type 2 diabetes and with microvascular and macrovascular complications. *JAMA* **2014**, *311*, 2297–2304. [CrossRef]
47. Courcoulas, A.P.; Patti, M.E.; Hu, B.; Arterburn, D.E.; Simonson, D.C.; Gourash, W.F.; Jakicic, J.M.; Vernon, A.H.; Beck, G.J.; Schauer, P.R.; et al. Long-Term Outcomes of Medical Management vs Bariatric Surgery in Type 2 Diabetes. *JAMA* **2024**, *331*, 654–664. [CrossRef]
48. De Brito, E.S.M.B.; Tustumi, F.; de Miranda Neto, A.A.; Dantas, A.C.B.; Santo, M.A.; Cecconello, I. Gastric Bypass Compared with Sleeve Gastrectomy for Nonalcoholic Fatty Liver Disease: A Systematic Review and Meta-analysis. *Obes. Surg.* **2021**, *31*, 2762–2772. [CrossRef] [PubMed]
49. Lee, Y.; Doumouras, A.G.; Yu, J.; Brar, K.; Banfield, L.; Gmora, S.; Anvari, M.; Hong, D. Complete Resolution of Nonalcoholic Fatty Liver Disease After Bariatric Surgery: A Systematic Review and Meta-analysis. *Clin. Gastroenterol. Hepatol.* **2019**, *17*, 1040–1060.e11. [CrossRef]

50. Lee, Y.H.; Johan, A.; Wong, K.K.; Edwards, N.; Sullivan, C. Prevalence and risk factors for obstructive sleep apnea in a multiethnic population of patients presenting for bariatric surgery in Singapore. *Sleep Med.* **2009**, *10*, 226–232. [CrossRef]
51. Kreitinger, K.Y.; Lui, M.M.S.; Owens, R.L.; Schmickl, C.N.; Grunvald, E.; Horgan, S.; Raphelson, J.R.; Malhotra, A. Screening for Obstructive Sleep Apnea in a Diverse Bariatric Surgery Population. *Obesity* **2020**, *28*, 2028–2034. [CrossRef] [PubMed]
52. Smith, P.L.; Gold, A.R.; Meyers, D.A.; Haponik, E.F.; Bleecker, E.R. Weight loss in mildly to moderately obese patients with obstructive sleep apnea. *Ann. Intern. Med.* **1985**, *103*, 850–855. [CrossRef] [PubMed]
53. Currie, A.C.; Kaur, V.; Carey, I.; Al-Rubaye, H.; Mahawar, K.; Madhok, B.; Small, P.; McGlone, E.R.; Khan, O.A. Obstructive sleep apnea remission following bariatric surgery: A national registry cohort study. *Surg. Obes. Relat. Dis.* **2021**, *17*, 1576–1582. [CrossRef]
54. Pillar, G.; Peled, R.; Lavie, P. Recurrence of sleep apnea without concomitant weight increase 7.5 years after weight reduction surgery. *Chest* **1994**, *106*, 1702–1704. [CrossRef] [PubMed]
55. Sampol, G.; Munoz, X.; Sagales, M.T.; Marti, S.; Roca, A.; Dolors de la Calzada, M.; Lloberes, P.; Morell, F. Long-term efficacy of dietary weight loss in sleep apnoea/hypopnoea syndrome. *Eur. Respir. J.* **1998**, *12*, 1156–1159. [CrossRef] [PubMed]
56. Jastreboff, A.M.; Aronne, L.J.; Ahmad, N.N.; Wharton, S.; Connery, L.; Alves, B.; Kiyosue, A.; Zhang, S.; Liu, B.; Bunck, M.C.; et al. Tirzepatide Once Weekly for the Treatment of Obesity. *N. Engl. J. Med.* **2022**, *387*, 205–216. [CrossRef] [PubMed]
57. Gastaldelli, A.; Cusi, K.; Fernandez Lando, L.; Bray, R.; Brouwers, B.; Rodriguez, A. Effect of tirzepatide versus insulin degludec on liver fat content and abdominal adipose tissue in people with type 2 diabetes (SURPASS-3 MRI): A substudy of the randomised, open-label, parallel-group, phase 3 SURPASS-3 trial. *Lancet Diabetes Endocrinol.* **2022**, *10*, 393–406. [CrossRef] [PubMed]
58. Malhotra, A.; Bednarik, J.; Chakladar, S.; Dunn, J.P.; Weaver, T.; Grunstein, R.; Fietze, I.; Redline, S.; Azarbarzin, A.; Sands, S.A.; et al. Tirzepatide for the treatment of obstructive sleep apnea: Rationale, design, and sample baseline characteristics of the SURMOUNT-OSA phase 3 trial. *Contemp. Clin. Trials* **2024**, *141*, 107516. [CrossRef] [PubMed]
59. Zhao, F.; Zhou, Q.; Cong, Z.; Hang, K.; Zou, X.; Zhang, C.; Chen, Y.; Dai, A.; Liang, A.; Ming, Q.; et al. Structural insights into multiplexed pharmacological actions of tirzepatide and peptide 20 at the GIP, GLP-1 or glucagon receptors. *Nat. Commun.* **2022**, *13*, 1057. [CrossRef]
60. Jastreboff, A.M.; Kaplan, L.M.; Frias, J.P.; Wu, Q.; Du, Y.; Gurbuz, S.; Coskun, T.; Haupt, A.; Milicevic, Z.; Hartman, M.L.; et al. Triple-Hormone-Receptor Agonist Retatrutide for Obesity—A Phase 2 Trial. *N. Engl. J. Med.* **2023**, *389*, 514–526. [CrossRef]
61. Sanyal, A.J. Retatrutide NAFLD—Phase 2 trial results in subset of patients with obesity and NAFLD. In Proceedings of the American Diabetes Association Meeting, San Diego, CA, 23–26 June 2023.
62. Rosenstock, J.; Frias, J.; Jastreboff, A.M.; Du, Y.; Lou, J.; Gurbuz, S.; Thomas, M.K.; Hartman, M.L.; Haupt, A.; Milicevic, Z.; et al. Retatrutide, a GIP, GLP-1 and glucagon receptor agonist, for people with type 2 diabetes: A randomised, double-blind, placebo and active-controlled, parallel-group, phase 2 trial conducted in the USA. *Lancet* **2023**, *402*, 529–544. [CrossRef] [PubMed]
63. Pamidi, S.; Wroblewski, K.; Stepien, M.; Sharif-Sidi, K.; Kilkus, J.; Whitmore, H.; Tasali, E. Eight Hours of Nightly Continuous Positive Airway Pressure Treatment of Obstructive Sleep Apnea Improves Glucose Metabolism in Patients with Prediabetes. A Randomized Controlled Trial. *Am. J. Respir. Crit. Care Med.* **2015**, *192*, 96–105. [CrossRef] [PubMed]
64. Labarca, G.; Reyes, T.; Jorquera, J.; Dreyse, J.; Drake, L. CPAP in patients with obstructive sleep apnea and type 2 diabetes mellitus: Systematic review and meta-analysis. *Clin. Respir. J.* **2018**, *12*, 2361–2368. [CrossRef] [PubMed]
65. Ng, S.S.S.; Wong, V.W.S.; Wong, G.L.H.; Chu, W.C.W.; Chan, T.O.; To, K.W.; Ko, F.W.S.; Chan, K.P.; Hui, D.S. Continuous Positive Airway Pressure Does Not Improve Nonalcoholic Fatty Liver Disease in Patients with Obstructive Sleep Apnea. A Randomized Clinical Trial. *Am. J. Respir. Crit. Care Med.* **2021**, *203*, 493–501. [CrossRef] [PubMed]
66. Chen, L.D.; Lin, L.; Zhang, L.J.; Zeng, H.X.; Wu, Q.Y.; Hu, M.F.; Xie, J.J.; Liu, J.N. Effect of continuous positive airway pressure on liver enzymes in obstructive sleep apnea: A meta-analysis. *Clin. Respir. J.* **2018**, *12*, 373–381. [CrossRef]
67. Van de Graaff, W.B. Thoracic influence on upper airway patency. *J. Appl. Physiol.* **1988**, *65*, 2124–2131. [CrossRef] [PubMed]
68. Schwab, R.J.; Gupta, K.B.; Gefter, W.B.; Metzger, L.J.; Hoffman, E.A.; Pack, A.I. Upper airway and soft tissue anatomy in normal subjects and patients with sleep-disordered breathing. Significance of the lateral pharyngeal walls. *Am. J. Respir. Crit. Care Med.* **1995**, *152*, 1673–1689. [CrossRef]
69. Schwartz, A.R.; Eisele, D.W.; Smith, P.L. Pharyngeal airway obstruction in obstructive sleep apnea: Pathophysiology and clinical implications. *Otolaryngol. Clin. N. Am.* **1998**, *31*, 911–918. [CrossRef]
70. Wang, S.H.; Keenan, B.T.; Wiemken, A.; Zang, Y.; Staley, B.; Sarwer, D.B.; Torigian, D.A.; Williams, N.; Pack, A.I.; Schwab, R.J. Effect of Weight Loss on Upper Airway Anatomy and the Apnea-Hypopnea Index. The Importance of Tongue Fat. *Am. J. Respir. Crit. Care Med.* **2020**, *201*, 718–727. [CrossRef]
71. Sands, S.A.; Eckert, D.J.; Jordan, A.S.; Edwards, B.A.; Owens, R.L.; Butler, J.P.; Schwab, R.J.; Loring, S.H.; Malhotra, A.; White, D.P.; et al. Enhanced Upper-airway Muscle Responsiveness is a Distinct Feature of Overweight/Obese Individuals without Sleep Apnea. *Am. J. Respir. Crit. Care Med.* **2014**, *190*, 930–937. [CrossRef]
72. Chirinos, J.A.; Gurubhagavatula, I.; Teff, K.; Rader, D.J.; Wadden, T.A.; Townsend, R.; Foster, G.D.; Maislin, G.; Saif, H.; Broderick, P.; et al. CPAP, weight loss, or both for obstructive sleep apnea. *N. Engl. J. Med.* **2014**, *370*, 2265–2275. [CrossRef] [PubMed]
73. Alotaibi, M.; Shao, J.; Pauciulo, M.W.; Nichols, W.C.; Hemnes, A.R.; Malhotra, A.; Kim, N.H.; Yuan, J.X.; Fernandes, T.; Kerr, K.M.; et al. Metabolomic Profiles Differentiate Scleroderma-PAH from Idiopathic PAH and Correspond with Worsened Functional Capacity. *Chest* **2022**, *163*, 204–215. [CrossRef] [PubMed]

74. Ambroselli, D.; Masciulli, F.; Romano, E.; Catanzaro, G.; Besharat, Z.M.; Massari, M.C.; Ferretti, E.; Migliaccio, S.; Izzo, L.; Ritieni, A.; et al. New Advances in Metabolic Syndrome, from Prevention to Treatment: The Role of Diet and Food. *Nutrients* **2023**, *15*, 640. [CrossRef] [PubMed]
75. Harrison, S.A.; Bedossa, P.; Guy, C.D.; Schattenberg, J.M.; Loomba, R.; Taub, R.; Labriola, D.; Moussa, S.E.; Neff, G.W.; Rinella, M.E.; et al. A Phase 3, Randomized, Controlled Trial of Resmetirom in NASH with Liver Fibrosis. *N. Engl. J. Med.* **2024**, *390*, 497–509. [CrossRef] [PubMed]

Disclaimer/Publisher's Note: The statements, opinions and data contained in all publications are solely those of the individual author(s) and contributor(s) and not of MDPI and/or the editor(s). MDPI and/or the editor(s) disclaim responsibility for any injury to people or property resulting from any ideas, methods, instructions or products referred to in the content.

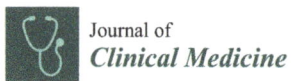

Review

Achieving Better Understanding of Obstructive Sleep Apnea Treatment Effects on Cardiovascular Disease Outcomes through Machine Learning Approaches: A Narrative Review

Oren Cohen [1], Vaishnavi Kundel [1], Philip Robson [2], Zainab Al-Taie [3], Mayte Suárez-Fariñas [3,†] and Neomi A. Shah [1,*,†]

1. Department of Medicine, Division of Pulmonary, Critical Care and Sleep Medicine, Icahn School of Medicine at Mount Sinai, New York, NY 10029, USA; oren.cohen@mountsinai.org (O.C.); vaishnavi.kundel@mssm.edu (V.K.)
2. Biomedical Engineering and Imaging Institute, Icahn School of Medicine at Mount Sinai, New York, NY 10029, USA; philip.robson@mountsinai.org
3. Center for Biostatistics, Department of Population Health Science and Policy, Icahn School of Medicine at Mount Sinai, New York, NY 10029, USA; zainab.al-taie@mountsinai.org (Z.A.-T.); mayte.suarezfarinas@mssm.edu (M.S.-F.)
* Correspondence: neomi.shah@mssm.edu; Tel.: +1-212-241-5900
† These authors contributed equally to this work.

Abstract: Obstructive sleep apnea (OSA) affects almost a billion people worldwide and is associated with a myriad of adverse health outcomes. Among the most prevalent and morbid are cardiovascular diseases (CVDs). Nonetheless, randomized controlled trials (RCTs) of OSA treatment have failed to show improvements in CVD outcomes. A major limitation in our field is the lack of precision in defining OSA and specifically subgroups with the potential to benefit from therapy. Further, this has called into question the validity of using the time-honored apnea–hypopnea index as the ultimate defining criteria for OSA. Recent applications of advanced statistical methods and machine learning have brought to light a variety of OSA endotypes and phenotypes. These methods also provide an opportunity to understand the interaction between OSA and comorbid diseases for better CVD risk stratification. Lastly, machine learning and specifically heterogeneous treatment effects modeling can help uncover subgroups with differential outcomes after treatment initiation. In an era of data sharing and big data, these techniques will be at the forefront of OSA research. Advanced data science methods, such as machine-learning analyses and artificial intelligence, will improve our ability to determine the unique influence of OSA on CVD outcomes and ultimately allow us to better determine precision medicine approaches in OSA patients for CVD risk reduction. In this narrative review, we will highlight how team science via machine learning and artificial intelligence applied to existing clinical data, polysomnography, proteomics, and imaging can do just that.

Keywords: obstructive sleep apnea; cardiovascular disease; machine learning; artificial intelligence; heterogeneity of treatment effects; ethics in machine learning and artificial intelligence

Citation: Cohen, O.; Kundel, V.; Robson, P.; Al-Taie, Z.; Suárez-Fariñas, M.; Shah, N.A. Achieving Better Understanding of Obstructive Sleep Apnea Treatment Effects on Cardiovascular Disease Outcomes through Machine Learning Approaches: A Narrative Review. *J. Clin. Med.* **2024**, *13*, 1415. https://doi.org/10.3390/jcm13051415

Academic Editor: Silvano Dragonieri

Received: 31 January 2024
Revised: 13 February 2024
Accepted: 17 February 2024
Published: 29 February 2024

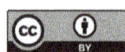

Copyright: © 2024 by the authors. Licensee MDPI, Basel, Switzerland. This article is an open access article distributed under the terms and conditions of the Creative Commons Attribution (CC BY) license (https:// creativecommons.org/licenses/by/ 4.0/).

1. Introduction

Obstructive sleep apnea (OSA) affects almost one billion people worldwide and 24 million people in the United States alone [1]. Despite the magnitude of this disorder, there remains a considerable knowledge gap in how we address its implications. The belief that all OSA patients require treatment has been questioned due to the lack of concrete evidence supporting this stance [2,3]. For instance, while continuous positive airway pressure (CPAP) enhances measures of sleepiness, blood pressure, and overall quality of life [4,5], its positive influence on cardiovascular disease (CVD) risk has not been consistently demonstrated, especially among nonsleepy OSA patients [6–8]. This inconsistency in outcomes suggests that the OSA population is heterogeneous and that not all patients derive equal benefits from CPAP.

Moreover, there is an absence of clinical risk-prediction tools specifically for CVD in OSA patients, though there are ongoing efforts within this domain [9,10]. Clinicians find it challenging to prioritize treatment for those at elevated risk, underscoring the need for more sophisticated, data-driven solutions. The current challenges focus on optimizing treatment plans, discerning those at increased risk of primary and recurrent CVD events, and identifying those patients who might benefit from interventions like CPAP for CVD risk mitigation. The significance of developing machine learning (ML)/artificial intelligence (AI)-based prediction tools for CVD risk reduction especially in asymptomatic OSA patients cannot be overstated. Randomized clinical trials (RCTs), unfortunately, do not always provide clarity on the full scope of treatment benefits. Though the major RCTs have not shown significant advantages of CPAP in decreasing CVD events in nonsleepy OSA patients, we speculate that this may be partially due to heterogeneity in treatment responses, i.e., not everyone with OSA will experience CVD risk reduction when CPAP is applied.

ML and AI present promising avenues for advancing our understanding and treatment of OSA. Both the National Institutes of Health (NIH) and the American Heart Association (AHA) have recognized the potential of ML/AI for advancing our understanding of how sleep disorders impact cardiovascular health and the need for fine-tuning treatment personalization [11,12]. Incorporating ML into medical research has led to the discovery of novel causal contributors to adverse outcomes [13,14]. For example, in the PARADIGM registry, ML models outperformed conventional statistical models and atherosclerotic CVD risk scores in identifying individuals at risk of rapid progression of coronary atherosclerosis [15]. In the Multi-Ethnic Study of Atherosclerosis (MESA), ML more accurately predicted the CVD event rate compared to traditional risk scores [16]. The heterogeneity of OSA disease presentations, risk factors, overlapping comorbidities, and treatment outcomes make it an ideal condition for the application of ML/AI. Vast clinical, biomedical, and polysomnographic information in OSA patients often remains underutilized in current analyses due to the magnitude of and interdependencies within the data. There has been significant interest and progress in employing ML/AI to develop more effective diagnostic and monitoring programs for OSA. However, striking the right balance between ideal methods and practical constraints is essential in this pursuit. Furthermore, the application of ML in sleep medicine opens new avenues of investigation into the issue of treatment heterogeneity. Current projects within our group are applying ML to RCT data to develop advanced decision tools to identify nonsleepy OSA patient subgroups with differential treatment responses, a task that has been challenging using traditional methodologies. Furthermore, new advanced AI technologies, such as transformer-based neural networks, can augment ML-based applications. Transformers can effectively process raw image data, such as computed tomography (CT) scans of the face, oral cavity, or chest, or polysomnographic (PSG) data, enabling the automated recognition and categorization of prevalent sleep apnea-related patterns.

However, a major hurdle of ML/AI is the "black box" phenomenon, where the process from input to outcome remains obscured. This opaqueness can deter trust in the system, particularly for clinicians, researchers, and educators unfamiliar with ML/AI and its strengths and weaknesses. Thoroughly evaluating the output of ML is just as crucial as crafting the model itself, especially when considering its potential integration into clinical practice. Addressing this requires a team-science approach, blending the expertise of clinicians, data scientists, statisticians, and clinical bioinformaticians. The objective is to produce robust, high-performance prediction models that can be readily translated into clinical practice.

This review will focus on the crucial role of ML/AI in achieving a more patient-centered diagnosis of OSA by replacing traditional diagnostic metrics, as well as its application in understanding treatment heterogeneity. We believe that harnessing state-of-the-art ML/AI techniques to analyze extensive OSA datasets will usher in the long-awaited era of personalized medicine for OSA.

2. Statistical Methodology and Machine Learning Algorithms

ML, a subset of AI, uses computer algorithms to identify complex interactions in large, multidimensional datasets that might elude human analysis. There are currently three important forms of ML/AI currently in use: supervised, unsupervised, and reinforcement learning frameworks. Supervised approaches are characterized by their ability to learn the underlying relationships between predictor variables and known outcomes [17]. These types of analyses can be used in medicine for risk assessment, diagnosis, and predicting treatment outcomes. This category includes both models that are intuitive and easy to interpret, such as linear models and decision trees, as well as those that capture more complex interactions between predictor and outcome variables. Simpler models offer intuitive and more easily interpretable predictions based on patient features, but they often lack robustness and are sensitive to random perturbations in the data. More complex algorithms, including the support vector machine, random forest, and deep learning, can be very powerful and robust but difficult to understand. For example, a random forest model built using data from the Sleep Heart Health Study was more accurate in predicting 10-year CVD risk than the Framingham Risk Score (FRS) [18]. However, it is not possible to understand all the ways in which variables within the model interact to produce its predictions. Therefore, using such a model, it is not easy to identify specific clinical features to target for intervention. Users can only feed a patient's data into the model to obtain a risk prediction. Conversely, for the FRS, each variable and its weighted importance (i.e., the number of points it contributes to the score) are published. Thus, a clinician can assess which variables from an individual patient's history are contributing to a given score and tally their score manually. An ensemble method such as random forests improves the algorithm accuracy by stabilizing the model performance through averaging the outcomes of multiple decision trees. However, explaining the interaction between features within the model can still be problematic. Lastly, even more advanced methods like survival forests use similar ensemble methods but focus on time-to-event data, providing a measure of risk over time [19].

Unsupervised learning attempts to learn patterns from seemingly random data within large datasets [20]. This takes on two main forms: (1) the clustering of participants based on underlying data and (2) dimensionality reduction, which uncovers a smaller number of hidden features that best represent and summarize the data without loss of information. Clustering methods are useful for identifying disease phenotypes and subgroups with similar characteristics, and have evolved from commonly used methods, such as latent class analysis (LCA), hierarchical clustering, and K-means clustering, to more advanced deep learning-based approaches. A study by Bailly et al. represents a prime example of clustering within OSA utilizing multiple data domains, including clinical and PSG data, from a large European database [21]. Using LCA, the authors found eight distinct phenotypes among 23,139 OSA patients. Further, they found that the rate of CPAP prescription varied between groups, with overweight men and women having some of the lowest prescription rates (57% and 49%, respectively), while younger/sleepier obese patients as well as older obese men had the highest rates of CPAP prescription (94% and 93%, respectively). The second category of unsupervised learning, dimensionality reduction, includes methods such as the linear principal component analysis (PCA), the nonlinear uniform manifold approximation and projection (UMAP), and more complex deep learning-based autoencoders. These types of analyses are useful for identifying a parsimonious list of features that represent the data while reducing the redundancy present with other methods, such as clustering. PSG is a great example of high-dimensional data capturing a multitude of physiologic signals. Dimensionality reduction techniques allow us to combine and pare down this information. For example, PCA can be applied to clinical [22] and/or PSG [23] data to reduce the number of features, and combined with clustering methods to identify unique patient subgroups from immense streams of data, which would be missed by conventional clinical scores and traditional PSG criteria.

While both the aforementioned supervised and unsupervised ML methods are static, reinforcement learning is a dynamic learning method by which an algorithm continues to evolve using feedback from past experiences to improve its performance [24]. Autotitrating CPAP is an excellent candidate for the application of reinforcement learning. Currently, autotitrating CPAP responds to flow limitation from a fixed scanning window. However, using the principles of reinforcement learning, it is possible to develop a system that could also learn patterns within or across nights to better optimize continuous pressure adjustment adapted to an individual patient in a certain position at a given time during sleep. This technique has not been utilized as much within sleep medicine as yet. However, there is great potential for its application in the future.

Lastly, though not a separate category of ML, transfer learning is another technique that must be mentioned and can be used in combination with any of the above forms of ML. Transfer learning is the application of models designed for one task/environment to another, enabling more rapid development of ML in a new setting [25,26]. As AI continues to advance, existing ML/AI models trained on large comprehensive datasets offer researchers and clinicians a strong foundation for creating new, more specialized, and effective diagnostic and treatment decision tools in other datasets. For example, a supervised learning model that was developed in a large clinical cohort predominantly comprised of white males may perform poorly if applied directly to other cohorts. Transfer learning allows us to retrain and adjust this existing model in a cohort that has a higher percentage of women and racial/ethnic diversity. Transfer learning can also improve ML performance when applied to smaller cohorts in a phenotypic subgroup; for example, as it uses the robust model initially developed within a larger population but tailored to this subgroup. Not only does transfer learning accelerate the development process, but it also produces more precise and efficient solutions, particularly in these types of data-limited scenarios.

3. Applying Machine Learning and Artificial Intelligence to Obstructive Sleep Apnea Data Domains

3.1. Assessment of Clinical Data

While the power of ML really shines when analyzing high-dimensional data, such as PSG, or handling multiple large data streams, it can still be useful in developing risk-prediction tools based solely on clinical data. Holfinger et al. used several supervised learning approaches, including the support vector machine, random forest, and artificial neural networks, to predict OSA diagnosis within the clinic-based SAGIC and Sleep Heart Health Cohorts using only age, sex, BMI, and race [27]. The authors were able to show better performance than a logistic regression model and similar performance to the STOP-BANG score, which requires more features. We must pause here, though, to highlight that the use of race in such models must be performed cautiously. Further, both cohorts used within these ML algorithms had very limited numbers of some historically and persistently excluded racial and ethnic groups. This issue of bias and ethics in ML/AI will be discussed further in a later section. Unsupervised ML approaches have also been helpful in the clinical domain. Mazzotti et al. used LCA to uncover four unique symptom phenotypes within OSA patients: "disturbed sleep", "minimally symptomatic", "moderately sleepy", and "excessively sleepy" [28]. Survival analysis within these groups identified the "excessively sleepy" phenotype as having the highest risk of incident CVD. A similar analysis using LCA was performed within the Icelandic Sleep Apnoea Cohort, finding clusters with "disturbed sleep", "minimally symptomatic", and "excessive daytime sleepiness" [29]. These examples highlight the ways in which both supervised and unsupervised ML approaches can predict risk using a parsimonious list of features and uncover hidden relationships within clinical data.

3.2. Harnessing the Power of Polysomnography

The field of OSA is undergoing a paradigm shift [30,31]. Over the last several decades physicians and researchers have predominantly focused on the AHI as the primary, and often sole, measure of OSA severity, attempting to understand clinical outcomes based on this metric alone [32]. However, the AHI is a hypothesis-driven measure of OSA severity [33], developed with only the underlying disease process in mind and without consideration for disease effects on relevant outcomes [34]. This process of disease classification and study without the consideration of broader disease implications is outdated, lacking in patient-centeredness [35], and contributes to overdiagnosis. Though the AHI has been useful, it has ultimately reached its limits.

In the new age of OSA precision medicine and data-driven science, novel metrics to grade the disease severity and subtype using an individualized patient-centered approach have gained a foothold [36,37]. Four major OSA endotypes have been developed and described, including pharyngeal collapsibility, loop gain, arousal threshold, and airway dilator muscle compensation [38,39]. These distinct endotypes have been shown to be scalable using cloud-based algorithms [40] and can be used as relevant features within ML-based decision trees for personalized treatment selection [41–43]. There are emerging data demonstrating their utility in assessing favorability for alternative therapies such as hypoglossal nerve stimulation [44] and even blood pressure response to the CPAP treatment of OSA [45]. However, these endotypes were developed to better characterize the physiology underlying OSA-related respiratory events, not clinical outcomes such as symptoms or CVD risk.

To better understand OSA in the context of patient-centered outcomes, we can apply novel mathematical methods to identify the physiologic and clinical consequences of OSA-related respiratory events across an entire night and even breath-by-breath [46,47]. Physiologic responses to OSA events can be divided into several separate, though interconnected, axes, including arousal, sympathetic, hypoxemic, and ventilatory. Using these responses, we can better predict CVD morbidity and mortality [48–50]. Further, novel measures such as the pulse rate response—a surrogate for sympathetic tone—have been shown to predict CVD benefit after OSA treatment [51]. The automation of these measures will allow for greater application and combination of these features with additional clinical variables within ML models to better predict disease outcomes and treatment response.

As mentioned above, PSG data are an excellent candidate for ML/AI applications given the high dimensionality and multiple data signals. Automated scoring algorithms for PSG developed in the last two decades have shown promise in replacing manual scoring [52]. Deep-learning techniques like neural networks have been used to detect apneas and hypopneas in real time during PSG [53]. Further, the detection of these events can be achieved even in pared-down PSG signal data, such as a single respiratory channel [54] or limited EEG [55]. Layering automated analysis of physiologic responses on top of existing automation of traditional scoring will allow for a deeper understanding of patient-level data and the identification of additional features that contribute to meaningful disease outcomes in future research. For example, neural networks can meaningfully predict patient-relevant outcomes, such as daytime sleepiness [56]. Going beyond OSA itself, the data contained within a PSG and processed via neural networks can predict mortality, with much of the risk attributable to sleep fragmentation [57]. Though, it would seem from recent data that OSA-event-related arousals alone do not provide additional information regarding incident CVD [58]. Thus, there is a wealth of information available within the PSG. By applying modern machine- and deep-learning approaches to analyze PSG signals, we may finally be able to understand the complex links between OSA and health outcomes, such as CVD. Further, these robust analytical processes may allow for the more accurate assessment of OSA from wearable devices in the home sleep testing arena.

3.3. Proteomics to Predict Cardiovascular Disease Risk in OSA

While there have been significant advances in the physiologic endotyping and clinical phenotyping of OSA, the pathobiological mechanisms underlying OSA morbidity remain elusive. Gaining a comprehensive understanding of how physiological processes associated with respiratory events result in biological responses leading to cardiometabolic and neurocognitive dysfunction is key [59]. To better understand this disease complexity, it is important to elucidate molecular and proteomic biomarkers contributing to the basic mechanisms underlying OSA. Proteomics refers to the set of 'big data' technologies applied to discover protein biomarkers associated various disease states. Such analyses can be performed using a "shotgun" approach to identify all measured proteins/metabolites, or using a targeted approach centered on a group of proteins [60]. Either way, the combination of "omics"-based strategies and ML methods have the potential to revolutionize sleep medicine and boost our understanding of pathobiological pathways in OSA.

Advanced immunoassays, such as the Olink® inflammation and CVD biomarker panels (Olink® Bioscience, Uppsala, Sweden), allow for the exploration of personalized immunophenotyping. Olink® is a proteomics array that measures plasma biomarkers reflecting inflammation, immune response, cell adhesion, and tissue remodeling using a proximity extension assay. The Olink® platform has been used in several studies to identify proteins associated with various CVDs [61–63]. This panel has also been used in OSA patients to identify subgroups based on differential inflammatory protein expression. For example, in a recent post hoc analysis of the ISAACC study [8], Zapater et al. analyzed the proteomic profiles in 86 OSA patients admitted for acute coronary syndrome, divided into those with and without recurrent CVD events [64]. Using a supervised random forest algorithm to select relevant proteins and generate a predictive model of recurrent CVD, the authors identified 38 (of 276) cardiovascular and inflammatory proteins that were differentially expressed between the two groups. Additionally, 12 proteins emerged as predictive biomarkers, of which 3 were identified as having the highest contribution to prediction of recurrent CVD events among this cohort of OSA patients. These proteins included CXCL16, STK4, and TFPI, which are implicated in cell proliferation, communication and apoptosis, and regulation/response to inflammation and immune systems. Another study used the same proteomics panel to investigate the association between OSA severity and changes in inflammatory protein expression profiles in a cohort of women [65]. There was no significant association between OSA and protein expression after adjusting for age and BMI, though severe OSA during rapid eye movement (REM) sleep was negatively associated with Axin 1 (a protein involved in tumor suppression/regulation [66]). Severe REM OSA was also associated with reductions in Sirtuin-2 (a protein involved in metabolic regulation and adipogenesis inhibition [67,68]). In a subsequent study among men by Ljunggren et al., this REM OSA effect was not observed [69]. However, among men, an oxygen desaturation index $\geq$30 was associated with increased plasma levels of eight inflammatory proteins, including interferon gamma and angiotensin-converting enzyme 2.

Kundel et al. recently used unsupervised analyses to uncover three unique clusters of OSA in 46 patients with low, intermediate, and high inflammatory protein expression using the Olink® panel [70]. In an exploratory analysis, the authors found a differential response to CPAP among the three clusters, with an increase in inflammatory protein expression in the "low inflammatory" cluster and a decrease in inflammatory protein expression in the "high inflammatory" cluster following three months of CPAP. Although the samples sizes were small (total n = 46), the results are hypothesis-generating, and may guide future studies in the pursuit of characterizing "at-risk" subgroups of OSA patients. A similar approach using the Olink® panel was applied to nasal lavage samples collected from patients with OSA before and after initiating CPAP. In this study, Cohen et al. identified 13 proteins that significantly decreased after CPAP in a subset of participants classified as having a high baseline inflammatory protein expression by unsupervised clustering methods [71]. Many of these proteins (e.g., MCP-4, OSM, LAP TGF-beta1, and VEGF-alpha) have been linked to immune cell differentiation, chemotaxis, airway inflammation, and vascular remodeling. Further validation of these results using a combination of omics with ML algorithms can help risk-stratify OSA patients for future clinical trials for CVD risk reduction.

Despite these advances, there remains a long road ahead in identifying reliable OSA biomarkers from the extensive array of options offered by proteomics. Sleep medicine has traditionally lagged behind in the integration of omics data, leaving a significant knowledge gap in our understanding of sleep disorders like OSA. The emerging landscape of OSA's association with inflammation and CVD risk demands a more comprehensive approach. Integrating ML and omics data can unlock crucial insights into the molecular underpinnings of OSA and its impact on CVD risk. Moreover, embracing unsupervised ML approaches will be imperative for uncovering novel biomarkers that may have been previously overlooked. By combining ML/AI and omics, we have the potential to revolutionize sleep research, allowing us to (1) identify distinct subgroups within OSA populations with or without an elevated CVD risk, and (2) monitor OSA treatment efficacy [72]. This holistic approach can pave the way for more personalized diagnostics and treatments in sleep medicine.

3.4. Image-Based Machine Learning in OSA

Multiple ML approaches can be applied to OSA-related imaging data. Morphometric analysis, used in facial recognition technology, employs ML to analyze distances and arrangements of facial landmarks. Researchers have used the morphometric analysis of facial landmarks based on both 2D [73] and 3D [74,75] photography to differentiate between those with and without OSA. In a similar approach, Tsuiki et al. [76] used AI to analyze oropharynx architectures on 2D cephalometric radiographs. Automation of these technologies will allow for anatomic phenotyping within OSA and has the potential to replace OSA screening or even traditional sleep studies for diagnosis.

One of the most frequently used image-based ML applications is the automated segmentation of anatomical structures or the automatic classification of an image into different representative groups (e.g., disease versus no disease). This application typically utilizes a convolutional neural network approach. This approach allows rapid and robust segmentation to facilitate the measurement of dimensions and volumes of anatomical structures of interest. Extracted metrics can subsequently be used in diagnostic decision trees or in risk stratification. In the setting of OSA, most attention has been given to segmenting features of the upper airway based on 3D CT and magnetic resonance imaging (MRI) data. Craniofacial and upper-airway morphometric features on CT imaging, including the upper airway length, the A point–nasion–B point (ANB) angle, and the gonion–gnathion–hyoid angle, have been associated with elevated CVD risk [77]. De Bataille et al. [78] and Shujaat et al. [79] have used ML in cone-beam CT imaging to measure airway volume. A number of groups have demonstrated the use of the ML-based analysis of MRI to automatically segment upper-airway structures, including the pharynx, tongue, and soft palate, that may facilitate large-scale epidemiological analyses in OSA patients in the future [80–82]. Molnar et al. [83] used an AI analysis based on pharyngeal adipose tissue thickness derived from MRI, sex, and neck and waist circumference to separate patients with airway obstruction from those without. In a novel approach to airway measures, ML-supported computational fluid dynamics analysis has been used to predict OSA-related airflows [84].

Image-based ML has also been applied to brain MRI scans in OSA patients. Pang et al. [85] used the support vector machine and random forest to accurately classify OSA based on diffusion tensor MRI scans of the brain. In another study, Liu et al. [86] used ML analysis of resting-state functional MRI (rs-fMRI) scans of the brain to identify OSA patients with and without cognitive impairment. Similarly, Shu et al. [87] used rs-fMRI and ML analyses to investigate cognitive impairment in OSA. Agarwal et al. [88] used a convolutional neural network analysis of brain MRI scans to predict whether OSA patients treated with CPAP would experience a negative neurological condition post-treatment. These studies highlight the potential for the image-based analysis of the related and downstream effects of OSA in a multiorgan setting. Similar ML-enabled analyses combining multimodality data may be applicable in the setting of assessing the relationships between OSA and CVD risk.

In an alternative image-based ML approach, radiomics analyzes the relationships between the intensities of spatially correlated pixels. Radiomic metrics can provide insight into subtle features, patterns, or textures in the image that may not be apparent to the human observer. Using the feature tracking—a form of radiomic analysis—of cardiac-phase MRI images, Li et al. [89] assessed left ventricular (LV) parameters among patients with OSA and controls. The authors found that OSA was associated with a higher LV mass index and indexed cellular volume of the myocardium, suggesting cellular hypertrophy. Currently, however, there is a paucity of studies utilizing image-based ML or radiomics to evaluate the impact of OSA on CVD and future CVD risk. This is despite the extensive use of cardiovascular imaging in patients with OSA. Given the potential of image-based ML in diagnosing and characterizing OSA, there is an untapped opportunity in leveraging existing imaging data, such as chest X-rays, coronary artery calcium imaging, and cardiac MRI, through AI-driven analyses. For example, by applying AI to this wealth of historical data, we could gain insights into how various treatments for OSA impact cardiovascular health. This approach could help refine treatment strategies and identify the most effective interventions for individual patients, ultimately reducing the risk of cardiovascular complications associated with OSA.

3.5. Adding Multiple Domains for Better Prediction

Though each data domain alone provides a considerable substrate for novel statistical and AI methodologies, the true capabilities of ML lie in its ability to combine information from multiple domains. Within the field of OSA, this includes not only PSG and information from wearable technologies, but also demographic, social, behavioral, clinical, biological, and imaging data. As discussed above, techniques such as random forest [90] have been developed to handle these tasks and remain among the most powerful analytical tools available [91]. Data-driven random forest-built prediction models using a multitude of data outperform older hypothesis-driven risk scores, such as the FRS for predicting cardiovascular outcomes [18]. Wallace et al. applied random forest techniques to multidimensional data, including sleep data, and were able to demonstrate the accurate prediction of 15-year mortality risk [92]. Though the strength of this tool is the unique integration of data, individual variable importance analyses can be performed to better understand which specific features drive an algorithm's predictions. For example, in this aforementioned study by Wallace et al., sleep efficiency on PSG and time with oxygen saturation less than 90% were among the most important isolated features. However, demographic and comorbid health domains as whole categories were even more predictive of mortality than sleep domains. As shown, ML/AI approaches represent a new frontier in risk prediction. These promising tools combining multiple data streams will allow us to finally manage, assess, and leverage the immense information available for OSA patients.

4. Future Perspectives: Understanding Cardiovascular Disease Outcomes after OSA Treatment—A Futuristic Approach Using Machine Learning

Harnessing ML/AI for personalized treatment in medicine, and particularly OSA, will be a game-changer for tailoring therapy to individual needs. As described above, one common ML/AI strategy involves using supervised approaches to estimate the likelihood of a particular health outcome. This estimation can help prioritize individuals who are at higher risk. This is particularly effective in medical settings, where preventative treatments can be implemented to mitigate these risks. However, it is important to note that being at high risk does not always translate to significant benefits from a treatment. Although understanding CVD risk in OSA patients may enhance the outcomes and adherence of CPAP therapy [93], these risk assessment approaches do not directly measure how treatment changes that risk. Imagine a scenario where two patients with OSA of similar severity and symptom profile receive the same treatment (e.g., CPAP). One patient experiences a remarkable improvement in symptoms and a reduction in CVD risk, while the other sees little to no improvement in sleepiness and no risk reduction in CVD. We currently have few tools to understand and address such variations in outcomes.

Traditionally, healthcare determinations are based on the average treatment effect (ATE) of an intervention derived from large high-quality RCTs comparing the intervention to a control. However, these ATEs estimate the intervention's effect for a hypothetical chimeric patient who is an amalgamation of all the unique participants within a study [94]. These ATEs do not fully encompass the range of patient differences and risk levels essential for pinpointing those most in need of a particular intervention or potentially others that may be harmed by an intervention. The central challenge in advancing precision medicine lies in transcending the mere estimation of ATEs and risk stratification to recognize the diversity of therapeutic responses to an intervention based on factors such as patient attributes, inherent risk, and treatment susceptibility [95]. Overcoming such challenges requires a change in paradigm. Instead of directly predicting treatment outcomes, we need to understand and identify the patterns defining the heterogeneity in patient responses to a given intervention. This shift in focus is vital for more personalized and effective healthcare decisions.

Emerging methods combining AI models and causal inference have been developed to identify patients where treatment modifies the outcome risk [96]. These methods, collectively termed heterogeneous treatment effect (HTE) analyses, measure the difference in potential outcomes for an individual if they were treated versus if they were not treated. Traditionally, RCTs include subgroup analysis to understand diverse therapeutic responses by iteratively focusing on specific variables. In the realm of OSA, classic examples include secondary analysis by disease severity or by CPAP adherence thresholds. However, this can lead to erroneous conclusions either due to multiple statistical testing or limited statistical power, particularly when subgroup samples are small [97]. HTE analyses represent a considerable methodological step forward by assessing conditional average treatment effects (CATEs). CATEs reveal the treatment effect for ML/HTE model-derived subgroups—or even individuals depending on the specific form of HTE analysis—contingent on baseline covariates.

The first methods to address HTE in the context of RCTs utilized model-based recursive partitioning (MBRP) [98,99]. MBRP combines decision trees with classical statistical models to address the heterogeneity in patient responses. MBPR starts by fitting a statistical model (e.g., logistic regression in the case of binary outcomes or the Cox model for time-to-event outcomes) with treatment as a covariate on a complete dataset. It then identifies the baseline covariate that most strongly modifies the treatment effect (i.e., has an interaction with treatment) and uses that feature to partition the population into two subgroups. The procedure is applied recursively within each subgroup until no promising variables by which to split participants are left, resulting in a decision tree. Ultimately, the product of this model-derived decision tree is discrete patient subgroups clustered by their differential responses to treatment. Further, inspection of the key factors identified as the tree's nodes (i.e., the variables used to partition subgroups at each decision point) may lead to new and previously unfathomable hypotheses regarding associated conditions and disease mechanisms. Our group is using MBRP in ongoing work to identify the effect of CPAP on CVD outcomes among OSA participants within large RCTs.

As previously described, though supervised ML decision trees are easily interpretable, they suffer from issues of overfitting and sensitivity to noise. For purposes of risk prediction, these decision trees were expanded into random forest models [90], which combine data from a multitude of trees to improve the model accuracy. Similarly in the realm of HTEs, decision tree-based HTE methods, like MBRP, have been developed into the MBRP forest [100] and causal forest [101,102]. These methods maintain the core framework of the random forest, including recursive partitioning, subsampling, and random splits. However, they are adapted to HTEs, maximizing the ability to predict the variability of treatment effects rather than model accuracy, as is performed for risk prediction in supervised learning.

These algorithms provide the foundation for developing more accurate and personalized treatment strategies, moving beyond mere associations to uncover the underlying causality.

Causal forest models also have an added benefit over decision tree-based HTE models, as they directly estimate the individual treatment effect (ITE). The ITE can then be used to create a prioritization rule ranking patients by their predicted treatment response on a continuum from potential harm to benefit. The ITE is therefore much more granular than the CATE produced by decision tree-based HTE methods, which estimates the treatment effect for a subgroup of patients [103,104]. These innovative methods go beyond mere risk prediction; they measure the potential outcomes for an individual as if they were treated compared to as if they were not. These mathematical manipulations essentially allow for the equivalent of an RCT analysis within each individual participant, despite that given individual not actually having received both an intervention and control. This level of precision represents a substantial evolution in ML applications within healthcare. The game-changer here is our newfound ability to identify precisely which patients will benefit most from a particular treatment, and to therefore prioritize patients for interventions based on their individual predicted treatment response. These tools will finally enable us to tailor treatment plans to each patient's unique needs and maximize the likelihood of successful outcomes.

Lastly, just as transfer learning can be applied to other forms of ML, it can also be used to broaden the generalizability of HTE models trained on RCT cohorts by transferring these models and retraining them in observational datasets. This technique has the power to balance the precise causal estimates obtained in ideal RCTs and apply them to a larger number of patients in a more pragmatic setting. Although this application is in its nascency in sleep medicine, it has great potential in the near term. Further, federated learning approaches orchestrate the training of several local models from heterogeneous datasets without the need for individual participant-level data integration [105]. This form of model integration abides by local privacy laws and protects participant data while maximizing the power of large datasets [106]. This method protects study participants while allowing for global collaboration, and creates better diversity, equity, and inclusion of populations from previously under-represented countries.

In summary, the progression of HTE methods from basic ML to advanced causal forest methods and ITEs will allow the field to craft increasingly personalized and effective treatment plans for patients with OSA with relevant outcomes in mind, including improving cardiovascular outcomes. These approaches can be utilized to weigh various treatment options and their specific impact on cardiovascular health, ensuring that patients receive the most suitable interventions based on their unique characteristics and expected treatment effects. These examples highlight the potential of ML applications in healthcare to enhance patient care and cardiovascular well-being in individuals with OSA, ushering in an era of truly personalized medicine, where the right treatment is administered to the right patient at the right time. Future studies should focus on integrating these innovative approaches to fully leverage the capability of ML/AI and advanced statistical methods, making individualized treatment the norm rather than the exception.

5. Ethics in Machine Learning and Artificial Intelligence

Ethics in AI is a deeply important and continually evolving domain of study and discourse. As AI systems become more integrated in healthcare, the ethical implications of their applications grow in magnitude. Key issues like safety, fairness, privacy, and accountability demand action from AI developers, healthcare entities, governments, and society at large.

Bias and fairness are prominent concerns in AI, as decision-making models can inadvertently reflect and amplify societal biases in their training datasets. Research disparities persist in sleep medicine, particularly in regards to race/ethnicity, socioeconomic factors, and gender. OSA research has historically centered on males due to their higher condition prevalence, especially using older AHI criteria. This tendency is further exacerbated by sex differences in symptom presentation, driving underdiagnosis in women. Such disparities in research translate to the under-representation of certain groups in the data collected and used to train AI models. Prior research has already shown that only a minority of sleep clinic patients with OSA would meet the criteria for the existing RCTs within our field including a large proportion of women [107]. When predicting CVD risk in OSA patients using ML, such nonrepresentative training data can hinder the equity of AI models' performance across diverse backgrounds. This could inadvertently prioritize or neglect certain demographics in risk assessments. For example, if training data lean heavily towards male OSA patients, the AI might be less accurate in assessing CVD risks for female patients due to different symptom presentations. Other biases, such as those pertaining to the variability of treatment and diagnostic criteria, must also be carefully considered. For example, patients may be on different treatments for OSA that can affect CVD risk. Further, the criteria and modality used to diagnose OSA and measure its severity might change over time or vary between institutions. Models that do not account for such heterogeneity and unbalances can inject bias into AI predictions.

To ensure fairness in AI determinations, biases must be audited and addressed before the deployment of AI models. It is crucial to train AI users and developers on the use of fairness toolkits, such AI Fairness [108]. Prospectively, the research community should ensure diversity, equity, and inclusion in studies and trials to mitigate upstream biases within clinical datasets used by AI. Biased AI predictions can result in serious ramifications, leading to either neglect or excessive medical interventions. Hence, consistent evaluation and recalibration of AI models are vital to maintain fairness and adapt to the evolving medical understanding of OSA and CVD outcomes.

Finally, complex AI models, especially in deep learning, often act as a "black box", obscuring their decision-making and hindering trust. For patients and clinicians impacted by these models, understanding AI-driven decisions is paramount, even if it compromises peak model efficiency. The AI community is advancing and standardizing "explainable AI" [109] techniques, introducing methods like SHapley Additive exPlanation (SHAP), Local Interpretable Model-agnostic Explanations (LIME), attention mechanisms, and visualization tools. These techniques help us to understand how AI is using input data to reach its decisions and predictions. The evolution of explainable AI demands domain-specific insights for distinct needs, emphasizing the crucial role of team science with representation from both the OSA research community and data science developers. Further, the integration of AI into society requires a multidisciplinary approach, involving not just computer scientists, but also ethicists, sociologists, psychologists, and policymakers. As AI continues to advance, its users must prioritize ethical considerations to ensure that the technology benefits humanity and does not inadvertently harm or disadvantage certain groups.

6. Conclusions

In conclusion, ML and AI are important tools that have been used and developed in many fields of science and medicine. Their use in OSA is particularly exciting given the emerging research in our field uncovering disease heterogeneity and variability in treatment effects. The myriad of physiologic, biologic, and clinical data available for patients with OSA in the digital age from electronic health records, PSG, imaging, and multiomics are ripe for data science techniques that can combine multiple domains and assess high-dimensional data to improve patient experience, risk prediction, and treatment outcomes. Advances within ML/AI will allow for more complex analyses tailored to answer specific research questions and generate hypotheses previously unfathomable. However, despite the enticing features of ML/AI, we must remain cautious and vigilant to not overstep or introduce bias, as these methods have the potential to worsen pre-existing disparities in sleep medicine. OSA researchers using these methodologies must be rigorous and uncompromising on quality and fairness. We hope that the application of ML/AI will not only help identify patients who will benefit from OSA treatment, but also those who may potentially be harmed, aligning with the principles of the Hippocratic oath.

Author Contributions: O.C., V.K., P.R., Z.A.-T., M.S.-F. and N.A.S. contributed to conceptualizing, writing, and editing this narrative review. All authors have read and agreed to the published version of the manuscript.

Funding: O.C. receives funding from the Stony Wold-Herbert Fund. N.A.S. receives funding from the American Sleep Medicine Foundation (250-SR-21).

Institutional Review Board Statement: Not applicable.

Informed Consent Statement: Not applicable.

Data Availability Statement: Not applicable.

Acknowledgments: We thank Kavya Devarakonda for reviewing this manuscript and providing key edits.

Conflicts of Interest: The authors declare no relevant conflicts of interest.

References

1. Benjafield, A.V.; Ayas, N.T.; Eastwood, P.R.; Heinzer, R.; Ip, M.S.M.; Morrell, M.J.; Nunez, C.M.; Patel, S.R.; Penzel, T.; Pépin, J.-L.; et al. Estimation of the global prevalence and burden of obstructive sleep apnoea: A literature-based analysis. *Lancet Respir. Med.* **2019**, *7*, 687–698. [CrossRef]
2. Punjabi, N.M.; Gottlieb, D.J. COUNTERPOINT: Should Asymptomatic OSA Be Treated in Patients with Significant Cardiovascular Disease? No. *Chest* **2022**, *161*, 607–611. [CrossRef]
3. Drager, L.F.; Bortolotto, L.A.; Figueiredo, A.C.; Krieger, E.M.; Lorenzi-Filho, G. Effects of continuous positive airway pressure on early signs of atherosclerosis in obstructive sleep apnea. *Am. J. Respir. Crit. Care Med.* **2007**, *176*, 706–712. [CrossRef]
4. Haentjens, P.; Van Meerhaeghe, A.; Moscariello, A.; De Weerdt, S.; Poppe, K.; Dupont, A.; Velkeniers, B. The impact of continuous positive airway pressure on blood pressure in patients with obstructive sleep apnea syndrome: Evidence from a meta-analysis of placebo-controlled randomized trials. *Arch. Intern. Med.* **2007**, *167*, 757–764. [CrossRef] [PubMed]
5. Giles, T.; Lasserson, T.; Smith, B.; White, J.; Wright, J.; Cates, C. Continuous positive airways pressure for obstructive sleep apnoea in adults. *Cochrane Database Syst. Rev.* **2006**, *1*, CD001106. [CrossRef]
6. McEvoy, R.D.; Antic, N.A.; Heeley, E.; Luo, Y.; Ou, Q.; Zhang, X.; Mediano, O.; Chen, R.; Drager, L.F.; Liu, Z.; et al. CPAP for prevention of cardiovascular events in obstructive sleep apnea. *N. Engl. J. Med.* **2016**, *375*, 919–931. [CrossRef] [PubMed]
7. Peker, Y.; Glantz, H.; Eulenburg, C.; Wegscheider, K.; Herlitz, J.; Thunström, E. Effect of Positive Airway Pressure on Cardiovascular Outcomes in Coronary Artery Disease Patients with Nonsleepy Obstructive Sleep Apnea. The RICCADSA Randomized Controlled Trial. *Am. J. Respir. Crit. Care Med.* **2016**, *194*, 613–620. [CrossRef] [PubMed]
8. Sánchez-de-la-Torre, M.; Sánchez-de-la-Torre, A.; Bertran, S.; Abad, J.; Duran-Cantolla, J.; Cabriada, V.; Mediano, O.; Masdeu, M.J.; Alonso, M.L.; Masa, J.F.; et al. Effect of obstructive sleep apnoea and its treatment with continuous positive airway pressure on the prevalence of cardiovascular events in patients with acute coronary syndrome (ISAACC study): A randomised controlled trial. *Lancet Respir. Med.* **2020**, *8*, 359–367. [CrossRef] [PubMed]
9. Grote, L.; Sommermeyer, D.; Zou, D.; Eder, D.N.; Hedner, J. Oximeter-based autonomic state indicator algorithm for cardiovascular risk assessment. *Chest* **2011**, *139*, 253–259. [CrossRef]
10. Sommermeyer, D.; Zou, D.; Eder, D.N.; Hedner, J.; Ficker, J.H.; Randerath, W.; Priegnitz, C.; Penzel, T.; Fietze, I.; Sanner, B.; et al. The use of overnight pulse wave analysis for recognition of cardiovascular risk factors and risk: A multicentric evaluation. *J. Hypertens.* **2014**, *32*, 276–285. [CrossRef] [PubMed]
11. Yeghiazarians, Y.; Jneid, H.; Tietjens, J.R.; Redline, S.; Brown, D.L.; El-Sherif, N.; Mehra, R.; Bozkurt, B.; Ndumele, C.E.; Somers, V.K. Obstructive Sleep Apnea and Cardiovascular Disease: A Scientific Statement From the American Heart Association. *Circulation* **2021**, *144*, E56–E67. [CrossRef]
12. National Institutes of Health Sleep Research Plan | NHLBI, NIH. 2021. Available online: https://www.nhlbi.nih.gov/all-publications-and-resources/2021-nih-health-sleep-research-plan (accessed on 12 September 2023).
13. Dey, D.; Gaur, S.; Ovrehus, K.A.; Slomka, P.J.; Betancur, J.; Goeller, M.; Hell, M.M.; Gransar, H.; Berman, D.S.; Achenbach, S.; et al. Integrated prediction of lesion-specific ischaemia from quantitative coronary CT angiography using machine learning: A multicentre study. *Eur. Radiol.* **2018**, *28*, 2655–2664. [CrossRef]
14. Motwani, M.; Dey, D.; Berman, D.S.; Germano, G.; Achenbach, S.; Al-Mallah, M.H.; Andreini, D.; Budoff, M.J.; Cademartiri, F.; Callister, T.Q.; et al. Machine learning for prediction of all-cause mortality in patients with suspected coronary artery disease: A 5-year multicentre prospective registry analysis. *Eur. Heart J.* **2017**, *38*, 500–507. [CrossRef]
15. Han, D.; Kolli, K.K.; Al'Aref, S.J.; Baskaran, L.; van Rosendael, A.R.; Gransar, H.; Andreini, D.; Budoff, M.J.; Cademartiri, F.; Chinnaiyan, K.; et al. Machine Learning Framework to Identify Individuals at Risk of Rapid Progression of Coronary Atherosclerosis: From the PARADIGM Registry. *J. Am. Heart Assoc.* **2020**, *9*, e013958. [CrossRef]
16. Ambale-Venkatesh, B.; Yang, X.; Wu, C.O.; Liu, K.; Hundley, W.G.; McClelland, R.; Gomes, A.S.; Folsom, A.R.; Shea, S.; Guallar, E.; et al. Cardiovascular Event Prediction by Machine Learning: The Multi-Ethnic Study of Atherosclerosis. *Circ. Res.* **2017**, *121*, 1092–1101. [CrossRef] [PubMed]

17. Sidey-Gibbons, J.A.M.; Sidey-Gibbons, C.J. Machine learning in medicine: A practical introduction. *BMC Med. Res. Methodol.* **2019**, *19*, 64. [CrossRef] [PubMed]
18. Li, A.; Roveda, J.M.; Powers, L.S.; Quan, S.F. Obstructive sleep apnea predicts 10-year cardiovascular disease–related mortality in the Sleep Heart Health Study: A machine learning approach. *J. Clin. Sleep Med.* **2022**, *18*, 497–504. [CrossRef] [PubMed]
19. Pickett, K.L.; Suresh, K.; Campbell, K.R.; Davis, S.; Juarez-Colunga, E. Random survival forests for dynamic predictions of a time-to-event outcome using a longitudinal biomarker. *BMC Med. Res. Methodol.* **2021**, *21*, 216. [CrossRef] [PubMed]
20. Deo, R.C. Machine Learning in Medicine. *Circulation* **2015**, *132*, 1920. [CrossRef] [PubMed]
21. Bailly, S.; Grote, L.; Hedner, J.; Schiza, S.; McNicholas, W.T.; Basoglu, O.K.; Lombardi, C.; Dogas, Z.; Roisman, G.; Pataka, A.; et al. Clusters of sleep apnoea phenotypes: A large pan-European study from the European Sleep Apnoea Database (ESADA). *Respirology* **2021**, *26*, 378–387. [CrossRef] [PubMed]
22. Vavougios, G.D.; Natsios, G.; Pastaka, C.; Zarogiannis, S.G.; Gourgoulianis, K.I. Phenotypes of comorbidity in OSAS patients: Combining categorical principal component analysis with cluster analysis. *J. Sleep Res.* **2016**, *25*, 31–38. [CrossRef] [PubMed]
23. Zinchuk, A.V.; Jeon, S.; Koo, B.B.; Yan, X.; Bravata, D.M.; Qin, L.; Selim, B.J.; Strohl, K.P.; Redeker, N.S.; Concato, J.; et al. Polysomnographic phenotypes and their cardiovascular implications in obstructive sleep apnoea. *Thorax* **2018**, *73*, 472–480. [CrossRef] [PubMed]
24. Rajpurkar, P.; Chen, E.; Banerjee, O.; Topol, E.J. AI in health and medicine. *Nat. Med.* **2022**, *28*, 31–38. [CrossRef] [PubMed]
25. Gahungu, N.; Shariar, A.; Playford, D.; Judkins, C.; Gabbay, E. Transfer learning artificial intelligence for automated detection of atrial fibrillation in patients undergoing evaluation for suspected obstructive sleep apnoea: A feasibility study. *Sleep Med.* **2021**, *85*, 166–171. [CrossRef] [PubMed]
26. Nasifoglu, H.; Erogul, O. Obstructive sleep apnea prediction from electrocardiogram scalograms and spectrograms using convolutional neural networks. *Physiol. Meas.* **2021**, *42*, 065010. [CrossRef] [PubMed]
27. Holfinger, S.J.; Lyons, M.M.; Keenan, B.T.; Mazzotti, D.R.; Mindel, J.; Maislin, G.; Cistulli, P.A.; Sutherland, K.; McArdle, N.; Singh, B.; et al. Diagnostic Performance of Machine Learning-Derived OSA Prediction Tools in Large Clinical and Community-Based Samples. *Chest* **2022**, *161*, 807–817. [CrossRef] [PubMed]
28. Mazzotti, D.R.; Keenan, B.T.; Lim, D.C.; Gottlieb, D.J.; Kim, J.; Pack, A.I. Symptom Subtypes of Obstructive Sleep Apnea Predict Incidence of Cardiovascular Outcomes. *Am. J. Respir. Crit. Care Med.* **2019**, *200*, 493–506. [CrossRef]
29. Ye, L.; Pien, G.W.; Ratcliffe, S.J.; Björnsdottir, E.; Arnardottir, E.S.; Pack, A.I.; Benediktsdottir, B.; Gislason, T. The different clinical faces of obstructive sleep apnoea: A cluster analysis. *Eur. Respir. J.* **2014**, *44*, 1600–1607. [CrossRef]
30. Won, C.H. When will we ditch the AHI? *J. Clin. Sleep Med.* **2020**, *16*, 1001–1003. [CrossRef]
31. Shahar, E. Apnea-hypopnea index: Time to wake up. *Nat. Sci. Sleep* **2014**, *6*, 51–56. [CrossRef]
32. Redline, S.; Budhiraja, R.; Kapur, V.; Marcus, C.L.; Mateika, J.H.; Mehra, R.; Parthasarthy, S.; Somers, V.K.; Strohl, K.P.; Gozal, D.; et al. The Scoring of Respiratory Events in Sleep: Reliability and Validity. *J. Clin. Sleep Med.* **2007**, *03*, 169–200. [CrossRef]
33. Malhotra, A.; Ayappa, I.; Ayas, N.; Collop, N.; Kirsch, D.; Mcardle, N.; Mehra, R.; Pack, A.I.; Punjabi, N.; White, D.P.; et al. Metrics of sleep apnea severity: Beyond the apnea-hypopnea index. *Sleep* **2021**, *44*, zsab030. [CrossRef] [PubMed]
34. Won, C.H.; Qin, L.; Selim, B.; Yaggi, H.K. Varying Hypopnea Definitions Affect Obstructive Sleep Apnea Severity Classification and Association With Cardiovascular Disease. *J. Clin. Sleep Med.* **2018**, *14*, 1987–1994. [CrossRef]
35. Randerath, W.; Bassetti, C.L.; Bonsignore, M.R.; Farre, R.; Ferini-Strambi, L.; Grote, L.; Hedner, J.; Kohler, M.; Martinez-Garcia, M.-A.; Mihaicuta, S.; et al. Challenges and perspectives in obstructive sleep apnoea: Report by an ad hoc working group of the Sleep Disordered Breathing Group of the European Respiratory Society and the European Sleep Research Society. *Eur. Respir. J.* **2018**, *52*, 1702616. [CrossRef] [PubMed]
36. Edwards, B.A.; Redline, S.; Sands, S.A.; Owens, R.L. More than the sum of the respiratory events: Personalized medicine approaches for obstructive sleep apnea. *Am. J. Respir. Crit. Care Med.* **2019**, *200*, 691–703. [CrossRef]
37. Malhotra, A.; Mesarwi, O.; Pepin, J.-L.; Owens, R.L. Endotypes and phenotypes in obstructive sleep apnea. *Curr. Opin. Pulm. Med.* **2020**, *26*, 609–614. [CrossRef]
38. Sands, S.A.; Edwards, B.A.; Terrill, P.I.; Taranto-Montemurro, L.; Azarbarzin, A.; Marques, M.; Hess, L.B.; White, D.P.; Wellman, A. Phenotyping Pharyngeal Pathophysiology using Polysomnography in Patients with Obstructive Sleep Apnea. *Am. J. Respir. Crit. Care Med.* **2018**, *197*, 1187–1197. [CrossRef]
39. Eckert, D.J.; White, D.P.; Jordan, A.S.; Malhotra, A.; Wellman, A. Defining phenotypic causes of obstructive sleep apnea. Identification of novel therapeutic targets. *Am. J. Respir. Crit. Care Med.* **2013**, *188*, 996–1004. [CrossRef]
40. Finnsson, E.; Ólafsdóttir, G.H.; Loftsdóttir, D.L.; Jónsson, S.; Helgadóttir, H.; Ágústsson, J.S.; Sands, S.A.; Wellman, A. A scalable method of determining physiological endotypes of sleep apnea from a polysomnographic sleep study. *Sleep* **2021**, *44*, zsaa168. [CrossRef]
41. Pépin, J.-L.; Eastwood, P.; Eckert, D.J. Novel avenues to approach non-CPAP therapy and implement comprehensive obstructive sleep apnoea care. *Eur. Respir. J.* **2022**, *59*, 2101788. [CrossRef]
42. Dutta, R.; Delaney, G.; Toson, B.; Jordan, A.S.; White, D.P.; Wellman, A.; Eckert, D.J. A Novel Model to Estimate Key Obstructive Sleep Apnea Endotypes from Standard Polysomnography and Clinical Data and Their Contribution to Obstructive Sleep Apnea Severity. *Ann. Am. Thorac. Soc.* **2021**, *18*, 656–667. [CrossRef]
43. Dutta, R.; Tong, B.K.; Eckert, D.J. Development of a physiological-based model that uses standard polysomnography and clinical data to predict oral appliance treatment outcomes in obstructive sleep apnea. *J. Clin. Sleep Med.* **2022**, *18*, 861–870. [CrossRef]

44. de Beeck, S.O.; Wellman, A.; Dieltjens, M.; Strohl, K.P.; Willemen, M.; Van de Heyning, P.H.; Verbraecken, J.A.; Vanderveken, O.M.; Sands, S.A.; the STAR Trial Investigators. Endotypic Mechanisms of Successful Hypoglossal Nerve Stimulation for Obstructive Sleep Apnea. *Am. J. Respir. Crit. Care Med.* **2021**, *203*, 746–755. [CrossRef]
45. Schmickl, C.N.; Orr, J.E.; Sands, S.A.; Alex, R.M.; Azarbarzin, A.; McGinnis, L.; White, S.; Mazzotti, D.R.; Nokes, B.; Owens, R.L.; et al. Loop Gain as a Predictor of Blood Pressure Response in Patients Treated for Obstructive Sleep Apnea. *Ann. Am. Thorac. Soc.* **2024**, *21*, 296–307. [CrossRef] [PubMed]
46. Parekh, A.; Tolbert, T.M.; Mooney, A.M.; Ramos-Cejudo, J.; Osorio, R.S.; Treml, M.; Herkenrath, S.-D.; Randerath, W.J.; Ayappa, I.; Rapoport, D.M. Endotyping Sleep Apnea One Breath at a Time: An Automated Approach for Separating Obstructive from Central Sleep-disordered Breathing. *Am. J. Respir. Crit. Care Med.* **2021**, *204*, 1452–1462. [CrossRef] [PubMed]
47. Turnbull, C.D.; Stradling, J.R. Endotyping, phenotyping and personalised therapy in obstructive sleep apnoea: Are we there yet? *Thorax* **2023**, *78*, 726–732. [CrossRef] [PubMed]
48. Labarca, G.; Vena, D.; Hu, W.-H.; Esmaeili, N.; Gell, L.; Yang, H.C.; Wang, T.-Y.; Messineo, L.; Taranto-Montemurro, L.; Sofer, T.; et al. Sleep Apnea Physiological Burdens and Cardiovascular Morbidity and Mortality. *Am. J. Respir. Crit. Care Med.* **2023**, *208*, 802–813. [CrossRef] [PubMed]
49. Azarbarzin, A.; Sands, S.A.; Younes, M.; Taranto-Montemurro, L.; Sofer, T.; Vena, D.; Alex, R.M.; Kim, S.-W.; Gottlieb, D.J.; White, D.P.; et al. The Sleep Apnea–Specific Pulse-Rate Response Predicts Cardiovascular Morbidity and Mortality. *Am. J. Respir. Crit. Care Med.* **2021**, *203*, 1546–1555. [CrossRef]
50. Solelhac, G.; Sánchez-de-la-Torre, M.; Blanchard, M.; Berger, M.; Hirotsu, C.; Imler, T.; Sánchez-de-la-Torre, A.; Haba-Rubio, J.; Marchi, N.A.; Bayon, V.; et al. Pulse Wave Amplitude Drops Index: A Biomarker of Cardiovascular Risk in Obstructive Sleep Apnea. *Am. J. Respir. Crit. Care Med.* **2023**, *207*, 1620–1632. [CrossRef]
51. Azarbarzin, A.; Zinchuk, A.; Wellman, A.; Labarca, G.; Vena, D.; Gell, L.; Messineo, L.; White, D.P.; Gottlieb, D.J.; Redline, S.; et al. Cardiovascular Benefit of Continuous Positive Airway Pressure in Adults with Coronary Artery Disease and Obstructive Sleep Apnea without Excessive Sleepiness. *Am. J. Respir. Crit. Care Med.* **2022**, *206*, 767–774. [CrossRef]
52. Malhotra, A.; Younes, M.; Kuna, S.T.; Benca, R.; Kushida, C.A.; Walsh, J.; Hanlon, A.; Staley, B.; Pack, A.l.; Pien, G.W. Performance of an automated polysomnography scoring system versus computer-assisted manual scoring. *Sleep* **2013**, *36*, 573–582. [CrossRef]
53. Choi, S.H.; Yoon, H.; Kim, H.S.; Kim, H.B.; Bin Kwon, W.; Oh, S.M.; Lee, Y.J.; Park, K.S. Real-time apnea-hypopnea event detection during sleep by convolutional neural networks. *Comput. Biol. Med.* **2018**, *100*, 123–131. [CrossRef]
54. ElMoaqet, H.; Eid, M.; Glos, M.; Ryalat, M.; Penzel, T. Deep Recurrent Neural Networks for Automatic Detection of Sleep Apnea from Single Channel Respiration Signals. *Sensors* **2020**, *20*, 5037. [CrossRef]
55. Zhao, X.; Wang, X.; Yang, T.; Ji, S.; Wang, H.; Wang, J.; Wang, Y.; Wu, Q. Classification of sleep apnea based on EEG sub-band signal characteristics. *Sci. Rep.* **2021**, *11*, 5824. [CrossRef] [PubMed]
56. Nikkonen, S.; Korkalainen, H.; Kainulainen, S.; Myllymaa, S.; Leino, A.; Kalevo, L.; Oksenberg, A.; Leppänen, T.; Töyräs, J. Estimating daytime sleepiness with previous night electroencephalography, electrooculography, and electromyography spectrograms in patients with suspected sleep apnea using a convolutional neural network. *Sleep* **2020**, *43*, zsaa106. [CrossRef]
57. Brink-Kjaer, A.; Leary, E.B.; Sun, H.; Westover, M.B.; Stone, K.L.; Peppard, P.E.; Lane, N.E.; Cawthon, P.M.; Redline, S.; Jennum, P.; et al. Age estimation from sleep studies using deep learning predicts life expectancy. *NPJ Digit. Med.* **2022**, *5*, 103. [CrossRef] [PubMed]
58. Azarbarzin, A.; Sands, S.A.; Han, S.; Sofer, T.; Labarca, G.; Stone, K.L.; Gottlieb, D.J.; Javaheri, S.; Wellman, A.; White, D.P.; et al. Relevance of cortical arousals for risk stratification in sleep apnea: A 3 cohort analysis. *J. Clin. Sleep Med.* **2023**, *19*, 1475–1484. [CrossRef]
59. Feliciano, A.; Torres, V.M.; Vaz, F.; Carvalho, A.S.; Matthiesen, R.; Pinto, P.; Malhotra, A.; Bárbara, C.; Penque, D. Overview of proteomics studies in obstructive sleep apnea. *Sleep Med.* **2015**, *16*, 437–445. [CrossRef]
60. Lebkuchen, A.; Freitas, L.S.; Cardozo, K.H.; Drager, L.F. Advances and challenges in pursuing biomarkers for obstructive sleep apnea: Implications for the cardiovascular risk. *Trends Cardiovasc. Med.* **2020**, *31*, 242–249. [CrossRef] [PubMed]
61. Lind, L.; Ärnlöv, J.; Lindahl, B.; Siegbahn, A.; Sundström, J.; Ingelsson, E. Use of a proximity extension assay proteomics chip to discover new biomarkers for human atherosclerosis. *Atherosclerosis* **2015**, *242*, 205–210. [CrossRef]
62. Kulasingam, A.; Hvas, A.-M.; Grove, E.L.; Funck, K.L.; Kristensen, S.D. Detection of biomarkers using a novel proximity extension assay in patients with ST-elevation myocardial infarction. *Thromb. Res.* **2018**, *172*, 21–28. [CrossRef] [PubMed]
63. Wallentin, L.; Eriksson, N.; Olszowka, M.; Grammer, T.B.; Hagström, E.; Held, C.; Kleber, M.E.; Koenig, W.; März, W.; Stewart, R.A.H.; et al. Plasma proteins associated with cardiovascular death in patients with chronic coronary heart disease: A retrospective study. *PLoS Med.* **2021**, *18*, e1003513. [CrossRef] [PubMed]
64. Zapater, A.; Gracia-Lavedan, E.; Torres, G.; Mínguez, O.; Pascual, L.; Cortijo, A.; Martínez, D.; Benítez, I.D.; De Batlle, J.; Henríquez-Beltrán, M.; et al. Proteomic profiling for prediction of recurrent cardiovascular event in patients with acute coronary syndrome and obstructive sleep apnea: A post-hoc analysis from the ISAACC study. *Biomed. Pharmacother.* **2023**, *158*, 114125. [CrossRef]
65. Ljunggren, M.; Theorell-Haglöw, J.; Freyhult, E.; Sahlin, C.; Franklin, K.A.; Malinovschi, A.; Janson, C.; Lindberg, E. Association between proteomics and obstructive sleep apnea phenotypes in a community-based cohort of women. *J. Sleep Res.* **2020**, *29*, e13041. [CrossRef] [PubMed]
66. Salahshor, S.; Woodgett, J.R. The links between axin and carcinogenesis. *J. Clin. Pathol.* **2005**, *58*, 225–236. [CrossRef] [PubMed]

67. Gomes, P.; Outeiro, T.F.; Cavadas, C. Emerging Role of Sirtuin 2 in the Regulation of Mammalian Metabolism. *Trends Pharmacol. Sci.* **2015**, *36*, 756–768. [CrossRef]
68. Lemos, V.; de Oliveira, R.M.; Naia, L.; Szegö, É.; Ramos, E.; Pinho, S.; Magro, F.; Cavadas, C.; Rego, A.C.; Costa, V.; et al. The NAD+-dependent deacetylase SIRT2 attenuates oxidative stress and mitochondrial dysfunction and improves insulin sensitivity in hepatocytes. *Hum. Mol. Genet.* **2017**, *26*, 4105–4117. [CrossRef]
69. Ljunggren, M.; Zhou, X.; Theorell-Haglöw, J.; Janson, C.; Franklin, K.A.; Emilsson, Ö.; Lindberg, E. Sleep Apnea Indices Associated with Markers of Inflammation and Cardiovascular Disease: A Proteomic Study in the MUSTACHE Cohort. *Ann. Am. Thorac. Soc.* **2024**, *21*, 165–169. [CrossRef]
70. Kundel, V.; Cohen, O.; Khan, S.; Patel, M.; Kim-Schulze, S.; Kovacic, J.; Suárez-Fariñas, M.; Shah, N.A. Advanced Proteomics and Cluster Analysis for Identifying Novel Obstructive Sleep Apnea Subtypes before and after Continuous Positive Airway Pressure Therapy. *Ann. Am. Thorac. Soc.* **2023**, *20*, 1038–1047. [CrossRef]
71. Cohen, O.; Kaufman, A.E.; Choi, H.; Khan, S.; Robson, P.M.; Suárez-Fariñas, M.; Mani, V.; Shah, N.A. Pharyngeal Inflammation on Positron Emission Tomography/Magnetic Resonance Imaging Before and After Obstructive Sleep Apnea Treatment. *Ann. Am. Thorac. Soc.* **2023**, *20*, 574–583. [CrossRef] [PubMed]
72. Brennan, H.L.; Kirby, S.D. The role of artificial intelligence in the treatment of obstructive sleep apnea. *J. Otolaryngol. Head Neck Surg.* **2023**, *52*, 7. [CrossRef] [PubMed]
73. Chen, Q.; Liang, Z.; Wang, Q.; Ma, C.; Lei, Y.; Sanderson, J.E.; Hu, X.; Lin, W.; Liu, H.; Xie, F.; et al. Self-helped detection of obstructive sleep apnea based on automated facial recognition and machine learning. *Sleep Breath.* **2023**, *27*, 2379–2388. [CrossRef] [PubMed]
74. Eastwood, P.; Gilani, S.Z.; McArdle, N.; Hillman, D.; Walsh, J.; Maddison, K.; Goonewardene, M.; Mian, A. Predicting sleep apnea from three-dimensional face photography. *J. Clin. Sleep Med.* **2020**, *16*, 493–502. [CrossRef] [PubMed]
75. Monna, F.; Ben Messaoud, R.; Navarro, N.; Baillieul, S.; Sanchez, L.; Loiodice, C.; Tamisier, R.; Joyeux-Faure, M.; Pépin, J.-L. Machine learning and geometric morphometrics to predict obstructive sleep apnea from 3D craniofacial scans. *Sleep Med.* **2022**, *95*, 76–83. [CrossRef] [PubMed]
76. Tsuiki, S.; Nagaoka, T.; Fukuda, T.; Sakamoto, Y.; Almeida, F.R.; Nakayama, H.; Inoue, Y.; Enno, H. Machine learning for image-based detection of patients with obstructive sleep apnea: An exploratory study. *Sleep Breath.* **2021**, *25*, 2297–2305. [CrossRef]
77. Zhang, L.; Zhang, X.; Li, Y.M.; Xiang, B.Y.; Han, T.; Wang, Y.; Wang, C. Association of Craniofacial and Upper Airway Morphology with Cardiovascular Risk in Adults with OSA. *Nat. Sci. Sleep* **2021**, *13*, 1689–1700. [CrossRef]
78. de Bataille, C.; Bernard, D.; Dumoncel, J.; Vaysse, F.; Cussat-Blanc, S.; Telmon, N.; Maret, D.; Monsarrat, P. Machine Learning Analysis of the Anatomical Parameters of the Upper Airway Morphology: A Retrospective Study from Cone-Beam CT Examinations in a French Population. *J. Clin. Med.* **2022**, *12*, 84. [CrossRef]
79. Shujaat, S.; Jazil, O.; Willems, H.; Van Gerven, A.; Shaheen, E.; Politis, C.; Jacobs, R. Automatic segmentation of the pharyngeal airway space with convolutional neural network. *J. Dent.* **2021**, *111*, 103705. [CrossRef]
80. Shahid, M.L.U.R.; Mir, J.; Shaukat, F.; Saleem, M.K.; Tariq, M.A.U.R.; Nouman, A. Classification of Pharynx from MRI Using a Visual Analysis Tool to Study Obstructive Sleep Apnea. *Curr. Med. Imaging* **2021**, *17*, 613–622. [CrossRef]
81. Ivanovska, T.; Daboul, A.; Kalentev, O.; Hosten, N.; Biffar, R.; Völzke, H.; Wörgötter, F. A deep cascaded segmentation of obstructive sleep apnea-relevant organs from sagittal spine MRI. *Int. J. Comput. Assist. Radiol. Surg.* **2021**, *16*, 579–588. [CrossRef]
82. Bommineni, V.L.; Erus, G.; Doshi, J.; Singh, A.; Keenan, B.T.; Schwab, R.J.; Wiemken, A.; Davatzikos, C. Automatic Segmentation and Quantification of Upper Airway Anatomic Risk Factors for Obstructive Sleep Apnea on Unprocessed Magnetic Resonance Images. *Acad. Radiol.* **2023**, *30*, 421–430. [CrossRef]
83. Molnár, V.; Lakner, Z.; Molnár, A.; Tárnoki, D.L.; Tárnoki, Á.D.; Kunos, L.; Jokkel, Z.; Tamás, L. The Predictive Role of the Upper-Airway Adipose Tissue in the Pathogenesis of Obstructive Sleep Apnoea. *Life* **2022**, *12*, 1543. [CrossRef] [PubMed]
84. Yeom, S.H.; Na, J.S.; Jung, H.-D.; Cho, H.-J.; Choi, Y.J.; Lee, J.S. Computational analysis of airflow dynamics for predicting collapsible sites in the upper airways: Machine learning approach. *J. Appl. Physiol.* **2019**, *127*, 959–973. [CrossRef]
85. Pang, B.; Doshi, S.; Roy, B.; Lai, M.; Ehlert, L.; Aysola, R.S.; Kang, D.W.; Anderson, A.; Joshi, S.H.; Tward, D.; et al. Machine learning approach for obstructive sleep apnea screening using brain diffusion tensor imaging. *J. Sleep Res.* **2023**, *32*, e13729. [CrossRef] [PubMed]
86. Liu, X.; Shu, Y.; Yu, P.; Li, H.; Duan, W.; Wei, Z.; Li, K.; Xie, W.; Zeng, Y.; Peng, D. Classification of severe obstructive sleep apnea with cognitive impairment using degree centrality: A machine learning analysis. *Front. Neurol.* **2022**, *13*, 1005650. [CrossRef]
87. Shu, Y.; Liu, X.; Yu, P.; Li, H.; Duan, W.; Wei, Z.; Li, K.; Xie, W.; Zeng, Y.; Peng, D. Inherent regional brain activity changes in male obstructive sleep apnea with mild cognitive impairment: A resting-state magnetic resonance study. *Front. Aging Neurosci.* **2022**, *14*, 1022628. [CrossRef] [PubMed]
88. Agarwal, C.; Gupta, S.; Najjar, M.; Weaver, T.E.; Zhou, X.J.; Schonfeld, D.; Prasad, B. Deep Learning Analyses of Brain MRI to Identify Sustained Attention Deficit in Treated Obstructive Sleep Apnea: A Pilot Study. *Sleep Vigil.* **2022**, *6*, 179–184. [CrossRef]
89. Li, T.; Ou, Q.; Zhou, X.; Wei, X.; Cai, A.; Li, X.; Ren, G.; Du, Z.; Hong, Z.; Cheng, Y.; et al. Left ventricular remodeling and systolic function changes in patients with obstructive sleep apnea: A comprehensive contrast-enhanced cardiac magnetic resonance study. *Cardiovasc. Diagn. Ther.* **2022**, *12*, 436–452. [CrossRef]
90. Breiman, L. Random forests. *Mach Learn.* **2001**, *45*, 5–32. [CrossRef]

91. Fernández-Delgado, M.; Cernadas, E.; Barro, S.; Amorim, D.; Fernández-Delgado, A. Do we Need Hundreds of Classifiers to Solve Real World Classification Problems? *J. Mach. Learn. Res.* **2014**, *15*, 3133–3181. Available online: http://www.mathworks.es/products/neural-network (accessed on 4 October 2023).
92. Wallace, M.L.; Coleman, T.S.; Mentch, L.K.; Buysse, D.J.; Graves, J.L.; Hagen, E.W.; Hall, M.H.; Stone, K.L.; Redline, S.; Peppard, P.E. Physiological sleep measures predict time to 15-year mortality in community adults: Application of a novel machine learning framework. *J. Sleep Res.* **2021**, *30*, e13386. [CrossRef] [PubMed]
93. Mendelson, M.; Duval, J.; Bettega, F.; Tamisier, R.; Baillieul, S.; Bailly, S.; Pépin, J.-L. The individual and societal prices of non-adherence to continuous positive airway pressure, contributors, and strategies for improvement. *Expert Rev. Respir. Med.* **2023**, *17*, 305–317. [CrossRef] [PubMed]
94. Yeh, R.W.; Kramer, D.B. Decision Tools to improve personalized care in cardiovascular disease: Moving the art of medicine toward science. *Circulation* **2017**, *135*, 1097–1100. [CrossRef] [PubMed]
95. Kravitz, R.L.; Duan, N.; Braslow, J. Evidence-based medicine, heterogeneity of treatment effects, and the trouble with averages. *Milbank Q.* **2004**, *82*, 661–687. [CrossRef] [PubMed]
96. Sanchez, P.; Voisey, J.P.; Xia, T.; Watson, H.I.; O'neil, A.Q.; Tsaftaris, S.A. Causal machine learning for healthcare and precision medicine. *R. Soc. Open Sci.* **2022**, *9*, 220638. [CrossRef] [PubMed]
97. Wang, R.; Lagakos, S.W.; Ware, J.H.; Hunter, D.J.; Drazen, J.M. Statistics in Medicine—Reporting of Subgroup Analyses in Clinical Trials. *N. Engl. J. Med.* **2007**, *357*, 2189–2194. [CrossRef]
98. Seibold, H.; Zeileis, A.; Hothorn, T. Model-Based Recursive Partitioning for Subgroup Analyses. *Int. J. Biostat.* **2016**, *12*, 45–63. [CrossRef] [PubMed]
99. Zhang, Z.; Seibold, H.; Vettore, M.V.; Song, W.-J.; François, V. Subgroup identification in clinical trials: An overview of available methods and their implementations with R. *Ann. Transl. Med.* **2018**, *6*, 122. [CrossRef]
100. Garge, N.R.; Bobashev, G.; Eggleston, B. Random forest methodology for model-based recursive partitioning: The mobForest package for R. *BMC Bioinform.* **2013**, *14*, 125. [CrossRef]
101. Athey, S.; Wager, S. Estimating Treatment Effects with Causal Forests: An Application. *Obs. Stud.* **2019**, *5*, 37–51. [CrossRef]
102. Cui, Y.; Kosorok, M.R.; Sverdrup, E.; Wager, S.; Zhu, R. Estimating heterogeneous treatment effects with right-censored data via causal survival forests. *J. R. Stat. Soc. Ser. B Stat. Methodol.* **2023**, *85*, 179–211. [CrossRef]
103. Robertson, S.E.; Steingrimsson, J.A.; Dahabreh, I.J. Regression-based estimation of heterogeneous treatment effects when extending inferences from a randomized trial to a target population. *Eur. J. Epidemiol.* **2023**, *38*, 123–133. [CrossRef]
104. Falet, J.-P.R.; Durso-Finley, J.; Nichyporuk, B.; Schroeter, J.; Bovis, F.; Sormani, M.-P.; Precup, D.; Arbel, T.; Arnold, D.L. Estimating individual treatment effect on disability progression in multiple sclerosis using deep learning. *Nat. Commun.* **2022**, *13*, 5645. [CrossRef]
105. Diao, E.; Ding, J.; Tarokh, V.; Hetero, F.L. Computation and Communication Efficient Federated Learning for Heterogeneous Clients. In Proceedings of the ICLR 2021—9th International Conference on Learning Representations, Virtual Event, Austria, 3–7 May 2021; Available online: https://arxiv.org/abs/2010.01264v3 (accessed on 28 January 2024).
106. Sheller, M.J.; Edwards, B.; Reina, G.A.; Martin, J.; Pati, S.; Kotrotsou, A.; Milchenko, M.; Xu, W.; Marcus, D.; Colen, R.R.; et al. Federated learning in medicine: Facilitating multi-institutional collaborations without sharing patient data. *Sci. Rep.* **2020**, *10*, 12598. [CrossRef] [PubMed]
107. Reynor, A.; McArdle, N.; Shenoy, B.; Dhaliwal, S.S.; Rea, S.C.; Walsh, J.; Eastwood, P.R.; Maddison, K.; Hillman, D.R.; Ling, I.; et al. Continuous positive airway pressure and adverse cardiovascular events in obstructive sleep apnea: Are participants of randomized trials representative of sleep clinic patients? *Sleep* **2022**, *45*, zsab264. [CrossRef] [PubMed]
108. Bellamy, R.K.E.; Dey, K.; Hind, M.; Hoffman, S.C.; Houde, S.; Kannan, K.; Lohia, P.; Martino, J.; Mehta, S.; Mojsilovic, A.; et al. AI Fairness 360: An Extensible Toolkit for Detecting, Understanding, and Mitigating Unwanted Algorithmic Bias. *IBM J. Res. Dev.* **2018**, *63*, 4:1–4:15. [CrossRef]
109. Ribeiro, M.; Singh, S.; Guestrin, C. "Why Should I Trust You?": Explaining the Predictions of Any Classifier. In Proceedings of the 2016 Conference of the North American Chapter of the Association for Computational Linguistics: Human Language Technologies, San Diego, CA, USA, 12–17 June 2016; pp. 97–101. [CrossRef]

Disclaimer/Publisher's Note: The statements, opinions and data contained in all publications are solely those of the individual author(s) and contributor(s) and not of MDPI and/or the editor(s). MDPI and/or the editor(s) disclaim responsibility for any injury to people or property resulting from any ideas, methods, instructions or products referred to in the content.

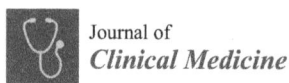

Article

Development and Internal Validation of a Prediction Model for Surgical Success of Maxillomandibular Advancement for the Treatment of Moderate to Severe Obstructive Sleep Apnea

Wouter P. Visscher [1,*,†], Jean-Pierre T. F. Ho [1,2,†], Ning Zhou [1,3], Madeline J. L. Ravesloot [4], Engelbert A. J. M. Schulten [5], Jan de Lange [1] and Naichuan Su [6]

1. Amsterdam UMC and Academic Centre for Dentistry Amsterdam (ACTA), Department of Oral and Maxillofacial Surgery/Oral Pathology, University of Amsterdam, 1105 AZ Amsterdam, The Netherlands
2. Department of Oral and Maxillofacial Surgery, Noordwest Ziekenhuisgroep, 1815 JD Alkmaar, The Netherlands
3. Academic Centre for Dentistry Amsterdam (ACTA), Department of Orofacial Pain and Dysfunction, University of Amsterdam and Vrije Universiteit Amsterdam, 1081 LA Amsterdam, The Netherlands
4. Department Otorhinolaryngology—Head and Neck Surgery, OLVG, 1061 AE Amsterdam, The Netherlands
5. Amsterdam UMC and Academic Centre for Dentistry Amsterdam (ACTA), Department of Oral and Maxillofacial Surgery/Oral Pathology, Vrije Universiteit Amsterdam, 1081 HV Amsterdam, The Netherlands
6. Academic Centre for Dentistry Amsterdam (ACTA), Department of Oral Public Health, University of Amsterdam and Vrije Universiteit Amsterdam, 1081 LA Amsterdam, The Netherlands
* Correspondence: w.p.visscher@amsterdamumc.nl; Tel.: +31-020-566-9111
† These authors contributed equally to this work.

Abstract: Background: Maxillomandibular advancement (MMA) has been shown to be the most effective surgical therapy for obstructive sleep apnea (OSA). Despite high success rates, there are patients who are considered as non-responders to MMA. In order to triage and inform these patients on their expected prognosis of MMA before the surgery, this study aimed to develop, internally validate, and calibrate a prediction model for the presence of surgical success for MMA in patients with OSA. Methods: A retrospective cohort study was conducted that included patients that had undergone MMA for moderate to severe OSA. Baseline clinical, polysomnographic, cephalometric, and drug-induced sleep endoscopy findings were recorded as potential predictors. Presence or absence of surgical success was recorded as outcome. Binary logistic regression analyses were conducted to develop the model. Performance and clinical values of the model were analyzed. Results: One hundred patients were included, of which sixty-seven (67%) patients reached surgical success. Anterior lower face height (ALFH) (OR: 0.93 [0.87–1.00], $p = 0.05$), superior posterior airway space (SPAS) (OR: 0.76 [0.62–0.92], $p < 0.05$), age (OR: 0.96 [0.91–1.01], $p = 0.13$), and a central apnea index (CAI) <5 events/hour sleep (OR: 0.16 [0.03–0.91], $p < 0.05$) were significant independent predictors in the model (significance level set at $p = 0.20$). The model showed acceptable discrimination with a shrunken area under the curve of 0.74, and acceptable calibration. The added predictive values for ruling in and out of surgical success were 0.21 and 0.32, respectively. Conclusions: Lower age at surgery, CAI < 5 events/hour, lower ALFH, and smaller SPAS were significant predictors for the surgical success of MMA. The discrimination, calibration, and clinical added values of the model were acceptable.

Keywords: obstructive sleep apnea; maxillomandibular advancement; prediction; surgical success

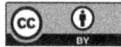

1. Introduction

Obstructive sleep apnea (OSA) is a breathing disorder which occurs during sleep and is characterized by recurrent obstruction (partial or complete) of the upper airway, resulting in hypopnea and/or apnea [1]. OSA results in hypoxemia, hypercapnia, and arousals from sleep. It is associated with cardiovascular and cognitive morbidity, a reduced quality of life, and premature death [2–6]. It is estimated that the prevalence of OSA in the general population is 9% to 38%, whilst prevalence percentages increase due to rising rates of obesity in addition to an aging population [7,8]. Polysomnography (PSG) is the gold standard test for the diagnosis of OSA. The diagnosis and severity of OSA have been largely quantified by the numeric calculation of the number of obstructive, central, and mixed apneas and hypopneas per hour of sleep (AHI). Severity, spanning three levels, is traditionally defined by the cut-offs 5–14, 15–29 and $\geq$30 events per hour defining mild, moderate and severe OSA, respectively, as suggested by the American Society of Sleep Medicine (AASM) [9].

Continuous positive airway pressure (CPAP) is considered the first treatment choice in patients with moderate to severe OSA [9]. However, a substantial proportion of patients experience problems tolerating CPAP, resulting in a reduced compliance to the therapy [10]. Alternatives for these patients usually consist of a mandibular advancement device (MAD) or surgical treatment, e.g., maxillomandibular advancement osteotomy (MMA) [11]. MMA has shown to be the most effective surgical therapy for OSA, excluding a tracheostomy, with a reported success rate of 85% [12]. However, despite the high success rates, there is a group of patients who are considered as non-responders to MMA [12]. It is thought that the presence of complete anteroposterior collapse at the level of the epiglottis and a minimal retro velar space might contribute to MMA failure [13,14]. However, only a few studies have assessed predictors for failure in MMA; therefore, drawing conclusions remains arbitrary.

In order to efficiently use the scarce medical resources, it is of utmost importance to triage the patients based on their expected prognosis of MMA before the surgeries. To ensure this, prediction models for surgical success are of vital importance. To date, no prediction models for the surgical success of MMA have been developed, further complicating preoperative clinical patient counseling and suitable candidate selection. This is because a prediction model helps to inform patients on their potential prognosis of the surgery and also aids clinicians during preoperative decision-making. Therefore, prediction models for the surgical success of MMA are warranted. Whilst we nowadays aim for tailor-made treatment (personalized medicine) for each individual patient, it is important that preoperative predictors for surgical success are identified. These predictors should lead to the development, validation, and implementation of a prediction model for the surgical success of MMA as a treatment of OSA in the future. Improving MMA candidate selection will not only contribute to improve appropriate care delivery, but also reduce morbidity and increase the therapeutic success of MMA. A broader goal is to better utilize the available healthcare costs by optimizing the cost-effectiveness of MMA as a treatment for OSA. Therefore, the aim of this study was to identify potential predictors for the surgical success of MMA (as defined by Sher's criteria [15]) in patients with OSA, and develop and internally validate a model for the prediction of surgical success.

2. Materials and Methods

The Medical Ethics Committee of the Amsterdam University Medical Centers (Amsterdam UMC, location Amsterdam Medical Center (AMC)) concluded that this study was exempted from the Medical Research Human Subjects Act (Reference number W22_061#22.093). The present study was carried out based on the Strengthening The Reporting of Observational studies in Epidemiology (STROBE) [16] statement and the Transparent Reporting of a multivariable prediction model for Individual Prognosis or Diagnosis (TRIPOD) statement [17].

2.1. Study Design and Participants Enrolment

The study was designed as a retrospective cohort study. The inclusion criteria were (1) patients with moderate to severe OSA, diagnosed by means of PSG (AHI $\geq$ 15/h); (2) age > 18 years old; (3) patients who underwent MMA as a treatment for OSA in the Amsterdam UMC location AMC, from September 2011 to September 2020; (4) an overnight level I or level II PSG was performed to measure the parameters relevant to OSA prior to surgery and at a minimum of 3 months postoperatively; (5) a standardized lateral cephalogram was performed prior to surgery and at a minimum of one week postoperatively; and (6) patients who were followed-up for at least 12 months on the outpatient clinic after MMA.

The non-inclusion criteria were as follows: (1) patients who did not undergo isolated MMA nor simultaneous upper airway surgery (e.g., uvulopalatopharyngoplasty, lateral pharyngoplasty, expansion sphincter pharyngoplasty, barbed reposition pharyngoplasty, tongue volume reduction surgery and/or hyoid bone suspension surgery); (2) patients who underwent a previous MMA osteotomy as a treatment for OSA; (3) patients with instable endocrine dysfunction prior to surgery (hypothyroidism, acromegaly and pituitary adenoma) and/or patients with craniofacial syndromes; and (4) patients who did not give permission for their data to be used for research purposes.

2.2. Treatment Protocol

All MMA osteotomies were performed by two experienced oral and maxillofacial surgeons dedicated to the treatment of OSA. MMA osteotomy consisted of a Le Fort I osteotomy of the maxilla with a Hunsuck-Dal Pont modification of the bilateral sagital split osteotomy (BSSO) of the mandible, as described by Obwegeser [18,19]. Subsequently, advancement of the maxillomandibular complex followed, and in a subgroup of patients additional counterclockwise rotation was performed [20]. After applying temporary maxillomandibular fixation by steel-wire ligatures or power chains and intraoperative splints, rigid internal fixation was applied [21,22]. Before the availability of three-dimensional planning, the surgery was planned two-dimensionally with manually fabricated intraoperative splints. In patients who had undergone more recent surgery, the surgery was virtually planned and involved three-dimensionally fabricated intraoperative splints [11].

2.3. Predictors

The potential predictors were extracted from the electronic patients' files, including patient-related variables, respiratory parameters assessed by PSG, drug-induced sleep endoscopy (DISE) findings, and cephalometric measurements. All the predictors were measured at baseline before the MMA. All the potential predictors in the present study were decided based on the previous literature [11,23,24] and the authors' clinical experience and knowledge.

2.3.1. Patient-Related Variables

The patient-related variables included gender, age, body mass index (BMI) at time of surgery, pre-existent physiological status by means of the ASA (American Society of Anesthesiology) classification score (ASA I, normal health; ASA II, mild systemic disease; ASA III, severe systemic disease; ASA IV, severe systemic disease that is a constant threat to life; ASA V, not expected to survive without operation) [25], history of upper airway surgery, excluding previous MMA, as a treatment for OSA (Yes or No), and the presence or absence of teeth (dentulous versus edentulous). Patients with 1–27 teeth (excluding the third molars) were classified as partially dentulous.

2.3.2. Respiratory Parameters

All patients underwent an overnight level I or level II PSG prior to surgery and a minimum of 3 months postoperatively. For scoring respiratory events, we adhered to the criteria of the American Academy of Sleep Medicine (AASM), with the use of the recommend rules for the scoring of hypopneas, i.e., (1) peak signal excursions drop by $\geq 30\%$ of pre-event baseline using nasal pressure (diagnostic study); (2) the duration of the $\geq 30\%$ drop in signal excursion is ≥ 10 s; and (3) $\geq 3\%$ oxygen desaturation from pre-event baseline and/or the event is associated with an arousal) [26]. The following data was obtained from PSG prior to surgery (baseline): AHI, central apnea index (CAI; presence of central apnea events was defined as a CAI $\geq$ 5 per hour sleep [27]), and presence of positional OSA (positional OSA was defined as a minimally two times higher AHI in supine position when compared to non-supine position [28]).

2.3.3. Cephalometric Variables

The lateral cephalograms were taken with the patients' head in a natural position with the mandibular condyle positioned in centric relation to the glenoid fossa. All cephalograms were analyzed by a single observer using Viewbox software (Viewbox 4, dHAL Software, Kifissia, Greece) [29]. For intra-observer reliability analyses, the observer repeated the measurements one month later in twenty cases that were randomly selected. In the present study, the following cephalometric data at baseline was obtained as the potential predictors: anterior lower face height, anterior total face height, presence of maxillomandibular deficiency (maxillomandibular deficiency was defined as sella-naison-A-point (SNA) angle $\leq$ 80.5° and/or sella-naison-B-point (SNB) angle $\leq$ 78.5°) [30], and superior posterior airway space (SPAS). An overview on the cephalometric variables and definitions is illustrated in Table 1. An overview of the landmarks, reference lines, and variables on cephalometry is illustrated in Figure 1.

Table 1. Cephalometric variables with definitions.

Variable	Definition
S-N	Distance between S and N
ATFH	Distance between N and Me
ALFH	Distance between ANS and Me
SNA	Angle from S to N to A
SNB	Angle from S to N to B
SPAS	Width of the posterior airway at the level of the midpoint of UT and PNS, parallel to line Go-B.

A, subspinale; ALFH, anterior lower face height; ANS, anterior nasal spine; ATFH, anterior total face height; B, supramentale; Go, gonion; Me, menon; N, nasion; PNS, posterior nasal spine; S, sella; S-N, sella-naison line; SPAS, superior posterior airway space; UT, uvula tip.

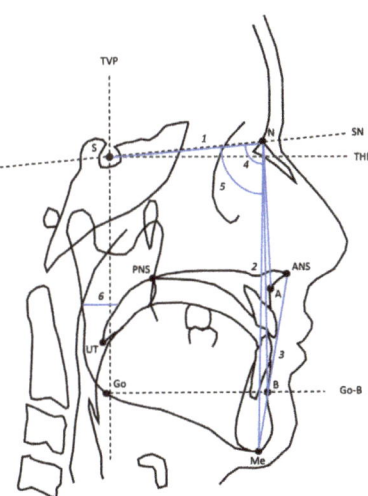

Figure 1. Landmarks, reference lines, and variables used from cephalometry. Landmarks: A, subspinale; ANS, anterior nasal spine; B, supramentale; Go, gonion; Me, menton; N, Nasion; PNS, posterior nasal spine; S, sella; UT, uvula tip; Reference lines: Go-B, gonion-supramentale; SN, sella-nasion; THP, true horizontal plane (through S, set at 7° from SN); TVP, true vertical plane (through S, set at 90° from THP). Variables: 1, S-N; 2, ATFH (anterior total face height, N-Me); 3, ALFH (anterior lower face height, ANS-Me); 4, SNA angle; 5, SNB angle; 6, SPAS (superior posterior airway space).

2.3.4. Drug-induced Sleep Endoscopy

In patients with previous unsuccessful CPAP and/or MAD therapy, DISE was performed prior to MMA osteotomy to assess the precise anatomic level(s) and pattern(s) of upper airway collapse. These patients underwent a standardized DISE procedure, of which the method is described in a previous study [27]. In order to quantify the observers' findings during DISE, the VOTE scoring system was used [28]. In the present study, we included data on presence/absence of concentric collapse at the velum and presence/absence of complete anteroposterior epiglottis collapse, both in supine position, as the potential predictors.

2.4. Outcomes

Changes in AHI at 3 to 12 months follow-up compared with the preoperative AHI were regarded as the primary outcome for surgical success. The outcome for surgical success was binary. The surgical success of MMA is considered 'present' if a patient's AHI was reduced by $\geq 50\%$ compared to the preoperative AHI, combined with a postoperative AHI < 20 events/h, as proposed by Sher et al. [15].

2.5. Statistical Analysis

2.5.1. Missing Data

The multiple imputation technique was used for the missing values. We created m = 35 imputed datasets with 10 iterations and used predictive mean matching (PMM) for imputing the missing values. All the potential predictors and the outcome variable were included in the imputation model.

2.5.2. Development of the Model

Screening of Potential Predictors and Modelling

The potential predictors for surgical success were determined based on clinical experience and previous literature by the research team. Multicollinearity of the potential predictors were assessed using the variance inflation factor (VIF). When a VIF value of a predictor was higher than 10 [31], collinearity was considered present and the predictor was excluded from the subsequent analysis.

To pre-screen the potential predictors, univariate binary logistic regression analysis was used to assess the association between each potential predictor and the outcome. The predictors with a p-value of ≤ 0.20 were selected for the subsequent multivariate analyses. Multivariate binary logistic regression analysis with backward selection (predictors with p-value of >0.20 were removed) was performed to further screen the potential predictors and develop the prediction model.

Shrinkage Factor

A global shrinkage factor was produced based on the bootstrapping procedure with 100 bootstrap samples. The shrinkage factor was used to shrink the regression coefficients of the predictors in order to prevent the overfitting of the prediction model [32,33].

Performance of the Prediction Model

The performance of the prediction model was assessed in aspects of calibration and discrimination. Calibration is defined as the agreement between predicted and observed outcomes [34]. The calibration of the model was assessed with the calibration plot by plotting the predicted individual outcomes against the observed actual outcomes. The patients were grouped into deciles based on their predicted probabilities of the outcomes. The prevalence of the outcome events in each decile is considered the observed probability. The mean of the individual predicted probabilities in each decile is considered the predicted probability. In the calibration plot, the agreement between predicted probabilities and observed probabilities across the range of the predicted risks was estimated. The overall calibration of the model was assessed with the overall observed–expected ratio (O:E ratio) [34].

The O:E ratio was defined as the ratio between the prevalence of the outcomes (observed) and the mean individual predicted probabilities of the outcomes (expected) within the cohort [35]. An O:E ratio between 0.8 and 1.2 indicates an acceptable overall calibration [36]. The calibration of the model was also assessed with the Hosmer–Lemeshow goodness-of-fit statistic test (HL test). A p-value of >0.10 of the HL test indicates that the model fits the observed data [37].

Discrimination is defined as the ability of the model to differentiate between those with and without the outcome events [34]. The discrimination of the model was assessed with the area under the receiver-operating characteristic curve (AUC). An AUC of 0.70 to 0.80 indicates an acceptable discrimination of the model, while an AUC of ≥ 0.80 indicates an excellent to outstanding discrimination of the model [38].

The optimal cutoff for the predicted probability of the model was defined as the predicted probability with the maximum sum of sensitivity and specificity in the receiver-operating characteristic curve (ROC).

Clinical (Added) Values

The clinical values of the model at the optimal cutoff for predicted probability were assessed using prevalence (prior probability) and posterior probabilities of the outcome events. The posterior probability was defined as positive predictive value (PPV) and negative predictive value (NPV). PPV was defined as the number of patients with the actual outcome events among the patients who were predicted to have the outcome events. NPV was defined as the number of patients without actual outcome events among the patients who were predicted to have no outcome events. The added predictive value of the model for ruling in an increased probability of the outcome events was defined as the PPV minus prevalence, while that for ruling out an increased probability of the outcome events was defined as the NPV minus complement of prevalence.

Score Chart and Line Chart

A clinical prediction rule for the outcome events was developed to provide an estimate for individual patients of their absolute probability of the outcome events. For the final multivariate binary logistic regression model, the individual probability (P) of the outcome events was predicted with the following formula:

$$P = 1 - 1/[1 + \exp(\text{constant} + \beta_1 X_1 + \ldots + \beta_i X_i)]$$

where β is the shrunken regression coefficient of a predictor in the models.

To facilitate the calculation of the predicted probability of the outcome events in individual patients, the multivariate logistic regression model was converted to a score chart. In the score chart, the score of each included predictor was produced by the shrunken regression coefficients being multiplied by -100 and subsequently rounded. A line chart was then developed to help determine the predicted probability of the outcome events.

All the statistical procedures mentioned above were performed via SPSS 27.0 (IBM, New York, NY, USA) and R software 4.0.4 ((R Development Core Team, Vienna, Austria).

3. Results

In the period of September 2011 to September 2020, 111 patients underwent MMA osteotomy for OSA. A total of 100 patients were eligible for analysis, of whom 82 (82%) were male. Eleven patients were excluded due to no patient approval for usage of their data for research purposes ($n = 3$), mild OSA ($n = 3$), no postoperative PSG performed ($n = 4$), and craniofacial syndrome ($n = 1$). Among the 100 eligible patients, mean age was 50.5 ($\pm$ 9.9) years and mean BMI was 29.8 (± 4.2) kg/m^2. The majority of patients were ASA II (56%), followed by ASA I (23%) and ASA III (21%). In ninety-eight (98%) patients, CPAP was an unsuccessful therapy and/or intolerance was noted. Two (2%) patients declined CPAP as first-choice therapy. Mean AHI prior to surgery was 52.9 ($\pm$ 21.4), and 16 (16%) patients had a CAI of ≥ 5 events per hour of sleep. A total of 67 (67%) patients had surgical success from treatment. The median preoperative percentage of total sleep time spent in supine position in the total population, the surgical success subgroup, and the surgical failure subgroup was 37.3% (interquartile range [IQR], 19.0–56.0), 36.3% (IQR, 16.7–56.1), and 44.0% (IQR, 25.5–54.6), respectively; after MMA, they were 37.0% (IQR, 17.0–53.0), 30.0% (IQR, 10.3–49.4), and 40.5% (IQR, 28.6–58.2), respectively. The median preoperative percentage of total sleep time spent in the rapid eye movement (REM) stage was 17.8% (IQR, 12.1–21.5), 17.8% (IQR, 12.1–21.5), and 18.3% (IQR, 12.1–21.7), respectively; after MMA, they were 22.5% (IQR, 15.8–27.2), 24.0% (IQR, 17.4–29.1), and 19.0% (IQR, 13.4–25.8), respectively. Preoperatively, the median ODI 3% in the total population, surgical success subgroup, and surgical failure subgroup was 51.0 (IQR, 34.4–66.6) events/hour, 48.7 (IQR, 35.3–68.9) events/hour, and 57.0 (IQR, 29.5–66.0) events/hour, respectively; postoperatively, they were 21.1 (IQR, 10.5–30.2) events/hour, 11.2 (IQR, 9.2–20.7) events/hour, and 33.6 (IQR, 25.8–50.3) events/hour, respectively. Further details on the baseline characteristics of the potential predictors and their distribution over the outcome are presented in Table 2 (Appendix A contains Table A1, which presents baseline characteristics without multiple imputation).

Table 2. Characteristics of the predictors and their distribution over the outcome based on the multiple imputation (n = 100).

Potential Predictors (n = 100)		Number (%) or Mean (±SD)	Surgical Success	
			Yes (±SD/%) (n = 67)	No (±SD/%) (n = 33)
Age		50.5 (9.9)	49.3 (9.8)	53.1 (9.7)
Gender	Male	82 (82.0)	54 (80.6)	28 (84.8)
	Female	18 (18.0)	13 (19.4)	5 (15.2)
BMI *		29.7 (27.4–32.2)	29.7 (27.4–32.4)	29.8 (28.2–32.0)
ASA classification score	I	23 (23.0)	17 (25.4)	6 (18.2)
	II	56 (56.0)	38 (56.7)	18 (54.5)
	III	21 (21.0)	12 (17.9)	9 (27.3)
Previous upper airway surgery	Yes	42 (42.0)	27 (40.3)	15 (45.5)
	No	58 (58.0)	40 (59.7)	18 (54.5)
Dentulous (full + partially) **	Yes	82.6 (82.6)	55.6 (83.0)	27 (81.8)
	No	17.4 (17.4)	11.4 (17)	6 (18.2)
Polysomnographic variables				
AHI pre-operative		52.9 (21.4)	54.2 (20.9)	50.3 (22.6)
Positional dependent OSA **	Yes	43.9 (43.9)	29.5 (44)	14.5 (43.9)
	No	56.1 (56.1)	37.5 (66)	18.5 (56.1)
CAI ≥ 5 events/hour **	Yes	16 (16)	7 (10.4)	9 (27.3)
	No	84 (84)	60 (89.6)	24 (72.7)
Cephalometric variables				
Anterior total face height **		123.9 (8.3)	122.8 (7.7)	126.1 (9.2)
Anterior lower face height **		73.0 (7.4)	72.0 (7.2)	75.0 (7.7)
SPAS **		8.3 (2.9)	7.7 (2.7)	9.6 (3.3)
Presence of maxillomandibular deficiency **	Yes	75.4 (75.4)	50.5 (75.4)	24.9 (75.5)
	No	24.6 (24.6)	16.5 (24.6)	8.1 (24.5)
DISE variables				
Concentric collapse velum **	Yes	30.5 (30.5)	17.7 (26.4)	12.9 (39.1)
	No	69.5 (69.5)	49.3 (73.6)	20.1 (60.9)
Complete anteroposterior epiglottis collapse **	Yes	24.2 (24.2)	15.9 (23.7)	8.3 (25.2)
	No	75.8 (75.8)	51.1 (76.3)	24.7 (74.8)

AHI, apnea hypopnea index; ASA, American Society of Anesthesiologists; BMI, body mass index; CAI, central apnea index; DISE, drug-induced sleep endoscopy; OSA, obstructive sleep apnea; SPAS, superior posterior airway space; * values not normally distributed given as median and interquartile range (Q1-Q3); ** including imputed data due to missing values.

The VIF values of all the predictors were lower than 10, which indicated that the multicollinearity between the predictors was negligible. Therefore, all the predictors were included for further analysis. In the univariate binary logistic regression analyses, anterior total face height, anterior lower face height, SPAS, age, and presence of CAI $\geq$ 5 events/hour had a p-values of $\leq$0.20 and were included in the subsequent multivariate binary logistic regression analysis (Table 3). In the multivariate analysis, anterior lower face height, SPAS, age, and presence of CAI $\geq$ 5 events/hour remained in the final model with p-values of $\leq$0.20 (Table 3).

Table 3. Univariate and multivariate logistic regression analyses for the surgical success (n = 100).

		Univariate Logistic Regression			Multivariate Logistic Regression			
Predictors	Coding	B (SE)	OR (95%CI)	p-Value	B (SE)	Shrunken B	OR (95%CI)	p-Value
Intercept					14.258 (5.082)	11.6005		<0.01
Age		−0.041 (0.023)	0.959 (0.917–1.003)	0.070	−0.041 (0.027)	−0.033	0.96 (0.91–1.01)	0.13
Gender	Female Male	Ref. −0.299 (0.575)	0.742 (0.240–2.291)	0.604				
BMI		−0.004 (0.051)	0.996 (0.901–1.101)	0.941				
ASA classification score	I II III	Ref. −0.294 (0.554) −0.754 (0.648)	0.745 (0.251–2.209) 0.471 (0.132–1.676)	0.596 0.245				
Previous upper airway surgery	No Yes	Ref. −0.211 (0.429)	0.810 (0.349–1.879)	0.623				
Dentulous (full + partially)	No Yes	Ref. 0.082 (0.560)	1.085 (0.362–3.252)	0.884				
AHI pre-operative		0.009 (0.010)	1.009 (0.989–1.029)	0.389				
Positional dependent OSA	No Yes	Ref. 0.002 (0.451)	1.002 (0.414–2.428)	0.996				
CAI $\geq$ 5 events/hour	No Yes	Ref. −1.185 (0.636)	0.306 (0.088–1.065)	0.063	Ref. −1.830 (0.865)	−1.473	0.16 (0.03–0.91)	0.04
Anterior total face height		−0.048 (0.028)	0.953 (0.901–1.008)	0.091				
Anterior lower face height		−0.056 (0.032)	0.945 (0.888–1.006)	0.075	−0.071 (0.036)	−0.057	0.93 (0.87–1.00)	0.05
SPAS		−0.235 (0.083)	0.791 (0.672–0.931)	0.005	−0.280 (0.099)	−0.225	0.76 (0.62–0.92)	0.01
Presence of maxillomandibular deficiency	No Yes	Ref. −0.016 (0.558)	0.984 (0.329–2.945)	0.978				
Concentric collapse velum	No Yes	Ref. −0.587 (0.535)	0.556 (0.194–1.591)	0.273				
Complete anteroposterior epiglottis collapse	No Yes	Ref. −0.050 (0.612)	0.951 (0.285–3.169)	0.935				

AHI, apnea hypopnea index; ASA, American Society of Anesthesiologists; BMI, body mass index; CAI, central apnea index; DISE, drug-induced sleep endoscopy; OR, odds ratio; OSA, obstructive sleep apnea; SE, standard error; SPAS, superior posterior airway space.

The shrinkage factor of the model was 0.80. The original AUC of the model was 0.78 (95% confidence interval [95%CI]: 0.66 to 0.87) and the shrunken AUC of the model was 0.74. This indicated that the discrimination of the model was acceptable. The calibration plot (Figure 2) showed that most plotted dots were lying close to the diagonal line. Therefore, there was a good agreement between the predicted probabilities and actual probabilities of the outcomes. The O:E ratio was 1.01 (95%CI: 0.81 to 1.24), which indicated that the overall calibration of the model was excellent. The p-value of the HL test was 0.42, which showed that the model had good fit.

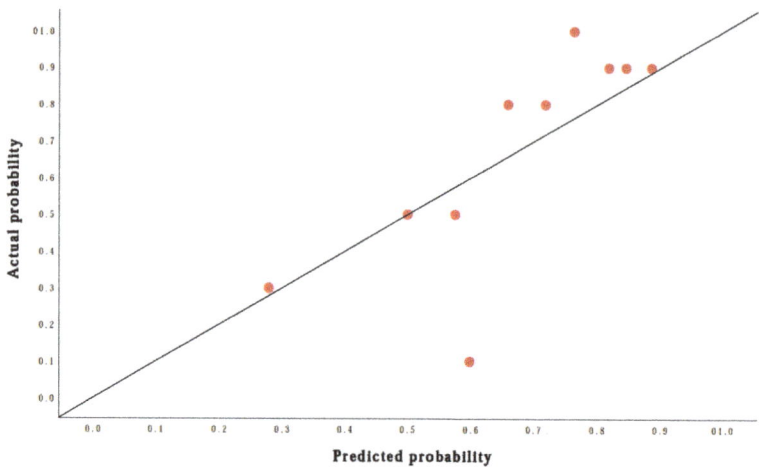

Figure 2. Calibration plot of the prediction model for surgical success. The diagonal line is what would result if the predicted probability of the model was the same as the actual probability of the model so that the prediction is neither underestimated nor overestimated. The red dots represent the deciles of the patients based on their predicted probabilities.

The optimal cutoff for the predicted probability of the model was 0.62. Table 4 presents the prevalence, sensitivity, specificity, PPV, and NPV of the model. The clinical added value of the model for ruling in the probability of surgical success was 0.21 (95%CI: 0.09 to 0.34) in addition to the prevalence, while that for ruling out the probability of surgical success was 0.32 (95%CI: 0.15 to 0.49) in addition to the complement of the prevalence.

Table 4. Clinical (added) values of the model (n = 100).

Outcome	Prevalence (95% CI)	Sensitivity (95% CI)	Specificity (95% CI)	PPV (95% CI)	NPV (95% CI)	Added Value for Ruling in the Outcome (95% CI)	Added Value for Ruling Out the Outcome (95% CI)
Surgical success	0.67 (0.57–0.76)	0.79 (0.68–0.88)	0.79 (0.62–0.90)	0.88 (0.78–0.95)	0.65 (0.49–0.79)	0.21 (0.09–0.34)	0.32 (0.15–0.49)

CI, confidence interval; NPV, negative predictive value; PPV, positive predictive value.

To enhance the clinical usefulness of the model, a score chart (Table 5) and a line chart (Figure 3) were produced. A clinician can easily calculate the sum score of a patient using the score chart and determine the corresponding predicted probability of surgical success based on a line chart using the sum score. The predicted probability of surgical success is lower when the sum score is higher. The cutoff of the sum score for the prediction of surgical success was 1111.

Table 5. Score chart for the prediction of surgical success.

Predictors		Score
Anterior lower face height		6
SPAS		23
Age		3
CAI ≥ 5 events/hour	No	0
	Yes	147
Sum score		

CAI, central apnea index; SPAS, superior posterior airway space.

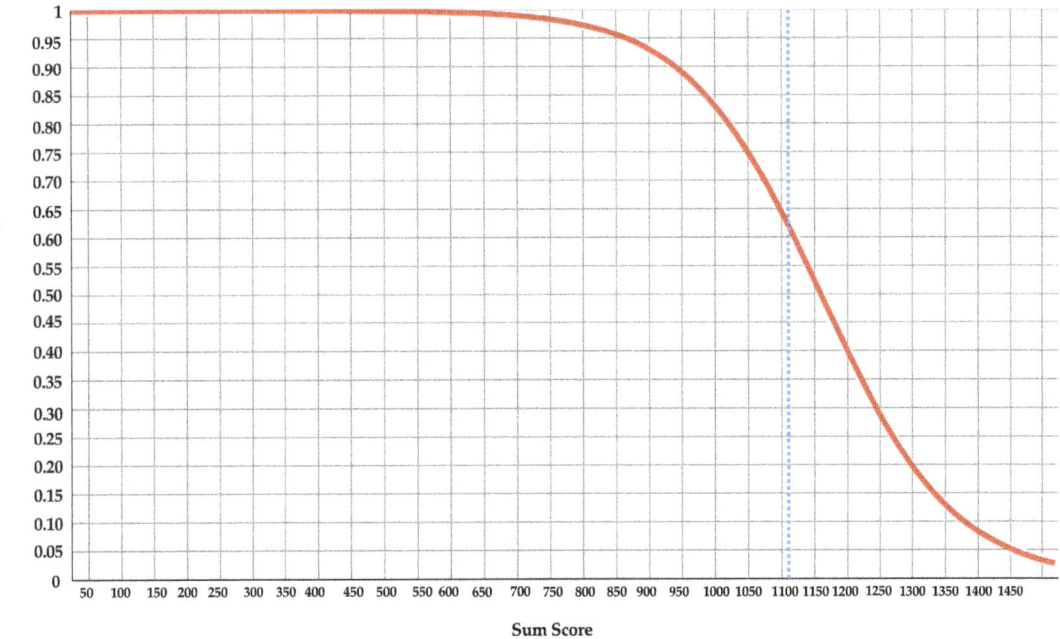

Figure 3. The line chart of the prediction model for surgical success. From the line chart, the exact predicted probability (%) of surgical success of an individual (Axis Y) can be determined based on the sum scores (Axis X) and the curve.

The algorithm for the calculation of a patient's sum score for surgical success is presented below:

Sum score = 6 ∗ anterior lower face height + 23 ∗ SPAS + 3 ∗ age + 147 ∗ CAI ≥ 5 events/hour

4. Discussion

In the present study, patients with a lower age at surgery, CAI < 5 events per hour, a lower anterior lower face height (ALFH), and a smaller superior posterior airway space (SPAS) may have a higher probability of obtaining surgical success. The prediction model for the surgical success of MMA was derived based on the predictors above, and the performance of the model may be acceptable. To the authors' best knowledge, this is the first study to develop a prediction model for the surgical success of MMA for the treatment of OSA with pre-operative patient data that can be utilized during daily clinical practice.

Clinicians frequently encounter the presence of central and/or mixed events on PSG in patients with OSA, which makes the treatment decision-making process more difficult [39]. The results presented in this study on the CAI and its role with respect to the surgical success of MMA are in line with a study by Markovey et al. [13], illustrating that a lower pre-operative CAI was a statistically significant predictor of surgical success (CAI pre-operatively in the success group was 0.6 versus 5.7 in the failure group, *p*-value = 0.005). Xie et al. studied the difference between patients with pure OSA (100% of the apneas are obstructive) and predominant OSA (presence of both central and obstructive apneas and the obstructive apneas account for >50% of the total number of apneas), and they reported lower breathing control stability in patients with predominant OSA [40]. Therefore, it is thought that in patients with a higher preoperative CAI, the lower breathing control stability might entail obstructive events, leading to lower surgical success rates. This present study also found that ALFH was significantly associated with surgical success. In a meta-analysis on craniofacial morphology in patients with OSA, the authors found a strong tendency towards an increased ALFH in adult patients with OSA [41]. A possible explanation for this altered craniofacial anatomy might be upper airway obstruction occurring as early as childhood [42]. However, to date, still little is known regarding the exact underlying mechanism of cephalometric measurements as predictors for surgical success. Despite the fact that the included predictors in the prediction model were significantly associated with surgical success, the causality between predictor and outcome was not assessed, and conclusions on causality cannot be drawn. Therefore, included predictors might not have a causal relation, whilst still being strong predictors for surgical success in the prediction model.

The original AUC of the model was 0.78, and the shrunken AUC of the model was 0.74, which indicates that the discrimination of the model was acceptable. The calibration plot (Figure 2) illustrates that there was a good agreement between the predicted probabilities and the actual probabilities of the outcomes. The added predictive value for ruling in surgical success was 0.21, whereas the added predictive value for ruling out surgical success was 0.32. These results denote that if the model predicts a patient to reach surgical success, the posterior probability of such patient to reach surgical success can be increased by 0.21 when compared with the prevalence of surgical success in the patient's group. If the model predicts a patient to have the absence of surgical success, such patient's posterior probability of an absence of surgical success can be increased by 0.32 when compared with the completement of prevalence of surgical success in the patient's group. Both these results denote that the clinical added values of the model were adequate for ruling in and ruling out surgical success.

In order to optimize the utilization of the model during daily clinical practice, calculation of the optimal cut-off value for predicted probability is needed for probability stratification. The optimal cut-off value is determined when both sensitivity and specificity are at their maximum, so false negative and false positive outcomes are at their lowest. The optimal cutoff for the predicted probability of surgical success was 0.62. Thus, in the event of a sum score lower than 1111, individuals were very likely to reach surgical success.

Of note is the fact that a prediction model might entail false positive and false negative outcomes. In the event of a false negative outcome, a patient and clinician might falsely waive MMA as the therapy of choice, which might worsen the patient's OSA and prognosis. On the other hand, a false positive outcome might lead to an incorrect indication for surgery, which entails comorbidity and the risks associated with surgery, such as bleeding, infection, and wound healing problems. Both false negative and false positive outcomes might result in an increase in costs and unfavorable health outcomes. The model presented in this study has a 35% and 12% risk of a false negative and false positive outcome, respectively. The percentage of false negative outcome can be regarded as moderately high. This indicates that when a patient is predicted to have failure of the surgery, clinicians need to be very cautious about the predicted results and should make the final decision based on their experience and other clinical examinations. This may avoid the false negatives to a large extent. In addition, as previously discussed, a false-negative outcome might entail incorrectly waiving MMA as the therapy of choice. However, the disadvantages of a false-positive outcome resulting in the incorrect indication for MMA may be more severe when compared to the incorrect waiving of MMA.

In order to increase surgical success rates, a prediction tool is warranted that aids surgeons in identifying responders and non-responders pre-operatively during patient counseling. If a patient is predicted to have a high probability of surgical success, this endorses the consideration for MMA as the therapy of choice. In addition, if a patient is predicted to have a low probability of surgical success, this will aid clinician and patient to be more cautious in choosing MMA as the therapy of choice and possibly search for other therapeutic options. When a patient with a low probability of surgical success is still determined to undergo MMA since he/she has no other therapeutic options left, the prediction might still help to inform the patient on the prognosis of their OSA, thereby shaping their expectations of MMA. The prediction model allows patients to be informed on their individual chances of surgical success rather than average group success rates.

For the presented study population, 67% of the included patients attained surgical success after MMA. These results are lower when compared with a recent review reporting surgical success rates of up to 85% [12]. We believe this is due to the fact that the patients included in this study had more multi-therapy resistant (complex) types of OSA, since these patients were referred to our academic hospital after the failure of one or more earlier therapies. This study included patients with moderate to severe OSA. This is because patients with mild OSA generally experience milder symptoms and therefore a lower burden of disease and a lower risk of untreated hypoxic burden compared to patients with moderate or severe OSA. Therefore, an invasive therapy such as MMA is not considered the therapy of choice in patients with mild OSA, and non-invasive therapies (i.e., CPAP or MAD therapy) resolve symptoms and obtain success of therapy in most cases [9]. The prediction model presented in this study can therefore solely be utilized for patients with moderate to severe OSA.

This study has some limitations. First, the retrospective design of the study entails higher proportions of missing data. The missing data was considered missing at random, and therefore the multiple imputation technique was used for the missing values. Ideally, a prospective study is preferred due to better control of the data. However, since imputation of missing values is considered superior to complete case analysis in the event of missing data, the potential bias in the results caused by the missing values were minimized [43]. Second, in a multivariate logistic regression analysis, an events per variable (EPV) value of 10 is widely advocated to obtain a reliable outcome [44,45]. The present study, however, did not meet the criterion because of the small sample size, which is a limitation. In order to reduce the number of predictors included in the multivariate analysis, we performed univariate analyses to pre-screen the predictors in the study. In addition, we used a less stringent threshold of p-value = 0.20 in modeling for the selection of potential predictors to avoid the incorrect exclusion of the important predictors due to the small sample size. In this way, the negative consequence caused by the sample size could be reduced to a large extent. Third, the cephalograms that were assessed in this study were all performed while the patients were awake and with a standard upright position. The data obtained on soft tissue measurements might therefore not be an accurate resemblance of the measurements of soft tissue during sleep in supine position. Nevertheless, it has been performed widely as a routine application prior to OSA surgery, and in the context of low costs and convenience, determining pharyngeal and skeletal anatomy by a cephalogram performed in the standard upright position is of added value. Because we did not have a different population, external validation of the model was not possible in our study, which is a limitation. Therefore, we recommend that the external validation of the model is warranted for future research. Fourth, the postoperative PSG was performed at the minimum of 3 months and at the maximum of 12 months. This difference in the timing of the follow-up PSG might influence the observed success rates of the patients, thus causing a bias in the results. However, several studies have illustrated that the decrease in AHI, and therefore surgical success, after MMA is stable over time [23,46], and it is therefore not likely that the postoperative PSG timing biased the final results in a major way. Last, the missing proportion of the DISE variables was 36%, which is relatively large. The main reason for the absence is that the DISE variables were not routinely collected in the clinical practice, and the variables were more likely to be collected when other alternative treatments for CPAP or MAD were indicated, when surgical options were indicated, or when the AHI was very high and initial therapy did not work. Therefore, we think the DISE variables are likely to be missing not at random, because the factors which may impact the absence of the variables were not adjusted in the imputation model. This may, to some extent, bias our results, which is another limitation.

5. Conclusions

The prediction model was developed for the surgical success of MMA as a surgical treatment for patients with moderate to severe OSA. A lower age at surgery, CAI < 5 events per hour, a lower anterior lower face height, and a smaller superior posterior airway space were significant predictors for the surgical success of MMA. The performance of the model terms of discrimination and calibration was acceptable. The clinical added values of the model were adequate for ruling in and ruling out surgical success of treatment. The model presented in this study may aid surgeons in identifying responders for MMA preoperatively. In addition, it improves preoperative patient counseling on the chances of reaching surgical success. However, prior to the implementation of the model in daily clinical practice, external validation is warranted.

Author Contributions: Conceptualization, W.P.V., J.-P.T.F.H., J.d.L. and N.S.; methodology, W.P.V., J.-P.T.F.H., J.d.L., M.J.L.R. and N.S.; software, W.P.V., N.S.; validation, W.P.V., J.-P.T.F.H., J.d.L. and N.S.; formal analysis, W.P.V., J.-P.T.F.H. and N.S.; investigation, W.P.V., J.-P.T.F.H., N.Z., M.J.L.R. and N.S.; writing—original draft preparation, W.P.V., J.-P.T.F.H. and N.S.; writing—review and editing, W.P.V., J.-P.T.F.H., J.d.L., M.J.L.R., N.Z., E.A.J.M.S. and N.S.; visualization, W.P.V.; supervision, W.P.V., J.-P.T.F.H. and J.d.L.; project administration, W.P.V. All authors have read and agreed to the published version of the manuscript.

Funding: This research received no external funding.

Institutional Review Board Statement: This study was exempted to the Medical Research Human Subjects Act: Reference number W22_061#22.093.

Informed Consent Statement: Informed consent was obtained from all subjects involved in the study.

Data Availability Statement: Not applicable.

Conflicts of Interest: The authors declare no conflict of interest.

Appendix A

Table A1. Characteristics of the predictors and their distribution over the outcome in the original data.

Potential Predictors		Number (%) or Mean (±SD)	Surgical Success		Missing Values (n)
			Yes (±SD/%) (n = 67)	No (±SD/%) (n = 33)	
Age (n = 100)		50.5 (9.9)	49.3 (9.8)	53.1 (9.7)	0
Gender (n = 100)	Male	82 (82.0)	54 (80.6)	28 (84.8)	0
	Female	18 (18.0)	13 (19.4)	5 (15.2)	
BMI (n = 100) *		29.7 (27.4–32.2)	29.7 (27.4–32.4)	29.8 (28.2–32.00)	0
ASA classification score (n = 100)	I	23 (23.0)	17 (25.4)	6 (18.2)	0
	II	56 (56.0)	38 (56.7)	18 (54.5)	
	III	21 (21.0)	12 (17.9)	9 (27.3)	
Previous upper airway surgery (n = 100)	Yes	42 (42.0)	27 (40.3)	15 (45.5)	0
	No	58 (58.0)	40 (59.7)	18 (54.5)	
Dentulous (full + partially) (n = 98)	Yes	81 (82.7)	54 (83.1)	27 (81.8)	2
	No	17 (17.3)	11 (16.9)	6 (18.2)	
Polysomnographic variables					
AHI pre-operative (n = 100)		52.9 (21.4)	54.2 (20.9)	50.3 (22.6)	0
Positional dependent OSA (n = 80)	Yes	34 (42.5)	22 (43.1)	12 (41.4)	20
	No	46 (57.5)	29 (56.9)	17 (58.6)	
CAI ≥ 5 events/hour (n = 84)	Yes	13 (15.5)	5 (9.1)	8 (27.6)	16
	No	71 (84.5)	50 (90.9)	21 (72.4)	
CAI (n = 84)		2.2 (3.5)	1.4 (2.4)	3.5 (4.8)	16

Table A1. Cont.

Potential Predictors		Number (%) or Mean (±SD)	Surgical Success		Missing Values (n)
			Yes (±SD/%) (n = 67)	No (±SD/%) (n = 33)	
		Cephalometric variables			
Anterior total face height (n = 82)		123.5 (8.4)	122.6 (7.6)	125.5 (9.6)	18
Anterior lower face height (n = 82)		72.8 (7.4)	71.9 (7.1)	74.8 (8.0)	18
SPAS (n = 95)		8.3 (2.9)	7.7 (2.7)	9.7 (3.1)	5
Presence of maxillomandibular deficiency (n = 82)	Yes	66 (80.5)	21 (65.6)	45 (90)	18
	No	16 (19.5)	11 (34.4)	5 (10)	
		DISE variables			
Concentric collapse velum (n = 64)	Yes	18 (28.1)	10 (23.8)	8 (33.3)	36
	No	46 (71.9)	32 (76.2)	14 (66.7)	
Complete anteroposterior epiglottis collapse (n = 64)	Yes	12 (18.8)	8 (19.0)	4 (18.2)	36
	No	52 (81.3)	34 (81.0)	18 (81.8)	

AHI, apnea hypopnea index; ASA, American Society of Anesthesiologists; BMI, body mass index; CAI, central apnea index; DISE, drug-induced sleep endoscopy; OSA, obstructive sleep apnea; SPAS, superior posterior airway space; * values not normally distributed given as median and interquartile range (Q1–Q3).

References

1. Malhotra, A.; White, D.P. Obstructive sleep apnoea. *Lancet* **2002**, *360*, 237–245. [CrossRef] [PubMed]
2. Young, T.; Finn, L.; Peppard, P.E.; Szklo-Coxe, M.; Austin, D.; Nieto, F.J.; Stubbs, R.; Hla, K.M. Sleep disordered breathing and mortality: Eighteen-year follow-up of the wisconsin sleep cohort. *Sleep* **2008**, *31*, 291–292.
3. Marshall, N.S.; Wong, K.K.H.; Liu, P.Y.; Cullen, S.R.J.; Knuiman, M.W.; Grunstein, R.R. Sleep apnea as an independent risk factor for all-cause mortality: The Busselton Health Study. *Sleep* **2008**, *31*, 1079–1085. [PubMed]
4. Shamsuzzaman, A.S.M.; Gersh, B.J.; Somers, V.K. Obstructive Sleep Apnea: Implications for Cardiac and Vascular Disease. *J. Am. Med. Assoc.* **2003**, *290*, 1906–1914. [CrossRef] [PubMed]
5. Kim, H.C.; Young, T.; Matthews, C.G.; Weber, S.M.; Woodard, A.R.; Palta, M. Sleep-disordered breathing and neuropsychological deficits: A population-based study. *Am. J. Respir. Crit. Care Med.* **1997**, *156*, 1813–1819. [CrossRef] [PubMed]
6. Baldwin, C.M.; Griffith, K.A.; Nieto, F.J.; O'Connor, G.T.; Walsleben, J.A.; Redline, S. The association of sleep-disordered breathing and sleep symptoms with quality of life in the sleep heart health study. *Sleep* **2001**, *24*, 96–105. [CrossRef]
7. Senaratna, C.V.; Perret, J.L.; Lodge, C.J.; Lowe, A.J.; Campbell, B.E.; Matheson, M.C.; Hamilton, G.S.; Dharmage, S.C. Prevalence of obstructive sleep apnea in the general population: A systematic review. *Sleep Med. Rev.* **2017**, *34*, 70–81. [CrossRef]
8. Peppard, P.E.; Young, T.; Barnet, J.H.; Palta, M.; Hagen, E.W.; Hla, K.M. Increased prevalence of sleep-disordered breathing in adults. *Am. J. Epidemiol.* **2013**, *177*, 1006–1014. [CrossRef]
9. Epstein, L.J.; Kristo, D.; Strollo, P.J.; Friedman, N.; Malhotra, A.; Patil, S.P.; Ramar, K.; Rogers, R.; Schwab, R.J.; Weaver, E.M.; et al. Clinical guideline for the evaluation, management and long-term care of obstructive sleep apnea in adults. *J. Clin. Sleep Med.* **2009**, *5*, 263–276.
10. Ravesloot, M.J.L.; de Vries, N. Reliable Calculation of the Efficacy of Non-Surgical and Surgical Treatment of Obstructive Sleep Apnea Revisited. *Sleep* **2011**, *34*, 105–110. [CrossRef]
11. Randerath, W.; de Lange, J.; Hedner, J.; Ho, J.P.T.F.; Marklund, M.; Schiza, S.; Steier, J.; Verbraecken, J. Current and novel treatment options for obstructive sleep apnoea. *ERJ Open Res.* **2022**, *8*, 00126–02022. [CrossRef]
12. Zhou, N.; Ho, J.P.T.F.; Huang, Z.; Spijker, R.; de Vries, N.; Aarab, G.; Lobbezoo, F.; Ravesloot, M.J.L.; de Lange, J. Maxillomandibular advancement versus multilevel surgery for treatment of obstructive sleep apnea: A systematic review and meta-analysis. *Sleep Med. Rev.* **2021**, *57*, 101471. [CrossRef] [PubMed]
13. Makovey, I.; Shelgikar, A.V.; Stanley, J.J.; Robinson, A.; Aronovich, S. Maxillomandibular Advancement Surgery for Patients Who Are Refractory to Continuous Positive Airway Pressure: Are There Predictors of Success? *J. Oral Maxillofac. Surg.* **2017**, *75*, 363–370. [CrossRef] [PubMed]
14. Teitelbaum, J.; Diminutto, M.; Comiti, S.; Pépin, J.L.; Deschaux, C.; Raphaël, B.; Bettega, G. Lateral cephalometric radiography of the upper airways for evaluation of surgical treatment of obstructive sleep apnea syndrome. *Rev. Stomatol. Chir. Maxillofac.* **2007**, *108*, 13–20. [CrossRef]
15. Sher, A.E.; Schechtman, K.B.; Piccirillo, J.F. The efficacy of surgical modifications of the upper airway in adults with obstructive sleep apnea syndrome. *Sleep* **1996**, *19*, 156–177. [CrossRef]
16. Cuschieri, S. The STROBE guidelines. *Saudi J. Anaesth.* **2019**, *13*, 31. [CrossRef] [PubMed]
17. Collins, G.S.; Reitsma, J.B.; Altman, D.G.; Moons, K.G.M. Transparent Reporting of a multivariable prediction model for Individual Prognosis Or Diagnosis (TRIPOD): The TRIPOD Statement. *Ann. Intern. Med.* **2015**, *162*, 55–63. [CrossRef]

18. Trauner, R.; Obwegeser, H. The surgical correction of mandibular prognathism and retrognathia with consideration of genioplasty. I. Surgical procedures to correct mandibular prognathism and reshaping of the chin. *Oral Surg. Oral Med. Oral Pathol.* **1957**, *10*, 677–689. [CrossRef]
19. Böckmann, R.; Meyns, J.; Dik, E.; Kessler, P. The Modifications of the Sagittal Ramus Split Osteotomy: A Literature Review. *Plast. Reconstr. Surg. Glob. Open* **2014**, *2*, e271. [CrossRef]
20. Liu, S.Y.C.; Awad, M.; Riley, R.W. Maxillomandibular Advancement: Contemporary Approach at Stanford. *Atlas Oral Maxillofac. Surg. Clin. North Am.* **2019**, *27*, 29–36. [CrossRef]
21. Kuik, K.; Ho, J.P.T.F.; de Ruiter, M.H.T.; Klop, C.; Kleverlaan, C.J.; de Lange, J.; Hoekema, A. Stability of fixation methods in large mandibular advancements after sagittal split ramus osteotomy: An in vitro biomechanical study. *Br. J. Oral Maxillofac. Surg.* **2021**, *59*, 466–471. [CrossRef] [PubMed]
22. Van Ewijk, L.J.; van Riet, T.C.T.; van der Tol, I.G.H.; Ho, J.P.T.F.; Becking, A.G. Power chains as an alternative to steel-wire ligatures in temporary maxillomandibular fixation: A pilot study. *Int. J. Oral Maxillofac. Surg.* **2022**, *51*, 975–980. [CrossRef] [PubMed]
23. Holty, J.-E.C.; Guilleminault, C. Maxillomandibular advancement for the treatment of obstructive sleep apnea: A systematic review and meta-analysis. *Sleep Med. Rev.* **2010**, *14*, 287–297. [CrossRef] [PubMed]
24. Zhou, N.; Ho, J.P.T.F.; de Vries, N.; Bosschieter, P.F.N.; Ravesloot, M.J.L.; de Lange, J. Evaluation of drug-induced sleep endoscopy as a tool for selecting patients with obstructive sleep apnea for maxillomandibular advancement. *J. Clin. Sleep Med.* **2022**, *18*, 1073–1081. [CrossRef] [PubMed]
25. Horvath, B.; Kloesel, B.; Todd, M.M.; Cole, D.J.; Prielipp, R.C. The Evolution, Current Value, and Future of the American Society of Anesthesiologists Physical Status Classification System. *Anesthesiology* **2021**, *135*, 904–919. [CrossRef] [PubMed]
26. Iber, C.; Chesson, A.Q.S. *The AASM Manual for the Scoring of Sleep and Associated Events: Rules, Terminology and Technical Specifications*; American Academy of Sleep Medicine: Westchester, IL, USA, 2007.
27. *American Academy of Sleep Medicine International Classification of Sleep Disorders—Third Edition (ICSD-3)*; American Academy of Sleep Medicine: Chicago, IL, USA, 2015.
28. Oksenberg, A.; Silverberg, D.S.; Arons, E.; Radwan, H. Positional vs Nonpositional Obstructive Sleep Apnea Patients: Anthropomorphic, Nocturnal Polysomnographic and Multiple Sleep Latency Test Data. *Chest* **1997**, *112*, 629–639. [CrossRef]
29. Livas, C.; Delli, K.; Spijkervet, F.K.L.; Vissink, A.; Dijkstra, P.U. Concurrent validity and reliability of cephalometric analysis using smartphone apps and computer software. *Angle Orthod.* **2019**, *89*, 889. [CrossRef]
30. Dantas, J.F.C.; de Carvalho, S.H.G.; Oliveira, L.S.D.A.F.; Barbosa, D.B.M.; de Souza, R.F.; Sarmento, V.A. Accuracy of Two Cephalometric Analyses in the Treatment of Patients with Skeletal Class III Malocclusion. *Braz. Dent. J.* **2015**, *26*, 186–192. [CrossRef]
31. Hair, J.F.J.; Anderson, R.E.; Tatham, R.L.; Black, W.C. *Multivariate Data Analysis*, 3rd ed.; Macmillan: New York, NY, USA, 1995.
32. Pavlou, M.; Ambler, G.; Seaman, S.R.; Guttmann, O.; Elliott, P.; King, M.; Omar, R.Z. How to develop a more accurate risk prediction model when there are few events. *BMJ* **2015**, *351*, h3868. [CrossRef]
33. Steyerberg, E.W.; Harrell, F.E.; Borsboom, G.J.J.M.; Eijkemans, M.J.C.; Vergouwe, Y.; Habbema, J.D.F. Internal validation of predictive models: Efficiency of some procedures for logistic regression analysis. *J. Clin. Epidemiol.* **2001**, *54*, 774–781. [CrossRef]
34. Steyerberg, E.W.; Vickers, A.J.; Cook, N.R.; Gerds, T.; Gonen, M.; Obuchowski, N.; Pencina, M.J.; Kattan, M.W. Assessing the performance of prediction models: A framework for traditional and novel measures. *Epidemiology* **2010**, *21*, 128–138. [CrossRef] [PubMed]
35. Siregar, S.; Groenwold, R.H.H.; de Heer, F.; Bots, M.L.; van der Graaf, Y.; van Herwerden, L.A. Performance of the original EuroSCORE. *Eur. J. Cardiothorac. Surg.* **2012**, *41*, 746–754. [CrossRef]
36. Debray, T.P.A.; Damen, J.A.A.G.; Snell, K.I.E.; Ensor, J.; Hooft, L.; Reitsma, J.B.; Riley, R.D.; Moons, K.G.M. A guide to systematic review and meta-analysis of prediction model performance. *BMJ* **2017**, *356*, 6460. [CrossRef] [PubMed]
37. Harrell, F.E.; Lee, K.L.; Mark, D.B. Multivariable prognostic models: Issues in developing models, evaluating assumptions and adequacy, and measuring and reducing errors. *Stat. Med.* **1996**, *15*, 361–387. [CrossRef]
38. Hosmer, D.W.; Lemeshow, S. Assessing the Fit of the Model. In *Applied Logistic Regression*, 2nd ed.; Wiley: Hoboken, NJ, USA, 2000; pp. 143–202. Available online: https://onlinelibrary.wiley.com/doi/full/10.1002/0471722146.ch5 (accessed on 3 October 2022).
39. Ho, J.P.T.F.; Zhou, N.; Verbraecken, J.; de Vries, N.; de Lange, J. Central and mixed sleep apnea related to patients treated with maxillomandibular advancement for obstructive sleep apnea: A retrospective cohort study. *J. Cranio Maxillofac. Surg.* **2022**, *50*, 537–542. [CrossRef]
40. Xie, A.; Bedekar, A.; Skatrud, J.B.; Teodorescu, M.; Gong, Y.; Dempsey, J.A. The heterogeneity of obstructive sleep apnea (predominant obstructive vs pure obstructive apnea). *Sleep* **2011**, *34*, 745–750. [CrossRef] [PubMed]
41. Neelapu, B.C.; Kharbanda, O.P.; Sardana, H.K.; Balachandran, R.; Sardana, V.; Kapoor, P.; Gupta, A.; Vasamsetti, S. Craniofacial and upper airway morphology in adult obstructive sleep apnea patients: A systematic review and meta-analysis of cephalometric studies. *Sleep Med. Rev.* **2017**, *31*, 79–90. [CrossRef] [PubMed]
42. Do Nascimento, R.R.; Masterson, D.; Trindade Mattos, C.; de Vasconcellos Vilella, O. Facial growth direction after surgical intervention to relieve mouth breathing: A systematic review and meta-analysis. *J. Orofac. Orthop.* **2018**, *79*, 412–426. [CrossRef]

43. Van der Heijden, G.J.M.G.; Donders, A.R.T.; Stijnen, T.; Moons, K.G.M. Imputation of missing values is superior to complete case analysis and the missing-indicator method in multivariable diagnostic research: A clinical example. *J. Clin. Epidemiol.* **2006**, *59*, 1102–1109. [CrossRef]
44. Ogundimu, E.O.; Altman, D.G.; Collins, G.S. Adequate sample size for developing prediction models is not simply related to events per variable. *J. Clin. Epidemiol.* **2016**, *76*, 175–182. [CrossRef]
45. Peduzzi, P.; Concato, J.; Kemper, E.; Holford, T.R.; Feinstem, A.R. A simulation study of the number of events per variable in logistic regression analysis. *J. Clin. Epidemiol.* **1996**, *49*, 1373–1379. [CrossRef] [PubMed]
46. Boyd, S.B.; Walters, A.S.; Waite, P.; Harding, S.M.; Song, Y. Long-Term Effectiveness and Safety of Maxillomandibular Advancement for Treatment of Obstructive Sleep Apnea. *J. Clin. Sleep Med.* **2015**, *11*, 699. [CrossRef] [PubMed]

Disclaimer/Publisher's Note: The statements, opinions and data contained in all publications are solely those of the individual author(s) and contributor(s) and not of MDPI and/or the editor(s). MDPI and/or the editor(s) disclaim responsibility for any injury to people or property resulting from any ideas, methods, instructions or products referred to in the content.

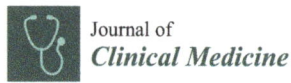

Review

The Present and Future of the Clinical Use of Physiological Traits for the Treatment of Patients with OSA: A Narrative Review

Yvonne Chu and Andrey Zinchuk *

Section of Pulmonary, Critical Care and Sleep Medicine, Department of Internal Medicine, Yale School of Medicine, 300 Cedar Street, The Anlyan Center, 455SE, New Haven, CT 06519, USA; yvonne.chu@yale.edu
* Correspondence: andrey.zinchuk@yale.edu

Abstract: People with obstructive sleep apnea (OSA) are a heterogeneous group. While many succeed in the treatment of their OSA, many others struggle with therapy. Herein, we discuss how anatomical and physiological factors that cause sleep apnea (OSA traits) impact treatment response and may offer an avenue for more precise care. These OSA traits, including anatomical (upper-airway collapsibility) and physiological (loop gain, airway muscle responsiveness, and arousal threshold) factors, may help determine who can succeed with continuous positive airway pressure, oral appliances, hypoglossal nerve stimulation, or pharmacotherapy. In the future, identifying OSA traits before initiating treatment may help guide the selection of the most effective and tolerable therapy modalities for each individual.

Keywords: OSA traits; upper airway collapsibility; loop gain; airway muscle responsiveness; arousal threshold; OSA therapy

Citation: Chu, Y.; Zinchuk, A. The Present and Future of the Clinical Use of Physiological Traits for the Treatment of Patients with OSA: A Narrative Review. *J. Clin. Med.* **2024**, *13*, 1636. https://doi.org/10.3390/jcm13061636

Academic Editor: Toru Oga

Received: 17 January 2024
Revised: 1 March 2024
Accepted: 1 March 2024
Published: 13 March 2024

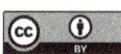

Copyright: © 2024 by the authors. Licensee MDPI, Basel, Switzerland. This article is an open access article distributed under the terms and conditions of the Creative Commons Attribution (CC BY) license (https://creativecommons.org/licenses/by/4.0/).

1. Introduction

Obstructive sleep apnea (OSA) is estimated to affect 1 billion adults aged 30–69 years worldwide [1], with prevalence increasing 2–3-fold in older adults (>65 years of age) compared to middle-aged adults [2,3]. Untreated OSA is associated with major causes of morbidity and mortality, including hypertension, strokes, coronary artery disease, metabolic syndrome, cognitive impairment, and mood disorders [4–6]. The timely diagnosis and treatment of OSA may have a role in mitigating the development or progression of these comorbid conditions [7]. Positive airway pressure (PAP) therapy is the gold standard and most efficacious therapy for OSA [8], and is prescribed to 80% of those diagnosed with OSA [9].

While PAP can eliminate airway obstruction in many patients, this "one size fits all" approach of PAP therapy for OSA has limitations. Long-term adherence to continuous positive airway pressure (CPAP) therapy is poor and varies widely. For example, adherence ranges from 50% in women aged 18–30 years to 80% in men aged 71–80 years [10]. Individuals from disadvantaged socioeconomic backgrounds struggle with PAP therapy even more (40% adherence) [11]. Numerous reasons for poor adherence have been identified, including claustrophobia, pressure intolerance, low self-efficacy or motivation for PAP use, and insomnia [12,13]. Despite advancements in PAP device technology, such as new masks and behavioral interventions, PAP adherence has not improved over the past 20 years [12,14]. Moreover, PAP therapy may not always be efficacious, with clinical cohorts and trials revealing that 25–30% of those using PAP therapy have a residual apnea–hypopnea index (AHI) score of >10/h [15,16]. Finally, patients do not consistently experience symptomatic relief with PAP therapy, and the lack of perceived symptomatic improvement is linked to poor PAP adherence [17]. As a result, many patients enter cycles of PAP trial and failure followed by attempts at non-PAP treatments [18]. This is, in part, because currently, there are no standardized methods to predict who will respond to PAP therapy and who will benefit from non-PAP therapies. New approaches in therapy decision-making are needed.

Emerging research shows that OSA is a heterogeneous disorder in terms of causes, presenting symptoms, and consequences [19–21]. Proposed models of susceptibility to OSA suggest that in addition to established anatomic causes (e.g., obesity, nasal obstruction, craniofacial structure, hyoid bone positioning, and upper airway edema), physiologic traits also predispose individuals to OSA. Tailoring OSA therapy based on the causes of sleep apnea in each individual has been proposed as a promising approach to precision medicine in OSA [21]. The overview of potential approaches to precision medicine in OSA, including factors beyond OSA's physiological traits, is highlighted in other reports [22–24].

The purpose of this manuscript is to review the anatomical and physiological contributors to OSA, describe the methods for their assessment, discuss potential applications based on current evidence, and highlight key obstacles in developing precision medicine approaches to OSA based on these traits. The key points of this manuscript are summarized in Table 1.

Table 1. Key points.

- The collapsibility of the upper airway, largely driven by anatomy, is a key determinant of OSA risk.
- When anatomic predisposition alone is not sufficient to cause OSA, physiologic traits such as a low arousal threshold (ArTH), high loop gain (LG), and poor upper airway muscle response (UAMR) can lead to OSA (Figure 1 and Figure 2).
- Retrospective analyses show that these traits can predict a response to current OSA treatments (Figure 3). For example, a high ArTH, low LG, and UAMR predict the success of oral appliance therapy.
- Measurements of the traits from clinical polysomnography require signal processing expertise and specialized arousal scoring. Point-of-care of care methods to estimate the traits exist (Table 2) but require prospective validation.
- Characterizing and targeting OSA traits that are failed by initial OSA therapy (e.g., CPAP) may offer one avenue to "rescue" treatments (Figure 4).
- Before evidence-based clinical use of traits to tailor therapy for OSA, several steps are critical, including the following:
  - (a) standardized and reliable methods of trait measurement,
  - (b) prospective, long-term (over 6 months) validation of the trait's utility in predicting outcomes of established OSA therapies (e.g., CPAP, oral appliances),
  - (c) prospective trials selecting first line therapy for each individual based on OSA traits, and
  - (d) once the above are established, implementation studies focused on ease of use, cost and applicability to diverse populations are required (see Sections 6 and 7).

2. OSA Traits

Four key traits contribute to the development of OSA [25]. These include increased upper-airway collapsibility, poor upper-airway dilator-muscle responsiveness, ventilatory-control instability (high loop gain), and a low arousal threshold. Different combinations and varying degrees of these traits may cause OSA in each individual [26].

One framework to understand how the four traits cause OSA examines upper-airway collapsibility (a surrogate of anatomic predisposition to collapse) as the key exposure (Figure 1). An upper airway that is not collapsible (i.e., an "open" airway) will result in the outcome of no OSA. In contrast, a highly collapsible airway (i.e., a "closed" airway) will consistently lead to OSA. For individuals with a "vulnerable" upper-airway anatomy (collapsibility between the "open" and "closed" airways), developing OSA (or no OSA) may depend on the modifying effects of the remaining physiological traits (loop gain, muscle responsiveness, arousal threshold) [26].

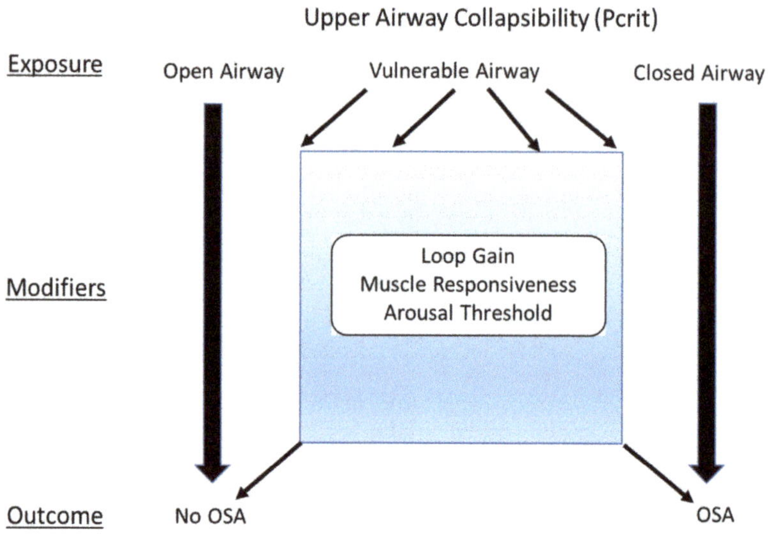

Figure 1. The interplay of the four key traits in predicting the outcome of OSA. In this conceptual framework, the upper airway collapsibility, measured by the critical closing pressure (P_{crit}) is the exposure. A very negative P_{crit} means the airway is non-collapsible (or an "open airway"), which results in no OSA phenotype. A high P_{crit}, on the other hand, means the airway is highly collapsible (or a "closed airway") and will inevitably result in the OSA phenotype. In between is the vulnerable airway, in which the modifying traits (loop gain, muscle responsiveness, and arousal threshold) can influence the phenotypic outcome of OSA vs. no OSA. The conceptual framework is adapted from Owens et al., Sleep 2015; 38: 961–70 [26].

2.1. Anatomic Contributions to Upper-Airway (UA) Collapsibility (the Exposure)

The concept of upper-airway collapsibility comes from the Starling resistor model, in which the airway "tube" spans from the posterior aspect of the nasal septum to the larynx [27,28]. This tube (airway) is susceptible to collapse because it has no rigid support. When the pressure surrounding the tube exceeds the pressure within the tube, collapse occurs. The critical closing pressure (P_{crit}) is the pressure within the tube equal to the surrounding pressure, and any increase in surrounding pressure beyond the P_{crit} results in collapse. The more negative the P_{crit}, the less collapsible the airway. For example, a P_{crit} of −5 cm water suggests a non-collapsible UA, while a P_{crit} of 5 cm water suggests a highly collapsible UA.

Factors that determine UA collapsibility are those that modify the airway diameter. These include obesity, which thickens the pharyngeal walls, and neck flexion, which also narrows the airway [29,30]. Similarly, low lung volume from abdominal obesity reduces tracheal traction, which is needed to unfold the airway and stiffen its walls [31]. Moving from the supine to lateral position results in a less collapsible airway and a lower P_{crit} [32]. Gender differences in airway collapsibility exist. Women have a less collapsible airway than BMI-matched men, in part due to having shorter airways (less opportunity for collapse) and a smaller cross-sectional area of the soft palate [33,34].

2.2. Physiological Contributors to OSA (the Effect Modifiers)
2.2.1. Ventilator Control Instability (High Loop Gain)

The respiratory system is composed of the ventilatory controller (chemoreceptors) and the ventilatory pump (the UA and the lungs) that are connected by a feedback loop (circulation). The arterial carbon dioxide level ($PaCO_2$) is a key determinant of ventilatory drive produced by the controller. In OSA, the decrease in ventilation (e.g., hypopnea) leads to a response (e.g., hyperpnea), the magnitude of which is determined by the individual's chemosensitivity to PaCO₂ changes. Because ventilatory drive affects not only the thoracic pump muscles (e.g., the diaphragm) but also the UA muscles [35], excessive $PaCO_2$ reductions from hyperpnea can result in airway collapse and obstructive events [36]. Thus, in individuals with OSA who have an overly sensitive ventilatory drive, the respiratory system can be unstable, cycling between hypopneas and hyperpneas [37] (Figure 2). Loop gain (LG) is a term describing how strongly a feedback loop system (i.e., respiratory system) responds to a disturbance. High LG represents ventilatory instability [37] and is considered an etiologic factor in one-third of patients with OSA [25].

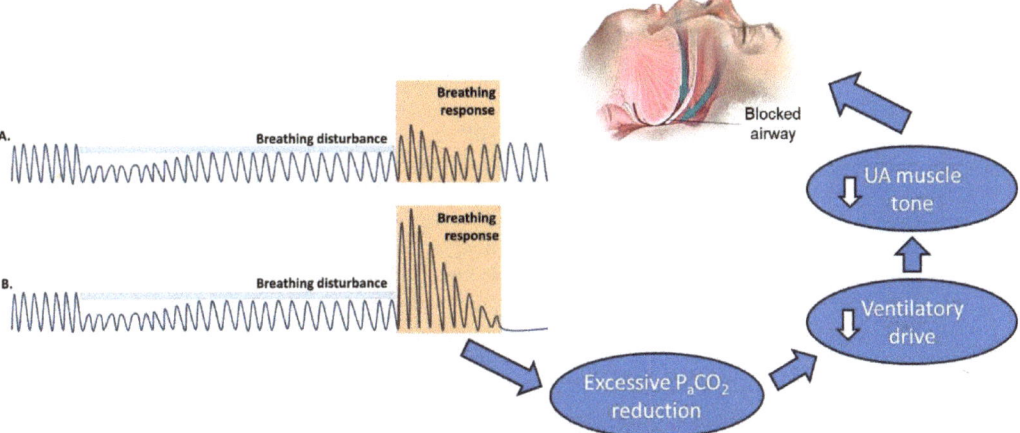

Figure 2. The pathogenesis of high-loop-gain OSA. In individuals with normal loop gain (e.g., flow tracing in (**A**)), the decrease in ventilation (hypopnea—"breathing disturbance" denoted as a blue bar) leads to an expected ventilatory response that is driven by the individual's chemosensitivity to PaCO₂ changes (a small rise in flow after the "breathing disturbance" is removed), before return to normal ventilation. Pathology arises in individuals with high loop gain (e.g., flow tracing in (**B**)); the same decrease in ventilation (hypopnea) leads to an exaggerated ventilatory response (hyperpnea) due to heightened chemosensitivity to PaCO₂ changes, resulting in the cycling between hypopneas/apneas and hyperpneas.

2.2.2. Pharyngeal Muscle Responsiveness

The upper-airway dilator muscles keep the upper airway patent, with the most studied dilator being the genioglossus. Muscle activity of the genioglossus declines from wake to sleep and furthermore from N2/N3 to REM sleep [38]. This decline may be the mechanism for REM-dependent OSA, especially in those who rely on the genioglossus to maintain airway patency during REM sleep [39]. While poor muscle responsiveness can result in OSA, vigorous muscle responsiveness may protect individuals from OSA. For example, in a study examining upper-airway muscle responsiveness (UAMR) between overweight/obese individuals with and without sleep apnea, the UAMR was 3-fold higher in those with obesity and no OSA [40], suggesting a protective effect. Progesterone increases genioglossus activity and dilates the airway [41]. Reduced levels of progesterone post-menopause may play a role in the pathogenesis of OSA in women.

2.2.3. Low Arousal Threshold

Arousal threshold (ArTH) measures the propensity to awaken from a respiratory stimulus (e.g., apnea). Arousals are necessary to reopen the UA and terminate obstructive events in some individuals [42,43]. A low ArTH (too easy of an arousability), however, has been postulated to lead to OSA [25]. This is partly because easy arousability may lead to frequent, short respiratory events. The resulting sleep fragmentation lowers the propensity for deeper, N3 sleep, during which sufficient ventilatory drive to the UA muscles may open the airway before a frank apnea or hypopnea develops. Similarly, ventilatory overshoot during arousal's opening of the UA lowers the $PaCO_2$ (and thus ventilatory stimuli for airway opening), promoting the recurrence of UA collapse [42]. A low ArTH is more common in individuals with REM-dependent OSA [44], and among those who are non-obese, older, and taking antidepressants [45]. Individuals with post-traumatic stress disorder may also have a lower ArTH, presumably due to their hyperadrenergic state [46].

2.2.4. Sex and Race Differences in Pathophysiology of OSA

A recent analysis of a diverse, multi-community cohort (Multi-Ethnic Study of Atherosclerosis, N = 1971; age range, 54–93 years) suggests that each of the four traits contribute differently to the pathophysiology of OSA in each sex and race/ethnicity [47]. For example, both increased UA collapsibility and reduced airway muscle responsiveness account for the majority of differences in AHI scores between males and females. Compared to white individuals with OSA, Black individuals exhibit lower AHI scores, potentially due to lower UA collapsibility despite having a higher LG. In contrast, UA collapsibility alone explained almost 90% of the differences in AHI scores between white individuals and individuals of Chinese ancestry, with adjustment for obesity.

Despite lower BMI rates among Asians, the prevalence of OSA is similar compared to Caucasian cohorts. Until recently, and as noted above, this has been attributed to greater craniofacial restriction (more predisposing anatomy) among Asian individuals [48]. Another analysis examined the role of the ArTH in OSA pathogenesis, comparing Caucasian (n = 163) and Chinese (n = 185) patients with OSA [49]. A low ArTH was a less common pathophysiological mechanism (28% vs. 49%) among Chinese versus Caucasian individuals with moderate-severe OSA, especially among those with mild craniofacial-anatomical restriction. In sum, findings from such studies suggest that OSA mechanisms vary across sex and race, which should be considered as investigators to assess the role of the traits in precision medicine in OSA.

2.2.5. Role of Comorbid Conditions in the Pathophysiology of OSA

Little data exist regarding the contribution of physiological traits to OSA in those with comorbid conditions. In a small study (n = 10) of non-hypercapnic chronic obstructive pulmonary disease (COPD) and OSA, UA collapsibility played a key role in OSA in only two individuals. The majority exhibited a high LG or a low ArTH, which were inversely correlated with markers of air trapping (high residual volume and residual volume to total lung capacity ratio) [50], suggesting that the worse the COPD severity, the lower the ArTH, resulting in fragmented sleep. Notably, ventilatory drive is reduced in REM sleep [51] and may explain the worsening of OSA in COPD overlap syndrome. In those with comorbid insomnia and OSA (COMISA), the UA is less collapsible and the ArTH is lower compared to those with OSA alone [52]. Notably, a low ArTH contributed to UA collapsibility in patients with COMISA only, and not those with OSA alone. Treating the underlying chronic insomnia in these patients may be key to the treatment of COMISA. In veterans with comorbid post-traumatic stress disorder (PTSD) and OSA, the presence of a low ArTH and insomnia predicted poor CPAP utilization, while a low ArTH alone was not a predictor [53]. More research is needed to assess the role of physiological traits in the pathogenesis of OSA and their impact on therapy selection among individuals with these and other comorbid conditions.

3. Measurement of OSA Traits

The gold standard for measuring physiologic OSA traits is invasive and is elegantly described by Eckert [54]. In brief, the measurement of upper-airway collapsibility, or the critical closing pressure (P_{crit}), involves the use of a pneumotachometer to assess flow and an esophageal pressure catheter [55] or a diaphragmatic electromyography (EMG) to assess ventilatory drive throughout the night during polysomnography with rapid CPAP pressure changes [56]. The LG and ArTH are determined from the ventilatory drive and responses to flow disturbances (CPAP pressure drops). For example, the ArTH reflects a median ventilatory drive just before an arousal from a series of CPAP drops (see Figure 3). Similarly, airway dilatory muscle responsiveness measurements require a surface EMG [57] of the tongue. Such methods are not practical outside of physiological research studies.

Advances in signal processing have enabled the development of an automated, non-invasive method for measuring OSA traits from a diagnostic PSG [58–60]. In brief, an in-laboratory polysomnogram is segmented into 7 min windows of non-REM sleep. The nasal pressure signal during a 7 min window is used to estimate the "baseline" eupneic non-obstructed ventilation (ventilatory drive (V_{drive})). LG is quantified as the V_{drive} response to ventilatory disturbance (e.g., hypopnea). The arousal threshold (ArTH) is calculated as the V_{drive} immediately preceding an arousal. To determine UA collapsibility ($1/V_{passive}$), a plot of the breath-by-breath values of ventilation and V_{drive} for NREM sleep is generated, and $V_{passive}$ is calculated as ventilation at the eupneic V_{drive}. Lower $V_{passive}$ values represent greater collapsibility (i.e., a higher P_{crit}). Pharyngeal muscle compensation (V_{comp}) is the difference between ventilation at an elevated V_{drive} (precisely, at the ArTH) and $V_{passive}$. The advantage of this approach is that it enables the measurement of OSA traits from a clinical polysomnography. This has led to an exponential growth in studies examining the traits and outcomes of OSA therapy. While promising, the method requires an understanding of signal processing and specialized arousal scoring, limiting its widespread use in clinical outcomes research.

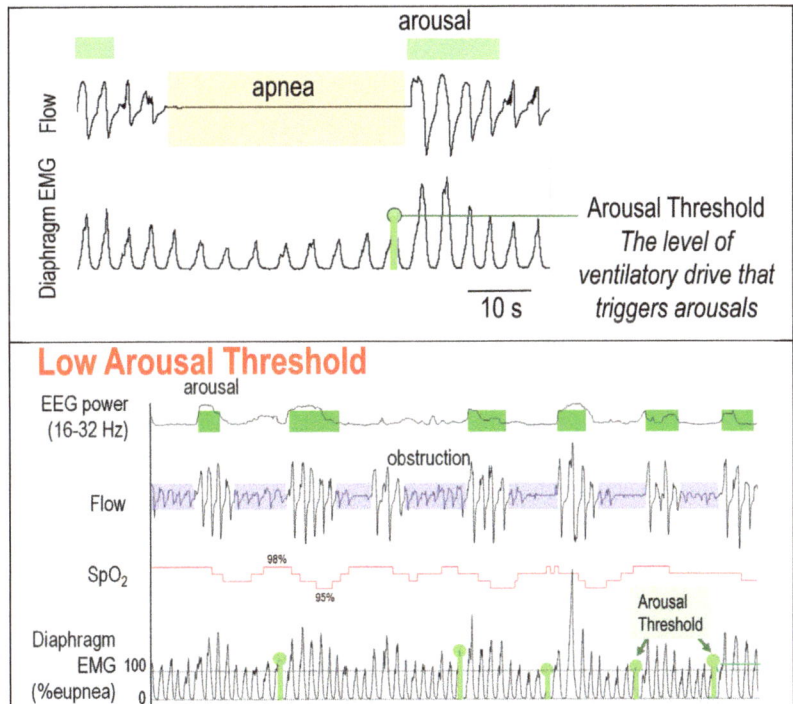

Figure 3. *Cont.*

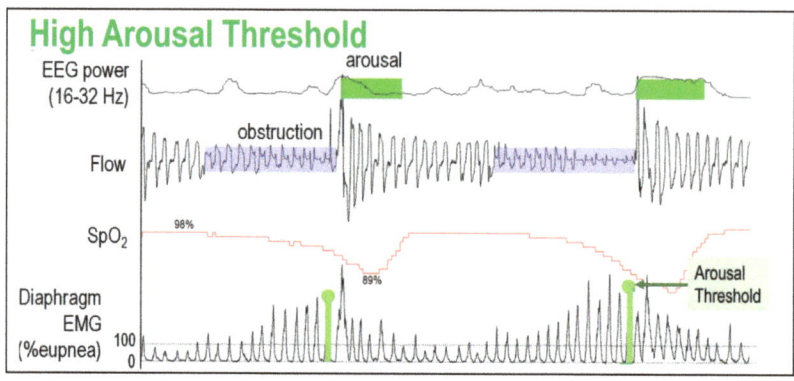

Figure 3. (**Top**) Determining ArTH from research polysomnography. Note that ventilator drive determined from the diaphragm EMG signal can be replaced by ventilatory drive (V_{drive}) from routine clinical polysomnography. OSA with low (**Middle**) and high (**Bottom**) ArTH. Note low ventilatory drive required for arousal (short vertical green bars within the diaphragm EMG signal), frequent respiratory events (purple), and minimal desaturations (red line) in low ArTH OSA in contrast to higher drive needed for and arousal (high vertical green bars within the diaphragm EMG signal), and less frequent and deeper obstructive events in high ArTH OSA. Images courtesy of Drs. Scott Sands and Laura Gell; top figure concept adapted from Gell LK et al. [61] Thorax 2022; 77: 707–716 online-supplement.

4. Point of Care Surrogate Measures of the Traits

Point of care (POC) tools based on routine clinical sleep study metrics to estimate the four OSA traits [62–65] have been developed. For example, Edwards et al. demonstrated that the therapeutic CPAP level on a titration study can discriminate a mildly from a moderately/severe collapsible UA. A therapeutic CPAP requirement of ≤8 cm of water was 89% sensitive and 84% specific for detecting a mildly collapsible airway [62].

The same group also showed that a simple clinical score can predict a low ArTH. A point is given for each: an apnea–hypopnea index (AHI) score of <30 events per hour, nadir oxygen saturation as measured by pulse oximetry > 82.5%), and the fraction of the AHI that are hypopneas ($F_{hypopneas}$) > 58.3%. A score of two or more predicts a low ArTH with 80% sensitivity and 88% specificity [65].

Methods to estimate LG from the AHI and from $F_{hypopneas}$ are less accurate [63]. LG can be effectively estimated using the formula LG = $2\pi/[2\pi DR - \sin(2\pi DR)]$ in those with treatment-emergent central sleep apnea (TE-CSA) [64]. Ten periodic breathing cycles with optimal CPAP during a titration study are needed. The DR is the ratio of the duration of the ventilatory phase (time from the end of one apnea to the start of the next) to the total cycle duration (time from the end of one apnea to the end of the next).

Dutta et al., developed a decision tree prediction model using standard metrics (e.g., AHI, REM AHI, and BMI) to predict the "good", "moderate", and "bad" levels of the four OSA traits [66]. If such tools are made user-friendly and are validated, they may offer a way for clinicians to derive these traits with clinical data.

Pattern recognition may also be useful when assessing ventilatory stability. For example, in contrast to the V-shaped pattern of oxygen desaturation seen in REM-related OSA, the "zipper-like" pattern of oxygen desaturation seen on hypnograms can be more consistent with the periodic breathing seen in NREM-predominant OSA, which is more likely to exhibit high LG [67,68].

In summary, while several promising POC tools to estimate the OSA traits exist (Table 2), they are limited by low accuracy, dependence on OSA severity (e.g., AHI score), or the requirement of PAP titration in the sleep laboratory. As with the promising non-invasive, automated methods to measure these traits [58,60], these tools also require prospective validation.

Table 2. Summary of Point of Care Clinical Tools for Measuring Traits.

Upper Airway Collapsibility: A CPAP requirement of ≤8 cm H_2O on titration PSG predicts a mildly collapsible airway (89% sensitive and 84% specific) [62].
Arousal Threshold: A point is given for each of the following: AHI < 30 events per hour, nadir oxygen saturation > 82.5%, and the fraction of the AHI that are hypopneas ($F_{hypopneas}$) > 58.3%. A score of 2 or more predicts a low ArTH (80% sensitive and 88% specific) [65].
Loop Gain: (1) $LG = 2\pi/[2\pi DR - \sin(2\pi DR)]$ on titration PSG with the presence of treatment-emergent central sleep apnea (TE-CSA) where DR is the ratio of the duration of the ventilatory phase (time from the end of one apnea to the start of the next) to the total cycle duration (time from the end of one apnea to the end of the next) [64]. (2) A "zipper-like" pattern of oxygen desaturation on hypnograms in NREM-predominant OSA suggest high LG [67,68].
Upper Airway Muscle Responsiveness: No published POC tool exist. A tool developed by Sands et al. [58] can be used to estimate UAMR and other traits from clinical PSG.

5. Precision Treatment of OSA Using the Traits

Here we will discuss the application of the OSA traits to improve the precision of OSA therapy approaches, in the order of most to least supported by available evidence: (1) predicting responses to established OSA therapies (see Figure 4), (2) guiding multi-modal therapy for OSA, and (3) targeting the traits to select initial therapy for OSA.

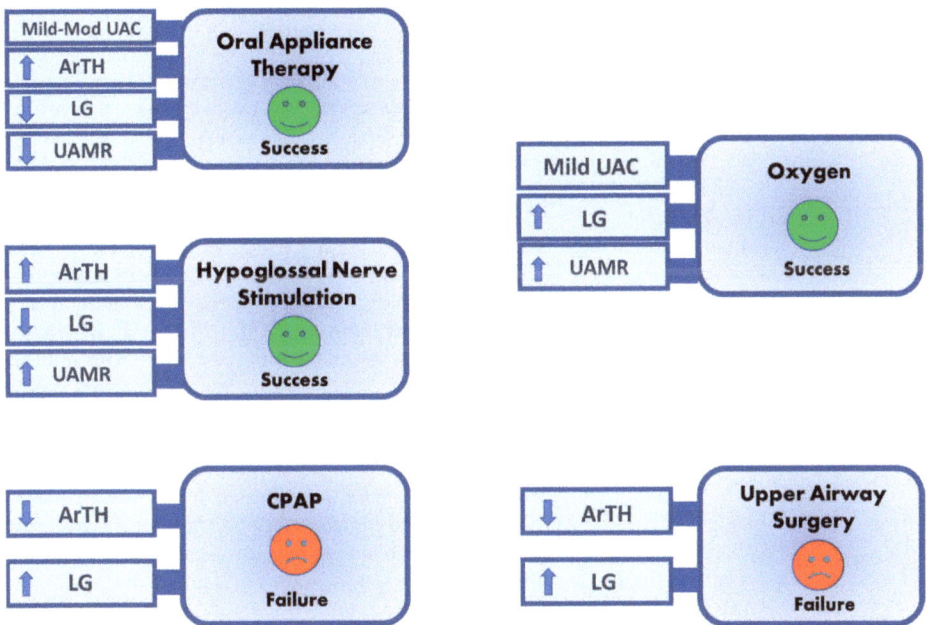

Figure 4. The traits predicting OSA treatment success and failure. Current evidence supporting the use of OSA traits to predict treatment response is summarized here. The identification of patients at risk of failure/success early on may lead to closer monitoring of the therapy and aid in the counseling of patients. ArTH = arousal threshold; LG = loop gain; UAC = upper-airway collapsibility; UAMR = upper-airway muscle responsiveness; up arrow = increased; down arrow = decreased.

5.1. Use of Traits to Predict Responses to OSA Therapy

Most of the literature on the OSA traits and OSA therapy focuses on predicting treatment response. OSA traits may help identify patients at risk of failure of a given treatment early on, prompting the provider to monitor treatment more closely and be prepared to use alternative or adjunctive therapies.

5.1.1. Conventional PAP therapy

CPAP and bilevel PAP therapy are considered conventional forms of PAP therapy. When assessed by the POC tool, a low ArTH was associated with PAP non-adherence (OR 4.4) at 3 months in a sleep clinic cohort [69]. Among non-obese veterans with OSA, a low ArTH (assessed by the POC tool) was also associated with a 45% reduction in long-term use of CPAP therapy. Such findings are consistent across populations and the measurements of OSA traits from polysomnography. In post-stroke patients, a reduction in ArTH of 8% and an increase in UA responsiveness of 33% were associated with a 1 h reduction in CPAP use [70]. Similarly, in patients with coronary artery disease and OSA, a phenotype of low ArTH and extremes of UA muscle responsiveness were associated with an over 2 h/night lower CPAP adherence [71]. In sum, close monitoring is prudent in those with a low ArTH during conventional PAP therapy. If PAP intolerance develops, interventions to improve adherence may be of benefit, including motivational interviewing [72,73], CBTi in those with comorbid insomnia [74], or a short course of a sedative hypnotic [75].

In cases of treatment emergent central sleep apnea, a high LG (>2) may predict persistence of TE-CSA in response to conventional PAP therapy at 1 month [64]. This may be considered when deciding on adaptive servo-ventilation (ASV) at the start of PAP therapy in those with TE-CSA.

5.1.2. Oral Appliance

Oral appliance therapy (OAT), most commonly the mandibular advancement device, can be an effective and tolerable OSA treatment. Several investigations have identified OSA traits that predict patient response to OAT. In a randomized cross-over study, those with mild UA airway collapsibility and a low/normal LG exhibited the highest AHI reductions with OAT [76,77]. In the largest study of 93 patients with AHI scores of $\geq$20/h, a lower LG, higher ArTH, moderate (non-mild and non-severe) UA collapsibility, and weaker dilator muscle compensation [78] predicted a greater AHI reduction. A model of OAT responders (AHI $\geq$ 50%) using these traits exhibited a positive predictive value (PPV) of 83% and a negative predictive value (NPV) of 58%. Notably, none of the clinical parameters, including age, BMI, sex, neck circumference, and REM/NREM AHI, were associated with a change in AHI score with OAT treatment. In summary, those with mild-to-moderate airway collapsibility, lower LG, higher ArTH, and weaker muscle compensation may be better candidates for OAT.

5.1.3. Upper Airway Surgery

UA collapsibility is reduced by surgery, including revised uvulopalatopharyngoplasty with uvula preservation, with or without concomitant transpalatal advancement (TA), pharyngoplasty, genioglossus advancement, and hyoid suspension. A high LG predicts the failure of upper airway surgery to achieve a $\geq$50% reduction in and <10/h post-surgical AHI [79]. Similarly, a low ArTH is associated with surgical failure [80]. Despite potential surgical improvements in UA collapsibility, the remaining abnormalities in LG and ArTH are not modifiable by surgery. Therefore, those with a high LG and/or low ArTH may be at high risk of residual OSA with upper airway surgery.

5.1.4. Hypoglossal Nerve Stimulation

Hypoglossal nerve stimulation is a rapidly growing option for individuals who are intolerant of CPAP therapy. HNS uses a cuff, implanted around the branches of the hypoglossal nerve, to stimulate the genioglossus, protruding it with each breath. Despite stringent selection criteria for this therapy (e.g., BMI < 32 kg/m², lack of complete concentric collapse on sleep endoscopy), about a third of those who are implanted achieve a <50% reduction in and a residual AHI score of ≥20/h [81]. A secondary analysis of the STAR trial of HNS revealed that a high ArTH, low LG, and increased UA muscle responsiveness [82] were associated responses to HNS. Notably, the trait relationships were complex. For example, the LG and ArTH were associated with HNS response in those with mild UA collapsibility. A multivariable prediction model of HNS responders using the OSA traits was better at ruling in success than avoiding failure (PPV and NPV of 83% and 61%, respectively).

5.1.5. Pharmacotherapy

The purpose of the below section is to provide a context of how pharmacotherapy may affect the OSA traits, rather than a comprehensive review of pharmacotherapy in OSA; this can be found elsewhere [83,84]. Notably, most pharmacotherapy studies do not target individuals based on OSA traits, but use OSA severity cut-offs. In addition to these studies, we highlight a few that select patients based on OSA traits.

Supplemental oxygen is a potential adjunctive therapy for OSA. In a physiologic study of six individuals with OSA, oxygen reduced both the LG and AHI score in those with a high LG, but not in those with a low LG [85]. In a larger (n = 36) single-night crossover RCT of oxygen for OSA, a high LG alone did not predict the response to oxygen [86]. However, a high LG in those with mild UA collapsibility and higher UA responsiveness were predictors of oxygen's success (≥50% AHI reduction).

The commonly prescribed sleep aid non-benzodiazepine GABA receptor agonists ("z-drugs"), specifically zolpidem 10 mg and eszopiclone 3 mg, appear to increase the ArTH in those with a low ArTH without impacting airway dilator muscle responsiveness, prolonging respiratory events or worsening hypoxemia [87,88]. A longer term, 1-month RCT of 7.5 mg zopiclone (a stereo-isomer of eszopiclone) in patients with OSA showed no effects on hypoxemia or sleepiness or driving simulator performance [89]. The effects on the AHI were inconsistent in these single-night physiologic studies and showed no changes in the 1-month trial [87–89]. While there is little effect on the AHI, sedative hypnotics may improve adherence to CPAP therapy [75], potentially by raising the ArTH.

Acetazolamide, a carbonic anhydrase inhibitor, has been studied in both OSA and CSA. Acetazolamide causes urinary excretion of bicarbonates with a metabolic acidosis, leading to respiratory compensation by way of increased ventilation. Notably, at this state, the efficiency of CO_2 excretion in the lungs is lower (i.e., acetazolamide lowers LG), which stabilizes breathing [90]. A systematic review that included 28 studies and 542 participants found that acetazolamide reduced AHI scores by 38% or 14/h in those with OSA or CSA compared to the controls. It also improved the SpO_2 nadir by 4 percent [91]. A dose of acetazolamide 500 mg twice daily was shown to reduce LG (with an interquartile range reduction from 2.4–5.4 to 1.4–3.5) [92] and reduce the NREM AHI (from 50/h to 24/h) in those with OSA. Acetazolamide had no significant effect on UA collapsibility, responsiveness or ArTH. Notably, baseline LG alone did not predict a response to acetazolamide [93].

Medications have been studied for their potential role in increasing UAMR. Increasing the endogenous levels of norepinephrine in a rat model showed increases in genioglossus muscle activity during NREM sleep [94]. In another study, a muscarinic receptor antagonist disinhibited hypoglossal motor neuron activity during REM sleep [95]. Therefore, upregulating norepinephrine activity during NREM and antimuscarinic activity in REM sleep exhibits potential to increase genioglossus muscle responsiveness throughout sleep. The combination of atomoxetine, a norepinephrine reuptake inhibitor, and oxybutynin, an antimuscarinic, has been studied in a randomized, placebo-controlled, double-blind, crossover trial comparing one night of 80 mg atomoxetine plus 5 mg oxybutynin (ato–oxy) to a placebo. Ato–oxy reduced AHI scores by 63%, increased genioglossus responsiveness 3-fold, and improved hypoxia [96]. While ato–oxy improved UA collapsibility and UA muscle responsiveness in a secondary analysis of this RCT, baseline traits did not predict a response to ato-oxy. In multivariate analyses, only the baseline AHI and $F_{hypopneas}$ predicted a response to ato-oxy [97]. A more recent, larger (*n* = 211), 4-week trial of atomoxetine and aroxybutynin showed a smaller but meaningful effect size (43% AHI reduction) [98]. Other combinations of noradrenergic-antimuscarinic therapies have been proposed and have undergone small trials, as nicely reviewed by Perger and colleagues [83]. They included reboxetine and oxybutynin, which demonstrated an improvement in UAMR and a 59% reduction in AHI scores at 1 week [99].

Dual orexin receptor antagonists (DORAs) are an emerging class of medications used to treat insomnia. The combination of atomoxetine-lemborexant has been studied in a small trial of 15 individuals with moderately collapsible upper airways. This combination did not significantly reduce the AHI [100]. Studies are needed to determine the potential role of DORAs in affecting the non-anatomical physiological traits and impact on OSA.

Precaution should be taken for the use of these pharmacologic agents in the growing population of older adults living with the OSA. They may be at a higher risk for adverse side effects. For example, Z-drugs may increase the risk of gait instability, falls, and fractures in older adults [101–103]. Acetazolamide may result in moderate to severe metabolic acidosis in older adults [104]. In an atomoxetine-oxybutynin combination, oxybutynin may increase the risk of delirium [105].

5.2. Use of Traits to Guide Multi-Modal Therapy for OSA

Multi-modal therapy is a cornerstone of the management of other chronic disorders (e.g., hypertension and diabetes mellitus), and the management of OSA is likely to be similar. One approach to multi-modal therapy may include addressing anatomic predisposition to OSA (UA collapsibility) alongside adjunctive or rescue therapies targeting physiological traits to improve treatment success.

5.2.1. Targeting Anatomy

Obesity is a key contributor to airway collapsibility. A weight reduction of 15–20% of the BMI in those with OSA significantly reduces P_{crit} (from 3.1 ± 4.2 to -2.4 ± 4.4 cm H_2O). If P_{crit} is sufficiently reduced to below -4 cm H_2O, there is a resolution of respiratory events [106]. Pharmacologic agents that have been shown to reduce the AHI by targeting obesity include liraglutide, semaglutide, naltrexone/bupropion, and orlistat, and by targeting fluid shifts include furosemide and spironolactone [83].

CPAP therapy may decrease P_{crit} by increasing both the retroglossal and retropalatal airway dimensions. A recent study of 14 participants shed light on the differences between mask interfaces from an anatomic-trait perspective. Each participant was titrated to a therapeutic pressure using both an oronasal and a nasal mask. Compared to the nasal mask, the oronasal mask was associated with a higher therapeutic CPAP requirement (+2.6 cm $H_2O \pm 0.5$ cm H_2O) and higher P_{crit} (+2.4 $\pm$ 0.5 cm H_2O) [107].

Oral appliance therapy reduces airway collapsibility in the retropalatal (23–29% reduction) and retroglossal (21–34% reduction) regions [108]. In a mechanistic study of 10 participants with OSA, oral appliance therapy reduced AHI scores from 25.0 ± 3.1 to 13.2 ± 4.5/h and significantly reduced P_{crit} in N2 and slow wave sleep (from -1.6 ± 0.4 to -3.9 ± 0.6 cm H_2O and -2.5 ± 0.7 to -4.7 ± 0.6 cm H_2O, respectively) [109].

Positional therapy is a treatment option for supine-predominant OSA, defined by a supine AHI that is $\geq$2X the non-supine AHI. Positional therapy techniques and devices can help a sleeping individual minimize time spent in the supine position. UC collapsibility (P_{crit}) decreases significantly when moving from a supine to a lateral position (supine Pcrit mean 2.5 cm H_2O, CI 1.4–3.6 to lateral PCrit mean 0.3 cm H_2O, CI −0.8–1.4) [110], with changes that remain significant regardless of the sleep stage [111]. The change in P_{crit} from a supine to a lateral position is comparable to that with oral appliance therapy [112]. The benefits of positional therapy may not be limited to improvement in airway collapsibility. Some studies [112] (but not all) [32] also show a reduction in LG. This is consistent with observations that central sleep apnea (a condition characterized by a high LG) is less severe in a lateral compared to a supine position [113,114].

5.2.2. Combination Therapy

Currently, combination therapy in OSA is considered a form of salvage treatment when the first-line therapy is inadequate. Several common clinical scenarios and potential "rescue" therapy approaches are shown in Figure 5. This approach may be promising in cases of inadequate efficacy (e.g., a high residual AHI score) or adherence, and reflects potential off-label use of some treatments (e.g., acetazolamide). To date, there are no algorithms utilizing OSA traits to address PAP failure. Notably, the approaches in Figure 5 are "off-label" and require validation in clinical trials. In addition, there are also individuals who are adherent to PAP therapy with a low residual AHI score who experience an inadequate treatment response due to persistent, excessive daytime sleepiness. The potential mechanisms of and therapy for residual hypersomnia secondary to OSA are described in detail by Javaheri et al. [115].

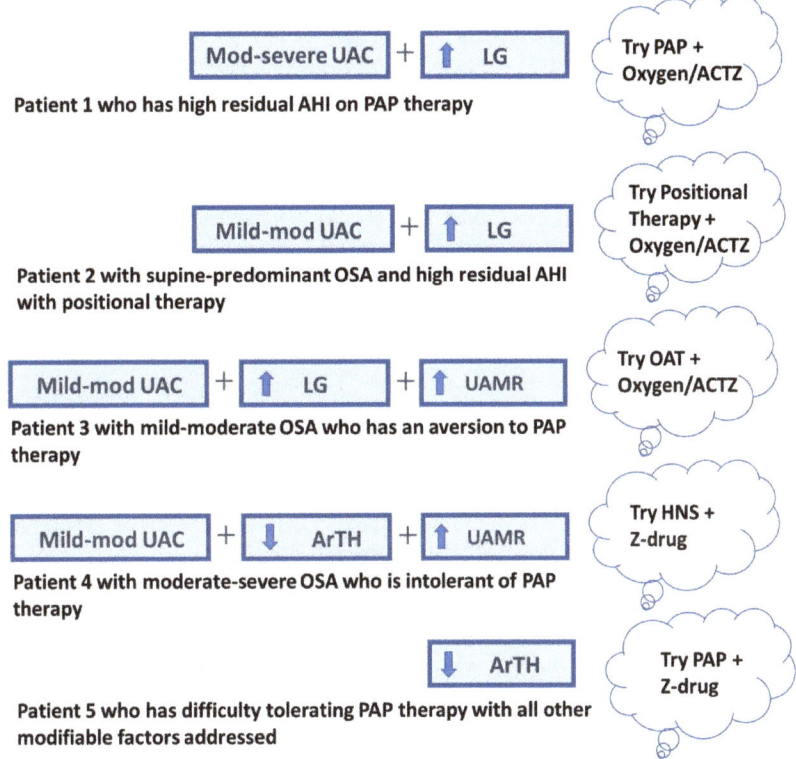

Figure 5. Examples of common patient scenarios in which the traits may be used to help select a "rescue" therapy. Patient 1 uses PAP therapy with good adherence, but data downloads show a high residual AHI score (e.g., AHI > 15/h). A review of this individual's CPAP titration study shows evidence of moderate-severe UA collapsibility (UAC) (i.e., CPAP requirement > 8 cm H_2O), and a high LG (NREM predominant OSA with "zipper" pattern on oximetry); therefore, a trial of oxygen and/or ACTZ with PAP therapy may be considered. Patient 2 is different from patient 1 in that this individual has mild-moderate UAC and supine-predominant OSA and a high LG (NREM predominant and a high LG (NREM predominant OSA with "zipper" pattern on oximetry); therefore,

and a high LG (NREM predominant OSA with "zipper" pattern on oximetry); therefore, a trial of oxygen and/or ACTZ with PAP therapy may be considered. Patient 2 is different from patient 1 in that this individual has mild-moderate UAC and supine-predominant OSA (supine AHI $\geq$ 2X the non-supine AHI), for which positional therapy is a potential first-line treatment. If this patient also fails positional therapy due to a high residual AHI score, oxygen and/or ACTZ can be added to positional therapy in a setting of high LG. Patient 3 is someone with mild-moderate OSA with an aversion to PAP therapy (e.g., claustrophobic with PAP) and chooses OAT. Due to a high LG and increased UAMR (see Table 2 for POC tool for LG, UAMR can be estimated using Sands et al. [58]), the predicted response to OAT alone will be inadequate; therefore, oxygen and/or ACTZ can be added. Patient 4 has moderate to severe OSA and was started on PAP therapy but ultimately discontinued therapy due to intolerance. The mild-to-moderate UAC and increased UAMR makes HNS a favorable option; however, with a low ArTH (as determined with the POC tool described in Table 2), HNS alone may not be effective at reducing the AHI. Therefore, a Z-drug can be used to raise the ArTH, in combination with HNS. Patient 5 has OSA and is using PAP therapy with difficulty tolerating therapy, frequently waking up from therapy, and is unable to keep the PAP interface on for the entire sleep duration. All other modifiable factors have been addressed (e.g., weight reduction, avoidance of alcohol, etc.). A review of the diagnostic sleep study reveals a low ArTH (see Table 2), and the addition of a Z-drug to PAP therapy can be considered. LG = loop gain; ACTZ = acetazolamide; ArTH = arousal threshold; HNS = hypoglossal nerve stimulation; OAT = oral appliance therapy; PAP = positive airway pressure; UAC = upper-airway collapsibility; UAMR = upper-airway muscle responsiveness; Z-drug = non-benzodiazepine GABA receptor agonist; up arrow = increased; down arrow = decreased.

Combining UA anatomy-targeted therapies can improve efficacy. For example, the combination of positional therapy and OAT is more efficacious than either positional therapy or OAT alone [116]. The combination of CPAP therapy with oral appliances can treat OSA when OAT alone is ineffective, while reducing CPAP requirement (~9 cm H_2O less with combined OAT and CPAP therapy than on CPAP therapy alone) [117]. Therefore, combination therapy may be a good option for those who are pressure intolerant.

Combining CPAP therapy with "z drugs" may improve adherence. A systemic review of eight studies showed an increase of 0.62 h of daily CPAP use and a 12% increase in the percentage of nights used compared to CPAP therapy alone. Eszopiclone had the most significant impact on adherence [118]. Notably, such studies include unselected patients with OSA. Some data suggest that hypnotics in those with a low ArTH might be of particular benefit [119]. A combination of a therapy to address UA collapsibility (e.g., CPAP or OAT) and a high LG (acetazolamide or oxygen) may be one way to improve the efficacy of OSA treatment [120,121].

A stepwise approach, addressing UA anatomy, followed by targeting physiological traits was examined in a study of 23 participants with OSA [122]. Participants who had a residual AHI score of >10/h with OAT alone (addressing UA anatomy) were included in a step-wise approach for additional therapy. The addition of expiratory positive airway pressure (EPAP) valve and positional therapy resulted in an AHI score of <10/h in 10 participants. A predictor of success was supine-dependent OSA. Of the remaining ten, five participants with high LG achieved therapeutic control with the addition of oxygen. Two with poor airway muscle responsiveness achieved control with atomoxetine-oxybutynin added to OAT, EPAP therapy, and positional therapy or oxygen. Of the remainder, two required CPAP therapy, and another was CPAP intolerant [122]. None of the participants qualified for the addition of a hypnotic. Three were lost to follow-up or declined further participation. While this was an exploratory study, it offers a perspective on how these traits may inform targeted combination therapy, a precision medicine approach in OSA.

5.3. Targeting Traits to Select Initial Therapy

Targeting the OSA traits to select the first-line therapy for each patient is the "holy grail" of physiology-based precision medicine to treat sleep apnea. For example, the combination of oxygen (lowering LG) and eszopiclone (raising the ArTH) may be effective in someone with mild UA collapsibility. In a randomized crossover study of this combination among those with an AHI score of $\geq$10/h, 9/20 participants responded to this combination (>50% reduction and <15/h residual AHI) in those with mild UA collapsibility [123]. Thus, in theory, carefully selecting individuals with mild-moderate UA collapsibility, high LG and a low ArTH for pharmacologic-only treatment may be viable. However, the baseline traits targeted by oxygen (LG) and eszopiclone (ArTH) in the above study did not predict treatment success, while a mild to moderately collapsible UA, and increased UA muscle responsiveness did. This highlights the complexity of targeting the OSA traits to select a first-line therapy in OSA. To date, no studies have prospectively targeted treatment based on a trait (or trait combinations) to assess effectiveness of a therapy.

6. Current Limitations

Physiological traits are promising for personalizing OSA therapy. However, several critical barriers exist. First, it is unclear to what degree each trait is a cause or a consequence of OSA. Hence, in this review, we use the term "trait" (a characteristic) and not "endotype" (pathogenic mechanism). For example, a low ArTH may be a phenotype (rather than an endotype) because the ArTH is lowered with the treatment of OSA and is more common in those with lower OSA severity [42]. Thus, a low ArTH may simply serve as a biomarker of treatment effectiveness (e.g., adherence). If the traits reflect OSA's consequences rather than causes, targeting them may not effectively eliminate UA obstruction (and may be the reason why baseline traits do not consistently predict a response to therapy targeting those traits). Second, an easy-to-use method that determines how much each trait, especially in combination with others, contributes to OSA in each individual is not yet available. Therefore, potential treatment decisions are based on arbitrary cut-offs of high versus low trait values or statistical models of a combination of traits. Such approaches are unlikely to be reproducible across patient cohorts, as prediction models in one cohort differ from models in another [77,78]. Finally, and most importantly, current studies of OSA traits and clinical outcomes are short-term, often lasting a single night, and most focus on the outcome of AHI reduction as a metric of success. Longitudinal studies examining patient-centered outcomes such as quality of life, function, and adverse consequences of OSA (e.g., endothelial function, blood pressure, neurocognition) are needed. If evidence supports targeting traits to improve patient-centered outcomes in OSA, studies assessing the implementation of a trait-based approach, including ease of use, cost, and applicability across demographic and social determinants of health, will be important.

7. Future Directions

Our vision for the future is for sleep providers to be able to routinely assess anatomic and non-anatomic contributors to OSA in clinical settings to (1) promote a shared decision-making process in selecting efficacious and tolerable therapy and (2) improve patient-centered outcomes.

In order for this vision to be realized, additional physiologic research as well as implementation science work are needed to address both the use of traits to predict treatment responses and to target traits for a more precise treatment approach. Below are the key challenges to be addressed:

(1) Standardized, reliable, and reproducible tools must be developed to measure the OSA traits using readily available clinical data (e.g., home respiratory polygraphy, wearables). Such tools should integrate how much each trait, or trait combination, contributes to OSA severity in each individual.
(2) A better understanding is required of how traits relate to clinical phenotypes (e.g., the ArTH and LG in those with OSA and insomnia) and their contributions to OSA

in those with common, co-morbid conditions (e.g., post-traumatic stress disorder, chronic obstructive pulmonary disease, opioid dependence).
(3) Studies are needed to determine the effect sizes of interventions targeting the OSA traits (e.g., acetazolamide for high LG) and their impact on OSA severity.
(4) Prospective validation of the traits (or their combinations) is needed to predict treatment responses to established therapies (e.g., randomization to a sedative-hypnotic vs. a placebo with CPAP based on the ArTH to assess the impact on CPAP adherence, daytime function, and quality of life).
(5) Longer-term (at least 3–6 months), randomized clinical trial studies on patient-centered outcomes are needed, for both prediction of outcomes and modification of the OSA traits to improve OSA outcomes. Studies should examine prognostic markers that are more effective than the AHI in assessing OSA alleviation (e.g., hypoxic burden, heart rate response), adherence, patient symptoms, function, and quality of life.
(6) Because little is known about the role of OSA traits in patient outcomes in non-white and non-male individuals, an assessment of traits in pathogenesis, clinical manifestations, and treatment outcomes in non-white and female populations is needed.

8. Summary

The interplay of the four key OSA traits, including UA airway collapsibility capturing anatomical predisposition and the remaining physiological traits of LG, ArTH, and upper-airway muscle responsiveness, can result in different pathways to OSA among individuals. These unique combinations offer a potential approach for precision medicine approach in OSA. For example, retrospective studies demonstrate that the traits predict treatment response of established therapies for OSA, including CPAP therapy, oral appliances, and hypoglossal nerve stimulation. Recent advances in the field show that these traits can be estimated from clinical data, including signal processing of polysomnography or even simple event-count-per-hour metrics such as the AHI, the fraction of hypopneas and the oxygen saturation nadir (Table 2). While not yet ready for "prime time", using these traits to select multi-modal rescue therapies for those failed by CPAP therapy can be a significant step towards improving the "one-size fits all" CPAP approach. The ultimate goal is to use these traits to select initial treatment. For now, the focus of the OSA field should include developing scalable and reliable methods for their assessment and longitudinal patient-centered validation of the OSA traits' utility for therapy selection (see Table 2).

Funding: This manuscript was supported by National Heart, Lung, and Blood Institute grant K23HL159259 (AZ).

Institutional Review Board Statement: Not applicable.

Informed Consent Statement: Not applicable.

Data Availability Statement: Not applicable.

Conflicts of Interest: The authors declare no conflict of interest.

References

1. Benjafield, A.V.; Ayas, N.T.; Eastwood, P.R.; Heinzer, R.; Ip, M.S.M.; Morrell, M.J.; Nunez, C.M.; Patel, S.R.; Penzel, T.; Pepin, J.L.; et al. Estimation of the global prevalence and burden of obstructive sleep apnoea: A literature-based analysis. *Lancet Respir. Med.* **2019**, *7*, 687–698. [CrossRef] [PubMed]
2. Young, T.; Skatrud, J.; Peppard, P.E. Risk factors for obstructive sleep apnea in adults. *JAMA* **2004**, *291*, 2013–2016. [CrossRef] [PubMed]
3. Young, T.; Palta, M.; Dempsey, J.; Skatrud, J.; Weber, S.; Badr, S. The occurrence of sleep-disordered breathing among middle-aged adults. *N. Engl. J. Med.* **1993**, *328*, 1230–1235. [CrossRef] [PubMed]
4. Levy, P.; Kohler, M.; McNicholas, W.T.; Barbe, F.; McEvoy, R.D.; Somers, V.K.; Lavie, L.; Pepin, J.L. Obstructive sleep apnoea syndrome. *Nat. Rev. Dis. Primers* **2015**, *1*, 15015. [CrossRef] [PubMed]
5. Gupta, M.A.; Simpson, F.C. Obstructive sleep apnea and psychiatric disorders: A systematic review. *J. Clin. Sleep Med.* **2015**, *11*, 165–175. [CrossRef]

6. Vanek, J.; Prasko, J.; Genzor, S.; Ociskova, M.; Kantor, K.; Holubova, M.; Slepecky, M.; Nesnidal, V.; Kolek, A.; Sova, M. Obstructive sleep apnea, depression and cognitive impairment. *Sleep Med.* **2020**, *72*, 50–58. [CrossRef]
7. Sircu, V.; Colesnic, S.I.; Covantsev, S.; Corlateanu, O.; Sukhotko, A.; Popovici, C.; Corlateanu, A. The Burden of Comorbidities in Obstructive Sleep Apnea and the Pathophysiologic Mechanisms and Effects of CPAP. *Clocks Sleep* **2023**, *5*, 333–349. [CrossRef]
8. Cao, M.T.; Sternbach, J.M.; Guilleminault, C. Continuous positive airway pressure therapy in obstuctive sleep apnea: Benefits and alternatives. *Expert. Rev. Respir. Med.* **2017**, *11*, 259–272. [CrossRef]
9. Hidden Health Crisis Costing America Billions. Underdiagnosing and Undertreating Obstructive Sleep Apnea Draining Healthcare System. American Academy of Sleep Medicine. Available online: http://www.aasmnet.org/sleep-apnea-economic-impact.aspx (accessed on 29 February 2024).
10. Patel, S.R.; Bakker, J.P.; Stitt, C.J.; Aloia, M.S.; Nouraie, S.M. Age and Sex Disparities in Adherence to CPAP. *Chest* **2021**, *159*, 382–389. [CrossRef]
11. Pandey, A.; Mereddy, S.; Combs, D.; Shetty, S.; Patel, S.I.; Mashaq, S.; Seixas, A.; Littlewood, K.; Jean-Luis, G.; Parthasarathy, S. Socioeconomic Inequities in Adherence to Positive Airway Pressure Therapy in Population-Level Analysis. *J. Clin. Med.* **2020**, *9*, 442. [CrossRef]
12. Bakker, J.P.; Weaver, T.E.; Parthasarathy, S.; Aloia, M.S. Adherence to CPAP: What Should We Be Aiming For, and How Can We Get There? *Chest* **2019**, *155*, 1272–1287. [CrossRef]
13. Crawford, M.R.; Espie, C.A.; Bartlett, D.J.; Grunstein, R.R. Integrating psychology and medicine in CPAP adherence--new concepts? *Sleep Med. Rev.* **2014**, *18*, 123–139. [CrossRef] [PubMed]
14. Rotenberg, B.W.; Murariu, D.; Pang, K.P. Trends in CPAP adherence over twenty years of data collection: A flattened curve. *J. Otolaryngol. Head. Neck Surg.* **2016**, *45*, 43. [CrossRef] [PubMed]
15. Gupta, A.; Shukla, G. Polysomnographic determinants of requirement for advanced positive pressure therapeutic options for obstructive sleep apnea. *Sleep Breath.* **2018**, *22*, 401–409. [CrossRef] [PubMed]
16. Mulgrew, A.T.; Lawati, N.A.; Ayas, N.T.; Fox, N.; Hamilton, P.; Cortes, L.; Ryan, C.F. Residual sleep apnea on polysomnography after 3 months of CPAP therapy: Clinical implications, predictors and patterns. *Sleep Med.* **2010**, *11*, 119–125. [CrossRef] [PubMed]
17. Wells, R.D.; Freedland, K.E.; Carney, R.M.; Duntley, S.P.; Stepanski, E.J. Adherence, reports of benefits, and depression among patients treated with continuous positive airway pressure. *Psychosom. Med.* **2007**, *69*, 449–454. [CrossRef] [PubMed]
18. Epstein, L.J.; Kristo, D.; Strollo, P.J., Jr.; Friedman, N.; Malhotra, A.; Patil, S.P.; Ramar, K.; Rogers, R.; Schwab, R.J.; Weaver, E.M.; et al. Clinical guideline for the evaluation, management and long-term care of obstructive sleep apnea in adults. *J. Clin. Sleep Med.* **2009**, *5*, 263–276.
19. Malhotra, A.; Mesarwi, O.; Pepin, J.L.; Owens, R.L. Endotypes and phenotypes in obstructive sleep apnea. *Curr. Opin. Pulm. Med.* **2020**, *26*, 609–614. [CrossRef]
20. Zinchuk, A.V.; Gentry, M.J.; Concato, J.; Yaggi, H.K. Phenotypes in obstructive sleep apnea: A definition, examples and evolution of approaches. *Sleep Med. Rev.* **2017**, *35*, 113–123. [CrossRef]
21. Edwards, B.A.; Redline, S.; Sands, S.A.; Owens, R.L. More than the Sum of the Respiratory Events: Personalized Medicine Approaches for Obstructive Sleep Apnea. *Am. J. Respir. Crit. Care Med.* **2020**, *200*, 691–703. [CrossRef]
22. Zinchuk, A.; Yaggi, H.K. Phenotypic Subtypes of OSA: A Challenge and Opportunity for Precision Medicine. *Chest* **2020**, *157*, 403–420. [CrossRef]
23. Martinez-Garcia, M.A.; Campos-Rodriguez, F.; Barbe, F.; Gozal, D.; Agusti, A. Precision medicine in obstructive sleep apnoea. *Lancet Respir. Med.* **2019**, *7*, 456–464. [CrossRef]
24. Sutherland, K.; Yee, B.J.; Kairaitis, K.; Wheatley, J.; de Chazal, P.; Cistulli, P.A. A Phenotypic Approach for Personalised Management of Obstructive Sleep Apnoea. *Curr. Otorhinolaryngol. Rep.* **2021**, *9*, 223–237. [CrossRef]
25. Eckert, D.J.; White, D.P.; Jordan, A.S.; Malhotra, A.; Wellman, A. Defining phenotypic causes of obstructive sleep apnea. Identification of novel therapeutic targets. *Am. J. Respir. Crit. Care Med.* **2013**, *188*, 996–1004. [CrossRef]
26. Owens, R.L.; Edwards, B.A.; Eckert, D.J.; Jordan, A.S.; Sands, S.A.; Malhotra, A.; White, D.P.; Loring, S.H.; Butler, J.P.; Wellman, A. An Integrative Model of Physiological Traits Can be Used to Predict Obstructive Sleep Apnea and Response to Non Positive Airway Pressure Therapy. *Sleep* **2015**, *38*, 961–970. [CrossRef]
27. Kazemeini, E.; Van de Perck, E.; Dieltjens, M.; Willemen, M.; Verbraecken, J.; Op de Beeck, S.; Vanderveken, O.M. Critical to Know Pcrit: A Review on Pharyngeal Critical Closing Pressure in Obstructive Sleep Apnea. *Front. Neurol.* **2022**, *13*, 775709. [CrossRef]
28. Gold, A.R.; Schwartz, A.R. The pharyngeal critical pressure. The whys and hows of using nasal continuous positive airway pressure diagnostically. *Chest* **1996**, *110*, 1077–1088. [CrossRef] [PubMed]
29. Kirkness, J.P.; Schwartz, A.R.; Schneider, H.; Punjabi, N.M.; Maly, J.J.; Laffan, A.M.; McGinley, B.M.; Magnuson, T.; Schweitzer, M.; Smith, P.L.; et al. Contribution of male sex, age, and obesity to mechanical instability of the upper airway during sleep. *J. Appl. Physiol.* **2008**, *104*, 1618–1624. [CrossRef]
30. Wilson, S.L.; Thach, B.T.; Brouillette, R.T.; Abu-Osba, Y.K. Upper airway patency in the human infant: Influence of airway pressure and posture. *J. Appl. Physiol. Respir. Environ. Exerc. Physiol.* **1980**, *48*, 500–504. [CrossRef] [PubMed]
31. Owens, R.L.; Malhotra, A.; Eckert, D.J.; White, D.P.; Jordan, A.S. The influence of end-expiratory lung volume on measurements of pharyngeal collapsibility. *J. Appl. Physiol.* **2010**, *108*, 445–451. [CrossRef] [PubMed]
32. Joosten, S.A.; Edwards, B.A.; Wellman, A.; Turton, A.; Skuza, E.M.; Berger, P.J.; Hamilton, G.S. The Effect of Body Position on Physiological Factors that Contribute to Obstructive Sleep Apnea. *Sleep* **2015**, *38*, 1469–1478. [CrossRef]

33. Jordan, A.S.; Wellman, A.; Edwards, J.K.; Schory, K.; Dover, L.; MacDonald, M.; Patel, S.R.; Fogel, R.B.; Malhotra, A.; White, D.P. Respiratory control stability and upper airway collapsibility in men and women with obstructive sleep apnea. *J. Appl. Physiol.* **2005**, *99*, 2020–2027. [CrossRef]
34. Malhotra, A.; Huang, Y.; Fogel, R.B.; Pillar, G.; Edwards, J.K.; Kikinis, R.; Loring, S.H.; White, D.P. The male predisposition to pharyngeal collapse: Importance of airway length. *Am. J. Respir. Crit. Care Med.* **2002**, *166*, 1388–1395. [CrossRef] [PubMed]
35. Haxhiu, M.A.; Mitra, J.; van Lunteren, E.; Prabhakar, N.; Bruce, E.N.; Cherniack, N.S. Responses of hypoglossal and phrenic nerves to decreased respiratory drive in cats. *Respiration* **1986**, *50*, 130–138. [CrossRef]
36. Badr, M.S.; Toiber, F.; Skatrud, J.B.; Dempsey, J. Pharyngeal narrowing/occlusion during central sleep apnea. *J. Appl. Physiol.* **1995**, *78*, 1806–1815. [CrossRef] [PubMed]
37. Giannoni, A.; Gentile, F.; Navari, A.; Borrelli, C.; Mirizzi, G.; Catapano, G.; Vergaro, G.; Grotti, F.; Betta, M.; Piepoli, M.F.; et al. Contribution of the Lung to the Genesis of Cheyne-Stokes Respiration in Heart Failure: Plant Gain Beyond Chemoreflex Gain and Circulation Time. *J. Am. Heart Assoc.* **2019**, *8*, e012419. [CrossRef]
38. Carberry, J.C.; Jordan, A.S.; White, D.P.; Wellman, A.; Eckert, D.J. Upper Airway Collapsibility (Pcrit) and Pharyngeal Dilator Muscle Activity are Sleep Stage Dependent. *Sleep* **2016**, *39*, 511–521. [CrossRef] [PubMed]
39. Eckert, D.J.; Malhotra, A.; Lo, Y.L.; White, D.P.; Jordan, A.S. The influence of obstructive sleep apnea and gender on genioglossus activity during rapid eye movement sleep. *Chest* **2009**, *135*, 957–964. [CrossRef]
40. Sands, S.A.; Eckert, D.J.; Jordan, A.S.; Edwards, B.A.; Owens, R.L.; Butler, J.P.; Schwab, R.J.; Loring, S.H.; Malhotra, A.; White, D.P.; et al. Enhanced upper-airway muscle responsiveness is a distinct feature of overweight/obese individuals without sleep apnea. *Am. J. Respir. Crit. Care Med.* **2014**, *190*, 930–937. [CrossRef]
41. Popovic, R.M.; White, D.P. Upper airway muscle activity in normal women: Influence of hormonal status. *J. Appl. Physiol.* **1998**, *84*, 1055–1062. [CrossRef]
42. Eckert, D.J.; Younes, M.K. Arousal from sleep: Implications for obstructive sleep apnea pathogenesis and treatment. *J. Appl. Physiol.* **2014**, *116*, 302–313. [CrossRef]
43. Remmers, J.E.; de Groot, W.J.; Sauerland, E.K.; Anch, A.M. Pathogenesis of upper airway occlusion during sleep. *J. Appl. Physiol. Respir. Environ. Exerc. Physiol.* **1978**, *44*, 931–938. [CrossRef]
44. Hoshino, T.; Sasanabe, R.; Murotani, K.; Hori, R.; Mano, M.; Nomura, A.; Konishi, N.; Baku, M.; Nishio, Y.; Kato, C.; et al. Estimated respiratory arousal threshold in patients with rapid eye movement obstructive sleep apnea. *Sleep Breath.* **2022**, *26*, 347–353. [CrossRef]
45. Zinchuk, A.; Edwards, B.A.; Jeon, S.; Koo, B.B.; Concato, J.; Sands, S.; Wellman, A.; Yaggi, H.K. Prevalence, Associated Clinical Features, and Impact on Continuous Positive Airway Pressure Use of a Low Respiratory Arousal Threshold Among Male United States Veterans With Obstructive Sleep Apnea. *J. Clin. Sleep Med.* **2018**, *14*, 809–817. [CrossRef] [PubMed]
46. McCall, C.A.; Watson, N.F. A Narrative Review of the Association between Post-Traumatic Stress Disorder and Obstructive Sleep Apnea. *J. Clin. Med.* **2022**, *11*, 415. [CrossRef] [PubMed]
47. Sands, S.A.; Alex, R.M.; Mann, D.; Vena, D.; Terrill, P.I.; Gell, L.K.; Zinchuk, A.; Sofer, T.; Patel, S.R.; Taranto-Montemurro, L.; et al. Pathophysiology Underlying Demographic and Obesity Determinants of Sleep Apnea Severity. *Ann. Am. Thorac. Soc.* **2023**, *20*, 440–449. [CrossRef] [PubMed]
48. Lee, R.W.; Vasudavan, S.; Hui, D.S.; Prvan, T.; Petocz, P.; Darendeliler, M.A.; Cistulli, P.A. Differences in craniofacial structures and obesity in Caucasian and Chinese patients with obstructive sleep apnea. *Sleep* **2010**, *33*, 1075–1080. [CrossRef]
49. Lee, R.W.W.; Sutherland, K.; Sands, S.A.; Edwards, B.A.; Chan, T.O.; Ng, S.S.S.; Hui, D.S.; Cistulli, P.A. Differences in respiratory arousal threshold in Caucasian and Chinese patients with obstructive sleep apnoea. *Respirology* **2017**, *22*, 1015–1021. [CrossRef] [PubMed]
50. Messineo, L.; Lonni, S.; Magri, R.; Pedroni, L.; Taranto-Montemurro, L.; Corda, L.; Tantucci, C. Lung air trapping lowers respiratory arousal threshold and contributes to sleep apnea pathogenesis in COPD patients with overlap syndrome. *Respir. Physiol. Neurobiol.* **2020**, *271*, 103315. [CrossRef]
51. Messineo, L.; Eckert, D.J.; Taranto-Montemurro, L.; Vena, D.; Azarbarzin, A.; Hess, L.B.; Calianese, N.; White, D.P.; Wellman, A.; Gell, L.; et al. Ventilatory Drive Withdrawal Rather Than Reduced Genioglossus Compensation as a Mechanism of Obstructive Sleep Apnea in REM Sleep. *Am. J. Respir. Crit. Care Med.* **2022**, *205*, 219–232. [CrossRef] [PubMed]
52. Brooker, E.J.; Landry, S.A.; Thomson, L.D.J.; Hamilton, G.S.; Genta, P.; Drummond, S.P.A.; Edwards, B.A. Obstructive Sleep Apnea Is a Distinct Physiological Endotype in Individuals with Comorbid Insomnia and Sleep Apnea (COMISA). *Ann. Am. Thorac. Soc.* **2023**, *10*, 1508–1515. [CrossRef]
53. El-Solh, A.A.; Lawson, Y.; Wilding, G.E. Impact of low arousal threshold on treatment of obstructive sleep apnea in patients with post-traumatic stress disorder. *Sleep Breath.* **2021**, *25*, 597–604. [CrossRef]
54. Eckert, D.J. Phenotypic approaches to obstructive sleep apnoea—New pathways for targeted therapy. *Sleep Med. Rev.* **2018**, *37*, 45–59. [CrossRef]
55. Issa, F.G.; Sullivan, C.E. Upper airway closing pressures in obstructive sleep apnea. *J. Appl. Physiol. Respir. Environ. Exerc. Physiol.* **1984**, *57*, 520–527. [CrossRef]
56. Wellman, A.; Eckert, D.J.; Jordan, A.S.; Edwards, B.A.; Passaglia, C.L.; Jackson, A.C.; Gautam, S.; Owens, R.L.; Malhotra, A.; White, D.P. A method for measuring and modeling the physiological traits causing obstructive sleep apnea. *J. Appl. Physiol.* **2011**, *110*, 1627–1637. [CrossRef]

57. O'Connor, C.M.; Lowery, M.M.; Doherty, L.S.; McHugh, M.; O'Muircheartaigh, C.; Cullen, J.; Nolan, P.; McNicholas, W.T.; O'Malley, M.J. Improved surface EMG electrode for measuring genioglossus muscle activity. *Respir. Physiol. Neurobiol.* **2007**, *159*, 55–67. [CrossRef]
58. Sands, S.A.; Edwards, B.A.; Terrill, P.I.; Taranto-Montemurro, L.; Azarbarzin, A.; Marques, M.; Hess, L.B.; White, D.P.; Wellman, A. Phenotyping Pharyngeal Pathophysiology using Polysomnography in Patients with Obstructive Sleep Apnea. *Am. J. Respir. Crit. Care Med.* **2018**, *197*, 1187–1197. [CrossRef] [PubMed]
59. Terrill, P.I.; Edwards, B.A.; Nemati, S.; Butler, J.P.; Owens, R.L.; Eckert, D.J.; White, D.P.; Malhotra, A.; Wellman, A.; Sands, S.A. Quantifying the ventilatory control contribution to sleep apnoea using polysomnography. *Eur. Respir. J.* **2015**, *45*, 408–418. [CrossRef] [PubMed]
60. Sands, S.A.; Terrill, P.I.; Edwards, B.A.; Taranto Montemurro, L.; Azarbarzin, A.; Marques, M.; de Melo, C.M.; Loring, S.H.; Butler, J.P.; White, D.P.; et al. Quantifying the Arousal Threshold Using Polysomnography in Obstructive Sleep Apnea. *Sleep* **2018**, *41*, zsx183. [CrossRef]
61. Gell, L.K.; Vena, D.; Alex, R.M.; Azarbarzin, A.; Calianese, N.; Hess, L.B.; Taranto-Montemurro, L.; White, D.P.; Wellman, A.; Sands, S.A. Neural ventilatory drive decline as a predominant mechanism of obstructive sleep apnoea events. *Thorax* **2022**, *77*, 707–716. [CrossRef] [PubMed]
62. Landry, S.A.; Joosten, S.A.; Eckert, D.J.; Jordan, A.S.; Sands, S.A.; White, D.P.; Malhotra, A.; Wellman, A.; Hamilton, G.S.; Edwards, B.A. Therapeutic CPAP Level Predicts Upper Airway Collapsibility in Patients With Obstructive Sleep Apnea. *Sleep* **2017**, *40*, zsx056. [CrossRef]
63. Schmickl, C.N.; Orr, J.E.; Kim, P.; Nokes, B.; Sands, S.; Manoharan, S.; McGinnis, L.; Parra, G.; DeYoung, P.; Owens, R.L.; et al. Point-of-care prediction model of loop gain in patients with obstructive sleep apnea: Development and validation. *BMC Pulm. Med.* **2022**, *22*, 158. [CrossRef]
64. Stanchina, M.; Robinson, K.; Corrao, W.; Donat, W.; Sands, S.; Malhotra, A. Clinical Use of Loop Gain Measures to Determine Continuous Positive Airway Pressure Efficacy in Patients with Complex Sleep Apnea. A Pilot Study. *Ann. Am. Thorac. Soc.* **2015**, *12*, 1351–1357. [CrossRef]
65. Edwards, B.A.; Eckert, D.J.; McSharry, D.G.; Sands, S.A.; Desai, A.; Kehlmann, G.; Bakker, J.P.; Genta, P.R.; Owens, R.L.; White, D.P.; et al. Clinical predictors of the respiratory arousal threshold in patients with obstructive sleep apnea. *Am. J. Respir. Crit. Care Med.* **2014**, *190*, 1293–1300. [CrossRef]
66. Dutta, R.; Delaney, G.; Toson, B.; Jordan, A.S.; White, D.P.; Wellman, A.; Eckert, D.J. A Novel Model to Estimate Key Obstructive Sleep Apnea Endotypes from Standard Polysomnography and Clinical Data and Their Contribution to Obstructive Sleep Apnea Severity. *Ann. Am. Thorac. Soc.* **2021**, *18*, 656–667. [CrossRef] [PubMed]
67. Zinchuk, A.; Yaggi, H.K. Treatment-Emergent Central Sleep Apnea. In *Complex Sleep Breathing Disorders*; Won, C., Ed.; Springer: Berlin/Heidelberg, Germany, 2021; pp. 92–94.
68. Joosten, S.A.; Landry, S.A.; Wong, A.M.; Mann, D.L.; Terrill, P.I.; Sands, S.A.; Turton, A.; Beatty, C.; Thomson, L.; Hamilton, G.S.; et al. Assessing the Physiologic Endotypes Responsible for REM- and NREM-Based OSA. *Chest* **2021**, *159*, 1998–2007. [CrossRef] [PubMed]
69. Wu, H.; Fang, F.; Wu, C.; Zhan, X.; Wei, Y. Low arousal threshold is associated with unfavorable shift of PAP compliance over time in patients with OSA. *Sleep Breath.* **2021**, *25*, 887–895. [CrossRef] [PubMed]
70. Zinchuk, A.V.; Redeker, N.S.; Chu, J.H.; Liang, J.; Stepnowsky, C.; Brandt, C.A.; Bravata, D.M.; Wellman, A.; Sands, S.A.; Yaggi, H.K. Physiological Traits and Adherence to Obstructive Sleep Apnea Treatment in Patients with Stroke. *Am. J. Respir. Crit. Care Med.* **2020**, *201*, 1568–1572. [CrossRef]
71. Zinchuk, A.V.; Chu, J.H.; Liang, J.; Celik, Y.; Op de Beeck, S.; Redeker, N.S.; Wellman, A.; Yaggi, H.K.; Peker, Y.; Sands, S.A. Physiological Traits and Adherence to Sleep Apnea Therapy in Individuals with Coronary Artery Disease. *Am. J. Respir. Crit. Care Med.* **2021**, *204*, 703–712. [CrossRef]
72. Bakker, J.P.; Wang, R.; Weng, J.; Aloia, M.S.; Toth, C.; Morrical, M.G.; Gleason, K.J.; Rueschman, M.; Dorsey, C.; Patel, S.R.; et al. Motivational Enhancement for Increasing Adherence to CPAP: A Randomized Controlled Trial. *Chest* **2016**, *150*, 337–345. [CrossRef] [PubMed]
73. Olsen, S.; Smith, S.S.; Oei, T.P.; Douglas, J. Motivational interviewing (MINT) improves continuous positive airway pressure (CPAP) acceptance and adherence: A randomized controlled trial. *J. Consult. Clin. Psychol.* **2012**, *80*, 151–163. [CrossRef]
74. Sweetman, A.; Lack, L.; Catcheside, P.G.; Antic, N.A.; Smith, S.; Chai-Coetzer, C.L.; Douglas, J.; O'Grady, A.; Dunn, N.; Robinson, J.; et al. Cognitive and behavioral therapy for insomnia increases the use of continuous positive airway pressure therapy in obstructive sleep apnea participants with comorbid insomnia: A randomized clinical trial. *Sleep* **2019**, *42*, zsz178. [CrossRef]
75. Lettieri, C.J.; Shah, A.A.; Holley, A.B.; Kelly, W.F.; Chang, A.S.; Roop, S.A.; Promotion, C.; Prognosis-The Army Sleep Apnea Program, T. Effects of a short course of eszopiclone on continuous positive airway pressure adherence: A randomized trial. *Ann. Intern. Med.* **2009**, *151*, 696–702. [CrossRef]
76. Antonaglia, C.; Vidoni, G.; Contardo, L.; Giudici, F.; Salton, F.; Ruaro, B.; Confalonieri, M.; Caneva, M. Low Arousal Threshold Estimation Predicts Failure of Mandibular Advancement Devices in Obstructive Sleep Apnea Syndrome. *Diagnostics* **2022**, *12*, 2548. [CrossRef]

77. Edwards, B.A.; Andara, C.; Landry, S.; Sands, S.A.; Joosten, S.A.; Owens, R.L.; White, D.P.; Hamilton, G.S.; Wellman, A. Upper-Airway Collapsibility and Loop Gain Predict the Response to Oral Appliance Therapy in Patients with Obstructive Sleep Apnea. *Am. J. Respir. Crit. Care Med.* **2016**, *194*, 1413–1422. [CrossRef]
78. Bamagoos, A.A.; Cistulli, P.A.; Sutherland, K.; Madronio, M.; Eckert, D.J.; Hess, L.; Edwards, B.A.; Wellman, A.; Sands, S.A. Polysomnographic Endotyping to Select Patients with Obstructive Sleep Apnea for Oral Appliances. *Ann. Am. Thorac. Soc.* **2019**, *16*, 1422–1431. [CrossRef]
79. Joosten, S.A.; Leong, P.; Landry, S.A.; Sands, S.A.; Terrill, P.I.; Mann, D.; Turton, A.; Rangaswamy, J.; Andara, C.; Burgess, G.; et al. Loop Gain Predicts the Response to Upper Airway Surgery in Patients With Obstructive Sleep Apnea. *Sleep* **2017**, *40*, zsx094. [CrossRef] [PubMed]
80. Li, Y.; Ye, J.; Han, D.; Cao, X.; Ding, X.; Zhang, Y.; Xu, W.; Orr, J.; Jen, R.; Sands, S.; et al. Physiology-Based Modeling May Predict Surgical Treatment Outcome for Obstructive Sleep Apnea. *J. Clin. Sleep Med.* **2017**, *13*, 1029–1037. [CrossRef] [PubMed]
81. Strollo, P.J., Jr.; Soose, R.J.; Maurer, J.T.; de Vries, N.; Cornelius, J.; Froymovich, O.; Hanson, R.D.; Padhya, T.A.; Steward, D.L.; Gillespie, M.B.; et al. Upper-airway stimulation for obstructive sleep apnea. *N. Engl. J. Med.* **2014**, *370*, 139–149. [CrossRef] [PubMed]
82. Op de Beeck, S.; Wellman, A.; Dieltjens, M.; Strohl, K.P.; Willemen, M.; Van de Heyning, P.H.; Verbraecken, J.A.; Vanderveken, O.M.; Sands, S.A.; Investigators, S.T. Endotypic Mechanisms of Successful Hypoglossal Nerve Stimulation for Obstructive Sleep Apnea. *Am. J. Respir. Crit. Care Med.* **2021**, *203*, 746–755. [CrossRef] [PubMed]
83. Perger, E.; Bertoli, S.; Lombardi, C. Pharmacotherapy for obstructive sleep apnea: Targeting specific pathophysiological traits. *Expert. Rev. Respir. Med.* **2023**, *17*, 663–673. [CrossRef]
84. Taranto-Montemurro, L.; Messineo, L.; Wellman, A. Targeting Endotypic Traits with Medications for the Pharmacological Treatment of Obstructive Sleep Apnea. A Review of the Current Literature. *J. Clin. Med.* **2019**, *8*, 1846. [CrossRef]
85. Wellman, A.; Malhotra, A.; Jordan, A.S.; Stevenson, K.E.; Gautam, S.; White, D.P. Effect of oxygen in obstructive sleep apnea: Role of loop gain. *Respir. Physiol. Neurobiol.* **2008**, *162*, 144–151. [CrossRef]
86. Sands, S.A.; Edwards, B.A.; Terrill, P.I.; Butler, J.P.; Owens, R.L.; Taranto-Montemurro, L.; Azarbarzin, A.; Marques, M.; Hess, L.B.; Smales, E.T.; et al. Identifying obstructive sleep apnoea patients responsive to supplemental oxygen therapy. *Eur. Respir. J.* **2018**, *52*, 1800674. [CrossRef]
87. Messineo, L.; Eckert, D.J.; Lim, R.; Chiang, A.; Azarbarzin, A.; Carter, S.G.; Carberry, J.C. Zolpidem increases sleep efficiency and the respiratory arousal threshold without changing sleep apnoea severity and pharyngeal muscle activity. *J. Physiol.* **2020**, *598*, 4681–4692. [CrossRef] [PubMed]
88. Eckert, D.J.; Owens, R.L.; Kehlmann, G.B.; Wellman, A.; Rahangdale, S.; Yim-Yeh, S.; White, D.P.; Malhotra, A. Eszopiclone increases the respiratory arousal threshold and lowers the apnoea/hypopnoea index in obstructive sleep apnoea patients with a low arousal threshold. *Clin. Sci.* **2011**, *120*, 505–514. [CrossRef] [PubMed]
89. Carter, S.G.; Carberry, J.C.; Cho, G.; Fisher, L.P.; Rollo, C.M.; Stevens, D.J.; D'Rozario, A.L.; McKenzie, D.K.; Grunstein, R.R.; Eckert, D.J. Effect of 1 month of zopiclone on obstructive sleep apnoea severity and symptoms: A randomised controlled trial. *Eur. Respir. J.* **2018**, *52*, 1800149. [CrossRef] [PubMed]
90. Schmickl, C.N.; Landry, S.; Orr, J.E.; Nokes, B.; Edwards, B.A.; Malhotra, A.; Owens, R.L. Effects of acetazolamide on control of breathing in sleep apnea patients: Mechanistic insights using meta-analyses and physiological model simulations. *Physiol. Rep.* **2021**, *9*, e15071. [CrossRef] [PubMed]
91. Schmickl, C.N.; Landry, S.A.; Orr, J.E.; Chin, K.; Murase, K.; Verbraecken, J.; Javaheri, S.; Edwards, B.A.; Owens, R.L.; Malhotra, A. Acetazolamide for OSA and Central Sleep Apnea: A Comprehensive Systematic Review and Meta-Analysis. *Chest* **2020**, *158*, 2632–2645. [CrossRef] [PubMed]
92. Edwards, B.A.; Sands, S.A.; Eckert, D.J.; White, D.P.; Butler, J.P.; Owens, R.L.; Malhotra, A.; Wellman, A. Acetazolamide improves loop gain but not the other physiological traits causing obstructive sleep apnoea. *J. Physiol.* **2012**, *590*, 1199–1211. [PubMed]
93. Edwards, B.A.; Connolly, J.G.; Campana, L.M.; Sands, S.A.; Trinder, J.A.; White, D.P.; Wellman, A.; Malhotra, A. Acetazolamide attenuates the ventilatory response to arousal in patients with obstructive sleep apnea. *Sleep* **2013**, *36*, 281–285. [CrossRef]
94. Chan, E.; Steenland, H.W.; Liu, H.; Horner, R.L. Endogenous excitatory drive modulating respiratory muscle activity across sleep-wake states. *Am. J. Respir. Crit. Care Med.* **2006**, *174*, 1264–1273. [CrossRef]
95. Grace, K.P.; Hughes, S.W.; Horner, R.L. Identification of the mechanism mediating genioglossus muscle suppression in REM sleep. *Am. J. Respir. Crit. Care Med.* **2013**, *187*, 311–319. [CrossRef]
96. Taranto-Montemurro, L.; Messineo, L.; Sands, S.A.; Azarbarzin, A.; Marques, M.; Edwards, B.A.; Eckert, D.J.; White, D.P.; Wellman, A. The Combination of Atomoxetine and Oxybutynin Greatly Reduces Obstructive Sleep Apnea Severity. A Randomized, Placebo-controlled, Double-Blind Crossover Trial. *Am. J. Respir. Crit. Care Med.* **2019**, *199*, 1267–1276. [CrossRef]
97. Taranto-Montemurro, L.; Messineo, L.; Azarbarzin, A.; Vena, D.; Hess, L.B.; Calianese, N.A.; White, D.P.; Wellman, A.; Sands, S.A. Effects of the Combination of Atomoxetine and Oxybutynin on OSA Endotypic Traits. *Chest* **2020**, *157*, 1626–1636. [CrossRef] [PubMed]
98. Schweitzer, P.K.; Taranto-Montemurro, L.; Ojile, J.M.; Thein, S.G.; Drake, C.L.; Rosenberg, R.; Corser, B.; Abaluck, B.; Sangal, R.B.; Maynard, J. The Combination of Aroxybutynin and Atomoxetine in the Treatment of Obstructive Sleep Apnea (MARIPOSA): A Randomized Controlled Trial. *Am. J. Respir. Crit. Care Med.* **2023**, *208*, 1316–1327. [CrossRef] [PubMed]

99. Perger, E.; Taranto Montemurro, L.; Rosa, D.; Vicini, S.; Marconi, M.; Zanotti, L.; Meriggi, P.; Azarbarzin, A.; Sands, S.A.; Wellman, A.; et al. Reboxetine Plus Oxybutynin for OSA Treatment: A 1-Week, Randomized, Placebo-Controlled, Double-Blind Crossover Trial. *Chest* **2022**, *161*, 237–247. [CrossRef] [PubMed]
100. Corser, B.; Eves, E.; Warren-McCormick, J.; Rucosky, G. Effects of atomoxetine plus a hypnotic on obstructive sleep apnea severity in patients with a moderately collapsible pharyngeal airway. *J. Clin. Sleep Med.* **2023**, *19*, 1035–1042. [CrossRef] [PubMed]
101. Allain, H.; Bentue-Ferrer, D.; Polard, E.; Akwa, Y.; Patat, A. Postural instability and consequent falls and hip fractures associated with use of hypnotics in the elderly: A comparative review. *Drugs Aging* **2005**, *22*, 749–765. [CrossRef] [PubMed]
102. Andrade, C. Sedative Hypnotics and the Risk of Falls and Fractures in the Elderly. *J. Clin. Psychiatry* **2018**, *79*, 18f12340. [CrossRef]
103. Amari, D.T.; Juday, T.; Frech, F.H.; Wang, W.; Wu, Z.; Atkins, N., Jr.; Wickwire, E.M. Falls, healthcare resources and costs in older adults with insomnia treated with zolpidem, trazodone, or benzodiazepines. *BMC Geriatr.* **2022**, *22*, 484. [CrossRef]
104. Heller, I.; Halevy, J.; Cohen, S.; Theodor, E. Significant metabolic acidosis induced by acetazolamide. Not a rare complication. *Arch. Intern. Med.* **1985**, *145*, 1815–1817. [CrossRef]
105. Nishtala, P.S.; Chyou, T.Y. Risk of delirium associated with antimuscarinics in older adults: A case-time-control study. *Pharmacoepidemiol. Drug Saf.* **2022**, *31*, 883–891. [CrossRef]
106. Schwartz, A.R.; Gold, A.R.; Schubert, N.; Stryzak, A.; Wise, R.A.; Permutt, S.; Smith, P.L. Effect of weight loss on upper airway collapsibility in obstructive sleep apnea. *Am. Rev. Respir. Dis.* **1991**, *144*, 494–498. [CrossRef]
107. Landry, S.A.; Mann, D.L.; Beare, R.; McIntyre, R.; Beatty, C.; Thomson, L.D.J.; Collet, J.; Joosten, S.A.; Hamilton, G.S.; Edwards, B.A. Oronasal vs Nasal Masks: The Impact of Mask Type on CPAP Requirement, Pharyngeal Critical Closing Pressure (P(crit)), and Upper Airway Cross-Sectional Areas in Patients With OSA. *Chest* **2023**, *164*, 747–756. [CrossRef]
108. Choi, J.K.; Hur, Y.K.; Lee, J.M.; Clark, G.T. Effects of mandibular advancement on upper airway dimension and collapsibility in patients with obstructive sleep apnea using dynamic upper airway imaging during sleep. *Oral. Surg. Oral. Med. Oral. Pathol. Oral. Radiol. Endod.* **2010**, *109*, 712–719. [CrossRef] [PubMed]
109. Ng, A.T.; Gotsopoulos, H.; Qian, J.; Cistulli, P.A. Effect of oral appliance therapy on upper airway collapsibility in obstructive sleep apnea. *Am. J. Respir. Crit. Care Med.* **2003**, *168*, 238–241. [CrossRef] [PubMed]
110. Ong, J.S.; Touyz, G.; Tanner, S.; Hillman, D.R.; Eastwood, P.R.; Walsh, J.H. Variability of human upper airway collapsibility during sleep and the influence of body posture and sleep stage. *J. Sleep Res.* **2011**, *20*, 533–537. [CrossRef] [PubMed]
111. Penzel, T.; Moller, M.; Becker, H.F.; Knaack, L.; Peter, J.H. Effect of sleep position and sleep stage on the collapsibility of the upper airways in patients with sleep apnea. *Sleep* **2001**, *24*, 90–95. [CrossRef] [PubMed]
112. Landry, S.A.; Beatty, C.; Thomson, L.D.J.; Wong, A.M.; Edwards, B.A.; Hamilton, G.S.; Joosten, S.A. A review of supine position related obstructive sleep apnea: Classification, epidemiology, pathogenesis and treatment. *Sleep Med. Rev.* **2023**, *72*, 101847. [CrossRef]
113. Szollosi, I.; Roebuck, T.; Thompson, B.; Naughton, M.T. Lateral sleeping position reduces severity of central sleep apnea/Cheyne-Stokes respiration. *Sleep* **2006**, *29*, 1045–1051. [CrossRef]
114. Pinna, G.D.; Dacosto, E.; Maestri, R.; Crotti, P.; Montemartini, S.; Caporotondi, A.; Guazzotti, G.; Bruschi, C. Postural changes in lung volumes in patients with heart failure and Cheyne-Stokes respiration: Relationship with sleep apnea severity. *Sleep Med.* **2023**, *101*, 154–161. [CrossRef]
115. Javaheri, S.; Javaheri, S. Update on Persistent Excessive Daytime Sleepiness in OSA. *Chest* **2020**, *158*, 776–786. [CrossRef] [PubMed]
116. Dieltjens, M.; Vroegop, A.V.; Verbruggen, A.E.; Wouters, K.; Willemen, M.; De Backer, W.A.; Verbraecken, J.A.; Van de Heyning, P.H.; Braem, M.J.; de Vries, N.; et al. A promising concept of combination therapy for positional obstructive sleep apnea. *Sleep Breath.* **2015**, *19*, 637–644. [CrossRef] [PubMed]
117. Liu, H.W.; Chen, Y.J.; Lai, Y.C.; Huang, C.Y.; Huang, Y.L.; Lin, M.T.; Han, S.Y.; Chen, C.L.; Yu, C.J.; Lee, P.L. Combining MAD and CPAP as an effective strategy for treating patients with severe sleep apnea intolerant to high-pressure PAP and unresponsive to MAD. *PLoS ONE* **2017**, *12*, e0187032. [CrossRef]
118. Wang, D.; Tang, Y.; Chen, Y.; Zhang, S.; Ma, D.; Luo, Y.; Li, S.; Su, X.; Wang, X.; Liu, C.; et al. The effect of non-benzodiazepine sedative hypnotics on CPAP adherence in patients with OSA: A systematic review and meta-analysis. *Sleep* **2021**, *44*, zsab077. [CrossRef]
119. Schmickl, C.N.; Lettieri, C.J.; Orr, J.E.; DeYoung, P.; Edwards, B.A.; Owens, R.L.; Malhotra, A. The Arousal Threshold as a Drug Target to Improve Continuous Positive Airway Pressure Adherence: Secondary Analysis of a Randomized Trial. *Am. J. Respir. Crit. Care Med.* **2020**, *202*, 1592–1595. [CrossRef] [PubMed]
120. Ni, Y.N.; Holzer, R.C.; Thomas, R.J. Acute and long-term effects of acetazolamide in presumed high loop gain sleep apnea. *Sleep Med.* **2023**, *107*, 137–148. [CrossRef] [PubMed]
121. Eskandari, D.; Zou, D.; Grote, L.; Hoff, E.; Hedner, J. Acetazolamide Reduces Blood Pressure and Sleep-Disordered Breathing in Patients With Hypertension and Obstructive Sleep Apnea: A Randomized Controlled Trial. *J. Clin. Sleep Med.* **2018**, *14*, 309–317. [CrossRef] [PubMed]

122. Aishah, A.; Tong, B.K.Y.; Osman, A.M.; Pitcher, G.; Donegan, M.; Kwan, B.C.H.; Brown, E.; Altree, T.J.; Adams, R.; Mukherjee, S.; et al. Stepwise Add-on and Endotype-informed Targeted Combination Therapy to Treat Obstructive Sleep Apnea: A Proof-of-Concept Study. *Ann. Am. Thorac. Soc.* **2023**, *20*, 1316–1325. [CrossRef]
123. Edwards, B.A.; Sands, S.A.; Owens, R.L.; Eckert, D.J.; Landry, S.; White, D.P.; Malhotra, A.; Wellman, A. The Combination of Supplemental Oxygen and a Hypnotic Markedly Improves Obstructive Sleep Apnea in Patients with a Mild to Moderate Upper Airway Collapsibility. *Sleep* **2016**, *39*, 1973–1983. [CrossRef] [PubMed]

Disclaimer/Publisher's Note: The statements, opinions and data contained in all publications are solely those of the individual author(s) and contributor(s) and not of MDPI and/or the editor(s). MDPI and/or the editor(s) disclaim responsibility for any injury to people or property resulting from any ideas, methods, instructions or products referred to in the content.

MDPI AG
Grosspeteranlage 5
4052 Basel
Switzerland
Tel.: +41 61 683 77 34
www.mdpi.com

Journal of Clinical Medicine Editorial Office
E-mail: jcm@mdpi.com
www.mdpi.com/journal/jcm

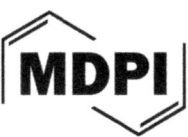

Disclaimer/Publisher's Note: The statements, opinions and data contained in all publications are solely those of the individual author(s) and contributor(s) and not of MDPI and/or the editor(s). MDPI and/or the editor(s) disclaim responsibility for any injury to people or property resulting from any ideas, methods, instructions or products referred to in the content.

www.ingramcontent.com/pod-product-compliance
Lightning Source LLC
LaVergne TN
LVHW070411100526
838202LV00014B/1439